Second Edition

THE INSTANT
EXAM REVIEW
for the USMLE
STEP 2

Second Edition

THE INSTANT EXAM REVIEW
for the USMLE
STEP 2

Joel S. Goldberg, DO
Assistant Professor of Medicine
Department of Medicine
Medical College of Pennsylvania and
Hahnemann University
Philadelphia, Pennsylvania

Medical Director
Gardendale Medical Center
Delaware County, Pennsylvania

Appleton & Lange
Stamford, Connecticut

96 97 98 99 00 / 10 9 8 7 6 5 4 3 2 1

Prentice-Hall International (UK) Limited, *London*
Prentice-Hall of Australia Pty. Limited, *Sydney*
Prentice-Hall Canada, Inc., *Toronto*
Prentice-Hall Hispanoamericana, S.A., *Mexico*
Prentice-Hall of India Private Limited, *New Delhi*
Prentice-Hall of Japan, Inc., *Tokyo*
Simon & Schuster Asia Pte. Ltd., *Singapore*
Editora Prentice-Hall do Brasil Ltda., *Rio de Janeiro*
Prentice Hall, *Upper Saddle River, New Jersey*

Library of Congress Cataloging-in-Publication Data

Goldberg, Joel S.
    The instant exam review for the USMLE step 2 / Joel S. Goldberg. —
2nd ed.
      p.   cm.
    Includes index.
    ISBN 0-8385-4328-6 (pbk. : alk. paper)
    1. Medicine—Examinations, questions, etc. 2. Medicine—Outlines,
syllabl, etc, I. Title.
    [DNLM: 1. Clinical Medicine—examination questions. 2. Clinical
Medicine—outlines. 3. Licensure, Medical—examination questions.
  WB 18.2 G6181 1996]
R834.5.G65 1996
610′.76—dc20
DNLM/DLC
for Library of Congress   95-52038
                                CIP

ISBN 0-8385-4328-6

90000

9 780838 543283

Acquisitions Editor: Marinita S. Timban
Production Service: Rainbow Graphics, Inc.

PRINTED IN THE UNITED STATES OF AMERICA

To my parents, Louis and Marion, a gift for the past . . .
To my wife, Mickey, a gift for the present . . .
To my son, Daniel, a gift for the future . . .

CONTENTS

CONTRIBUTORS

Alex I. Dever, MD
Attending Psychiatrist
Medical Center of Delaware
Wilmington, Delaware

Charles K. Field, MD
Assistant Professor in Surgery
Division of Vascular Surgery
Department of Surgery
Hahnemann University School of Medicine
Philadelphia, Pennsylvania

Joel S. Goldberg, DO
Assistant Professor of Medicine
Department of Medicine
Medical College of Pennsylvania and
    Hahnemann University School of Medicine
Philadelphia, Pennsylvania
Medical Director
Gardendale Medical Center
Delaware County, Pennsylvania

Richard Goldman, MD
Clinical Assistant Professor of Medicine
Division of Internal Medicine
Hahnemann University School of Medicine
Philadelphia, Pennsylvania
Attending Physician
Division of Internal Medicine
Department of Hematology/Oncology
Crozer–Chester Medical Center
Chester, Pennsylvania

Ralph P. Ierardi, MD
Vascular Surgery
Clinical Instructor in Surgery
Medical College of Pennsylvania and
    Hahnemann University School of Medicine
Philadelphia, Pennsylvania

Ancil A. Jones, MD
Clinical Assistant Professor
Division of Cardiology
Department of Internal Medicine
Hahnemann University Hospital
Philadelphia, Pennsylvania
Director, Cardiac Catheterization Laboratory
Division of Cardiology
Department of Medicine
Crozer–Chester Medical Center
Chester, Pennsylvania

Morris D. Kerstein, MD, FACS
Professor of Surgery
Medical College of Pennsylvania and
    Hahnemann University School of Medicine
Philadelphia, Pennsylvania

Charles A. Pohl, MD, FAAP
Inpatient Services Coordinator
Clinical Assistant Professor
Division of General Pediatrics
Department of Pediatrics
Thomas Jefferson University
Philadelphia, Pennsylvania

Hector Stella, MD
Resident
Department of Pulmonary Medicine
Medical College of Pennsylvania and
    Hahnemann University School of Medicine
Philadelphia, Pennsylvania

Arthur F. Tuch, MD
Attending Gastroenterologist
Division of Gastroenterology
Department of Internal Medicine
Crozer–Chester Medical Center
Chester, Pennsylvania

Robert S. Walter, MD, FAAP
Director Pediatric Residency Program
Assistant Professor
Division of General Pediatrics
Department of Pediatrics
Thomas Jefferson University
Philadelphia, Pennsylvania
Attending Pediatrician
Division of General Pediatrics
Department of Pediatrics
Alfred I. duPont Institute
Wilmington, Delaware

PREFACE

For the medical student, there has always been a tremendous volume of information to learn and review, coupled with a perpetually inadequate amount of time for study. In preparation for my own examinations, both as student and physician (including medical school examinations, the National Board Examination, and specialty board certification), I discovered a disconcerting fact—a concise, rapid-reading review book of pure key facts was unavailable.

It was with that discovery that the notion of creating such a text was born.

The Instant Exam Review for the USMLE Step 2, Second Edition is a fully revised comprehensive compendium of general medical knowledge in a revolutionary new format designed to cover directly and completely the "high impact" fact list of the United States Medical Licensing Examination. The text is very concise to allow the handbook to be read quickly, and the information presented comprises only the essential core facts necessary for exam success.

Please note that this text was not designed to teach general medicine, nor to be a substitute for accepted methods of student education. However, *The Instant Exam Review for the USMLE Step 2, Second Edition*, **was designed to be a unique study tool, to enable the student to pass the USMLE Step 2 exam.**

Remember, *The Instant Exam Review for the USMLE Step 2* does not list any test questions, but it does supply most of the answers!

Joel S. Goldberg, DO

ACKNOWLEDGMENTS

First and foremost, I wish to extend my appreciation to my first editor at Appleton & Lange, Ms. Jamie Kircher. It was through Jamie's keen perception and insight that my fledgling idea for *The Instant Exam Review* was first spotted. Jamie's continued assistance and support allowed my project to develop into a formal proposal that was accepted for publication, and ultimately, a substantial text that will assist medical students throughout the world. I would also like to thank my current editor, Marinita Timban, at Appleton & Lange for all her assistance through the development of this newly revised second edition.

I wish to thank my coauthors for their willingness to participate in this endeavor, despite their busy professional schedules, and the precious time they surely lost from their families and other activities during the laborious task of manuscript preparation.

Other individuals who provided assistance in completion, revision, or review of this project include John W. Boor, MD, Department of Neurology, Riddle Memorial Hospital, Media, Pennsylvania; S. Jay Hirsh, MD, Department of Urology, Crozer–Chester Medical Center, Chester, Pennsylvania; Robin J. O. Catlin, MD, Professor and Head, Department of Family Medicine, Louisiana State University Medical Center, New Orleans, Louisiana; Mark Kline, MD, Department of Pediatrics, Texas Children's Hospital, Houston, Texas; Marie Christine Durnan, MD, Department of Pediatrics, Texas Children's Hospital; Hector Stella, MD, Hahnemann University, Philadelphia, Pennsylvania; Jose Menoyo, MD, Hahnemann University; Bruce J. Rosen, MD, Department of Obstetrics and Gynecology, Crozer–Chester Medical Center, Chester, Pennsylvania; Doris Bartuska, MD, Chairman, Department of Endocrinology, Medical College of Pennsylvania, Philadelphia, Pennsylvania; Catherine Eissler, MD, and student reviewers Michael Yao and Tino Pena at Yale School of Medicine, New Haven, Connecticut.

Joel S. Goldberg, DO

INSTANT EXAM PREPARATION GUIDE

ORGANIZATION OF THIS BOOK

The Instant Exam Review for the USMLE Step 2 is divided into 19 chapters, and is formatted to follow the "high impact" fact list provided by the USMLE for the Step 2 examination.

Step 2 is a two-day, multiple-choice examination, including pediatrics, internal medicine, preventative medicine and public health, obstetrics and gynecology, psychiatry, and surgery. The Step 2 examination is constructed in an integrated content outline, which organizes clinical science material into three sections: physician task, population group, and disease process. The test items may describe clinical situations and require examinees to provide a diagnosis, mechanism of disease, preventive measures, and treatment. *The Instant Exam Review* provides review and study of these key issues.

HOW TO USE THIS BOOK

The Instant Exam Review is an innovative and practical study guide designed to be used in two ways. First, you can use it as a comprehensive study outline during the initial phase of USMLE Step 2 examination preparation. Second, you can use it as a quick review during the final few days and hours before the exam.

Using the Book as a Study Outline
The Instant Exam Review is an excellent companion to your third- and fourth-year study tools. Frequent review of the manual will assist in defining and remembering the core facts, so essential to both exam success and actual patient management.

When you begin to study, turn to the Contents to obtain an overview of this text. At this time, do not skip any chapters, but instead start at the beginning and read the book in its entirety. During the first reading of the text, concentrate on the essential facts noted under the sections including **Description, Pathology, Symptoms, Diagnosis,** and **Treatment.** Key terms and facts are highlighted in bold print.

Ask yourself questions after reading each section to enhance your retention of the facts. For example, after reading the paragraphs on Wilson's disease, ask yourself, "What are the key symptoms? How is the diagnosis made? What tests should be performed? What is the treatment?" This study method will refine your memory and help you to focus on the critical information needed for exam success.

Allow non-medical personnel to quiz you in the same fashion, while referring to the information under each section. This will provide a comprehensive review of the USMLE's "high impact" fact list and allow you to rapidly discover your areas of strength and weakness.

Use the extra space around items on each page to write in any terms or facts that you see as areas of weakness. Weak sections can be reviewed multiple times, building your knowledge base and confidence. Further study should be devoted to your areas of concern using textbooks listed in the bibliography or standard texts.

Throughout your third and fourth years you may find it useful to compile your own "pearls" in the spaces and margins of this book.

Using the Book as a Quick Review
In the final several weeks and days prior to your examination, *The Instant Exam Review* will serve as a rapid review tool. You will find this material represents the core of testing material and needed

medical facts, accessible in fewer than several hours of reading.

We have placed in bold print those terms and facts that are the key elements to master and represent prime examination topics. As your testing date approaches, scan only these phrases in each section, one chapter at a time, devoting more time to areas of weakness as necessary.

Use the spaces and margins of each page to jot down your own "pearls" as well as key points from other sources that you want to remember for the exam.

Second Edition

THE INSTANT EXAM REVIEW
for the USMLE
STEP 2

CHAPTER 1

Cardiovascular Medicine

ANCIL JONES, MD

I. ISCHEMIC HEART DISEASE

A. Stable Angina Pectoris

■ Description

Disagreeable chest discomfort, commonly substernal in location and often described as heaviness or squeezing. Can be felt anywhere from epigastrium to pharynx, arm(s), neck, or back. **Provoked by exertion** or **emotional upset, relieved within minutes** by rest.

■ Symptoms

The **relationship of symptoms to effort,** and **relief by cessation of activity,** is characteristic. Asymptomatic at rest.

■ Diagnosis

Dx by stress test b/c ECG is normal in absence of Sx

Typical symptoms, especially in presence of one or more risk factors. Exam often normal, as is electrocardiogram (ECG) in absence of prior myocardial infarction. Exercise stress testing. In selected cases, coronary angiography.

■ Pathology

Increase in myocardial demand for oxygen and nutrient substrate that **exceeds available supply.** Coronary blood supply restricted by arterial lumen narrowing due to **atherosclerotic plaque.** In some cases, excessive myocardial demand (eg, left ventricular hypertrophy due to aortic stenosis, thyrotoxicosis) can outpace blood supply through normal coronary arteries.

■ Treatment

Nitrates, beta blockers, calcium channel blockers. Percutaneous transluminal coronary angioplasty **(PTCA)** or **coronary artery bypass surgery** in patients with major ischemia, poorly controlled anginal symptoms.

B. Unstable Angina Pectoris

■ Description

Disagreeable **chest discomfort,** commonly **substernal** in location and often described as **heaviness** or squeezing. Can be felt anywhere from the epigastrium to pharynx, arm(s), neck, or back. Occurs unpredictably **at rest** or in a sharply and abruptly worsening pattern compared to previous stable angina. Duration of unstable angina attacks generally 15 minutes or less (an attack lasting hours suggests myocardial infarction).

■ Symptoms

Discomfort identical to stable angina pectoris, except occurs under conditions of rest or **minimal activity.** Unstable angina may occur *de novo* or in patient with known coronary artery disease (CAD). **Commonly** occurs at night or in early morning and may wake patient. May progress to acute myocardial infarction.

■ Diagnosis

Typical symptoms, especially in presence of one or more risk factors. Exam is often normal. The ECG may show ischemic ST-T abnormalities, especially if recorded during an attack. Exercise stress testing contraindicated. **Coronary angiography** in selected cases.

■ Pathology

Decrease in supply of coronary blood flow and oxygen to a level **below that required for baseline metabolic needs of myocardium.** Coronary blood flow is interrupted by **thrombus or platelet plug** developing on a **fissured or ulcerated atherosclerotic plaque.** Coronary vasospasm plays role in some patients. The transient ischemia of unstable angina is reversible.

■ **Treatment**

Nitrates, beta blockers, calcium channel blockers, aspirin, heparin. In selected patients, PTCA or coronary artery bypass surgery.

C. **Acute Myocardial Infarction**

■ **Description**

Clinical syndrome of ischemic myocardial necrosis. Amount of necrosis variable depending on quantity of myocardium affected by ischemia, collateral blood supply, and treatment administered within the first few hours of infarction.

■ **Symptoms**

Prolonged chest discomfort, most commonly substernal in location, but may be felt in arm(s), jaw, back, pharynx, epigastrium. Dyspnea, diaphoresis common. Syncope may occur.

■ **Diagnosis**

• ECG suggestive
• CPK mB, SGOT,
ξ LDH confirm

Typical history, especially in patient with one or more risk factors for CAD. Exam may disclose bradycardia, tachycardia, hypertension, cardiac gallop(s), congestive heart failure. The ECG is usually suggestive or diagnostic (ST elevation) of acute myocardial ischemia. Serial cardiac enzyme testing. [creatine phosphokinase (CPK) with myocardial isoenzyme, serum glutamic-oxaloacetic transaminase (SGOT), lactate dehydrogenase (LDH)] confirmatory.

■ **Pathology**

Caused by an abrupt decrease in coronary blood flow or, less commonly, by a severe and prolonged increase in myocardial oxygen need that cannot be met by available coronary arterial flow. Abrupt decrease in coronary artery flow can be due to thrombus formation

(most common) on fissured or ulcerated atherosclerotic plaque, hemorrhage into atherosclerotic plaque, coronary vasoconstriction (spasm), coronary artery embolus (rare), or shock. Tachycardia or sustained severe hypertension can cause prolonged increase in myocardial oxygen demand sufficient to cause myocardial necrosis. Irreversible necrosis can develop within 1 to 6 (variable) hours after onset of persistent ischemia.

■ **Treatment**

For patients with transmural MI (ST elevation on ECG) and no contraindication, thrombolytic therapy (streptokinase, tissue plasminogen activator, APSAC [t-PA]), nitrates, aspirin, heparin, beta blockers. PTCA may be used as alternative. Antiarrhythmic therapy as required. Coronary catheterization followed by cardiac surgery or PTCA may be required for complications of recurrent angina, cardiogenic shock, mitral regurgitation, ventricular septal defect, cardiac rupture, ventricular aneurysm.

D. **Risk Factors for Coronary Artery Disease**

■ **Description**

Risk factors for CAD have a strong statistical correlation with likelihood of developing clinical CAD, although strict proof of causation lacking. Multiple risk factors combine to significantly increase CAD risk compared to one factor alone.

— Hypercholesterolemia
— Cigarette smoking
— Hypertension
— Diabetes mellitus
— Family history of premature CAD (< 55 yr of age)
— Male sex (in patients < 55 to 60 yr of age) or premature menopause in females

E. Prevention of Coronary Artery Disease

Primary prevention—attempt to lower risk of CAD by risk-factor modification before clinical manifestations of CAD appear.

Secondary prevention—attempt to lower risk of repeat CAD event in patient who has already developed clinical manifestations of CAD (eg, angina, myocardial infarction).

Prevention efforts focus on modifiable risk factors:

- Cessation of cigarette smoking
- Control of hypertension
- Weight control
- Behavior modification
- Dietary modification
- Exercise
- Estrogen replacement in postmenopausal women

F. Cardiac Rehabilitation

■ **Description**

Physician-supervised **program of exercise and risk-factor modification** for patients with angina pectoris, prior myocardial infarction, or prior coronary bypass surgery.

■ **Goals**

Improvement in **exercise capacity** and **morale** of patients with CAD. Potential for improvement in survival through risk-factor modification.

II. HEART FAILURE

Congestive heart failure (CHF) is a serious clinical expression of myocardial or mechanical (valvular or structural) abnormalities of the heart. In many cases myocardial and mechanical dysfunction coexist. Because CHF is not a complete cardiac diagnosis, the underlying cause of the myocardial and/or mechanical problem must be sought.

A. Low-Output Heart Failure

■ **Description**

Inability of the heart to pump adequate blood to meet the metabolic needs of the body in the resting state or with day-to-day activities.

■ **Symptoms**

Left ventricular failure—**dyspnea, orthopnea, fatigue.** Exam shows LV gallops, cardiomegaly, pulmonary congestion.

Right ventricular failure—**edema, ascites, fatigue.** Exam shows RV gallops, neck vein distention, liver distention.

Signs and symptoms of LV failure and RV failure often coexist (**biventricular** CHF).

■ **Diagnosis**

History, exam. Chest x-ray, ECG, Doppler echocardiography. (EF<30%)

■ **Pathology**

Mechanical abnormalities of any cardiac valve (most commonly aortic or mitral) can limit cardiac output sufficiently to result in CHF.

Myocardial dysfunction can affect either **systolic (contractile)** or **diastolic (relaxation) function.** Often systolic and diastolic dysfunction coexist, although in some cases (eg, hypertrophic cardiomyopathy) diastolic dysfunction can dominate.

Left ventricle (LV) often affected alone early on, but in severe cases, right ventricle (RV) and LV usually both involved. Most common cause of RV failure is LV failure.

Systemic hypertension is the most common cause of CHF. Other etiologies are numerous and include coronary artery disease as well as **congenital heart disease, valvular diseases,** and **myocardial diseases.** (MI)

■ Treatment

Salt restriction, diuretic, digitalis in many cases. Vasodilators (eg, ACE inhibitors, nitrates, hydralazine) in some cases (predominantly regurgitant valve lesions, impaired LV contractile function; avoid in hypertrophic cardiomyopathy, stenotic valve lesions). Some patients with valve dysfunction appropriate for cardiac surgery.

treat underlying cause if possible!

B. High-Output Heart Failure

■ Description

Inability of the heart to pump adequate blood in face of a condition that requires an increased cardiac output to meet metabolic needs of the body.

■ Symptoms

Dyspnea, orthopnea, edema. May provoke angina in patients with coronary disease. On exam find pulmonary congestion, edema, neck vein distention. In contrast to patients with low-output CHF, patients with high-output CHF may have bounding pulses and hyperdynamic circulation.

■ Pathology

Persistent increased cardiac output leads to increased blood volume and salt retention, elevation of ventricular filling pressures, and CHF. Systemic vascular resistance (SVR) is reduced. Can occur in severe anemia, thyrotoxicosis, acute beriberi, Paget's disease, large arteriovenous fistula(e). Even mild high-output state may cause CHF in patients with other cardiac disease or in elderly.

■ Treatment

Salt restriction, diuretic. Treat underlying cause.

C. Acute Pulmonary Edema

■ Description

Abrupt increase in vascular volume of lungs causing impaired gas exchange and constituting a medical emergency. Most commonly occurs on cardiogenic basis, but can occur as a result of noncardiac disease.

■ Symptoms

May look just like MI!

Severe dyspnea and orthopnea, often of abrupt onset, with diaphoresis. May be accompanied by angina pectoris, especially in patients with coronary disease. On exam, tachypnea, tachycardia, marked pulmonary congestion (may cause wheezing or "cardiac asthma"), cardiac gallop(s). Failure of the RV may or may not be present.

■ Pathology

Cardiogenic pulmonary edema caused by elevation of pulmonary venous pressure (often precipitous) due to myocardial failure, valvular abnormality, or severe arrhythmia. Etiologic factors often coexist.

■ Treatment

(? to ↓ bp ?)

Elevation of head, diuretic, morphine, supplemental oxygen, nitrates. In severe cases mechanical ventilation may be needed. Treat arrhythmia, if present.

D. Cor Pulmonale

■ Description

Cardiac disease secondary to primary pulmonary disease.

■ Symptoms

Sx of RV failure

Dyspnea, edema, atrial arrhythmias, fatigue.

RV failure

On exam, RV gallop, RV heave, neck vein distention, ascites, tricuspid regurgitation, edema, hepatic congestion.

■ **Diagnosis**

Signs and symptoms of right ventricular failure in setting of severe pulmonary parenchymal or vascular disease. The ECG shows **right atrial and right ventricular hypertrophy. Echocardiography. Arterial blood gases.** Pulmonary function testing. Some patients may need **right heart catheterization** to confirm diagnosis and to assess response of pulmonary vasculature to vasodilators.

■ **Pathology**

Lung disease can affect the heart through abnormalities of pulmonary vasculature and severe hypoxia.

Severe hypoxia can lead to moderate or severe **pulmonary hypertension** by causing pulmonary vasoconstriction.

Obliteration of pulmonary vasculature sufficient to cause significant **pulmonary hypertension** can occur in pulmonary embolism, primary pulmonary hypertension (calcinosis, Raynaud's, esophageal dysfunction, sclerodactyly, telangiectasia) CREST syndrome.

■ **Treatment**

Diuretic. Antiarrhythmic therapy as needed. **Treat underlying condition. Oxygen supplement for severe hypoxia.**

III. CARDIAC ARRHYTHMIAS

A. Supraventricular Origin

1. Premature Beats

Premature atrial contraction (PAC)—an early beat originating from an atrial focus outside of the sinus node. Frequent PACs may lead to atrial tachycardia, atrial fibrillation, or atrial flutter.

Premature junctional contraction (PJC)—an early beat originating from the atrioventricular junction (AV node).

2. Tachycardias

Paroxysmal supraventricular (atrial) tachycardia—also called PSVT or PAT, is a regular tachycardia (usually 150 to 250 per min) of atrial or atrioventricular junction origin. Most common mechanism is re-entry within the atrioventricular junction, but may be due to automatic atrial focus or to re-entry involving atria and ventricles.

Non-paroxysmal junctional tachycardia—a regular tachycardia (usually ≤ 130 per min) due to increased rate of automaticity of the atrioventricular junction. Most commonly due to digitalis toxicity, acute myocardial infarction, or myocarditis.

Multifocal atrial tachycardia (MAT) — an irregular tachycardia (usually 120 to 200 per min) due to rapid atrial depolarizations with varying non-sinus P wave morphologies (at least three different contours). Usually associated with severe and decompensated lung disease.

Atrial fibrillation—a grossly irregular supraventricular rhythm (may be slow but usually rapid in untreated state) with coarse or fine atrial fibrillation waves and no identifiable P waves.

Atrial flutter—a supraventricular rhythm with identifiable ("sawtooth" ECG baseline) continuous atrial activity with atrial rate of 250 to 350 per minute. Ventricular rate depends on degree of block at atrioventricular junction. Ventricular rate of 150 per minute (2:1 AV block) is common.

B. Ventricular Origin

1. Premature Beats

Premature ventricular contraction (PVC)—an early beat originating from any portion of either ventricle. Found in a variety of diseases or in normal individuals, clinical significance de-

[handwritten top left] Sick sinus syndrome: bradycardia / tachycardia 40's 120's Rx: pacemaker

[handwritten top right] Torsades de pointes: type of Vtach hypocalc, hypoMg

cocaine
Rx: remove offending agent give iv Mg it goes away!

pends on underlying cardiac diagnosis.

2. Tachycardias

Ventricular tachycardia (VT)—consists of three or more consecutive ventricular beats originating from any portion of either ventricle. Usually paroxysmal and of abrupt onset and termination. May be sustained (over 30 beats in duration), non-sustained, monomorphic (each beat with similar or identical QRS morphology), or polymorphic (QRS morphology varies beat to beat). Can cause syncope, CHF, angina, or lead to ventricular fibrillation; P waves may or may not be identifiable.

[handwritten] → if pulseless Rx like Vfib!

Ventricular fibrillation (VF)—a grossly chaotic ventricular tachyarrhythmia (ventricular rate <250 per min or uncountable) without identifiable P waves. If not treated immediately, usually with direct current countershock (defibrillation), VF is rapidly fatal. Ventricular flutter, a ventricular tachyarrhythmia of 150 to 250 per minute without identifiable ST segments or T waves, has same clinical significance as VF.

C. Bradyarrhythmias

1. Sinus

Sinus arrest—failure of impulse formation in the sinus node. Asystole will result unless an escape rhythm (ectopic atrial, junctional, ventricular) develops.

Sinus bradycardia—an abnormally slow rate (< 50 to 60 per min) due to a slowing of the rate of depolarization of the sinus node. May be found in healthy individuals, but may be associated with vasovagal reaction, myocardial infarction (MI), drug therapy, brady-tachycardia syndrome, or aging. Usually asymptomatic, but can cause episodic weakness or syncope.

2. Heart Block

First-degree atrioventricular (AV) block—prolongation of the PR interval > .20 seconds in adults, usually due to slowing of conduction in the AV junction. May or may not be associated with bradycardia.

Second-degree AV block—intermittent failure of the cardiac impulse originating in the atria to reach the ventricles, is of two types:

Mobitz Type I—caused by block at the atrioventricular junction, is the most common type of second-degree heart block.

Mobitz Type II—caused by block at site distal to the AV junction. Less common than type I, but often a precursor to complete infranodal AV block.

Third-degree (complete) heart block—due to complete block of cardiac impulse at the AV junction, His bundle, or both right and left bundle branches. Atrial and ventricular activities are independent. The resultant escape QRS complex is generally regular and will be normal (narrow, originating from the AV junction) or wide (idioventricular, originating from the ventricles), depending on the level of block. This bradyarrhythmia can cause weakness, CHF, or syncope.

IV. MYOCARDIAL DISEASES

A. Congestive (Dilated) Cardiomyopathy

■ **Description**

Congestive (dilated) cardiomyopathy is a non-specific cardiac condition (multiple etiologies) and is characterized by dilated and poorly contractile ventricles. Atria are often dilated as well. **Right and left ventricles are often affected together;** however, the right or left ventricle may be affected predominantly, de-

[handwritten bottom] WPW - S waves - if present in flutter do NOT give digoxin b/c can cause Vfib! give verapamil or β-blockers

pending on the specific cause or stage of the disease process.

■ **Symptoms**

Dyspnea, palpitations, fatigue. Chest pain may occur, especially in ischemic disease. **Arrhythmias,** atrial and ventricular, are common. **Edema** may occur in advanced cases.

On exam, **cardiac enlargement, gallops, neck vein distention,** mitral and/or tricuspid **murmurs** (valve ring dilatation). *(regurgitant murmurs)*

■ **Diagnosis**

History, exam. Often with **LVH.** ECG may show Q waves suggestive of prior MI. **Chest x-ray** with cardiomegaly, pulmonary congestion. **Echocardiography** shows cardiac dilatation with reduced ventricular ejection fraction. Laboratory studies may confirm specific etiologies.

■ **Pathology**

Decreased ventricular contractility (systolic dysfunction) results in **reduced cardiac output** and/or **pulmonary congestion (CHF).** Basis for systolic dysfunction depends on etiology and, in some cases, is unknown. **Diastolic dysfunction** often coexists.

Etiologies are numerous:

1. Ischemic (CAD, prior myocardial infarction)
2. Systemic hypertension most common cause
3. Idiopathic (cause unknown)
4. Familial
5. Postpartum or peripartum
6. Alcoholic (toxic)
7. Chagas' heart disease (trypanosomiasis)
8. Radiation therapy
9. Beriberi (thiamine deficiency)
10. Drug induced (anthracyclines)

■ **Treatment**

Salt restriction, diuretic, digitalis, vasodilators. Specific etiologies may require special therapies.

ACE inhibitors

B. **Hypertrophic Cardiomyopathy**

■ **Description**

A form of cardiomyopathy characterized by a **hypertrophic and non-dilated left ventricle** in the absence of a systemic or coexisting cardiac condition, capable of producing LVH. Often **disproportionate hypertrophy of the ventricular septum,** which may produce variable amounts of obstruction in the left ventricular outflow tract. Right ventricle can be hypertrophied as well. May be **familial** or **sporadic.**

■ **Symptoms**

Dyspnea, chest pain, near-syncope or syncope, which can be caused by **arrhythmia** (ventricular tachycardia or atrial fibrillation) or LV outflow tract obstruction.

On exam, **systolic murmur** at lower left sternal border, **bifid carotid pulse** (in cases of LV outflow obstruction), S4. May have murmur of **mitral regurgitation.**

■ **Diagnosis**

Patient history, family history, and **exam.** With LVH, ECG may have pseudoinfarction pattern. Chest x-ray with cardiomegaly. **Doppler echocardiography usually diagnostic.**

■ **Pathology**

Evidence mounting for genetically determined abnormalities of cardiac muscle cells. **Diastolic dysfunction** causes pulmonary congestion, restriction to adequate left ventricular filling. **Dynamic obstruction to left ventricular outflow common,** but does not always occur.

Digoxin is contraindicated!

■ **Treatment**   *atenolol*

Beta blockers. Calcium channel blockers, pacing? Surgical incision of hypertrophied ventricular septum in severely obstructed patients when medical therapy inadequate.

C. Restrictive Cardiomyopathy

■ **Description**

A form of cardiomyopathy characterized by **non-compliant, poorly distensible ventricle(s)** on basis of infiltrative process. Ventricular systolic function often normal, and heart may not be enlarged. **Least common** form of cardiomyopathy.

■ **Symptoms**

Fatigue. Edema.

On exam, **neck vein distention,** edema, ascites, may mimic constrictive pericarditis.

■ **Diagnosis**

History, exam. Laboratory findings of underlying disease. Echocardiography may show endomyocardial fibroelastosis, if present.

■ **Pathology**

Any **infiltrative process** of myocardium that **results in interstitial fibrosis or thickening of heart wall** (not myocardial hypertrophy).

✓Amyloidosis
✓Sarcoidosis
✓Hemochromatosis
✓**Endomyocardial fibroelastosis** (may occur with or without idiopathic **hypereosinophilic syndrome)**
✓Glycogen storage disease

■ **Treatment**

Diuretic. Treat underlying disease. Prednisone for restrictive cardiomyopathy related to hypereosinophilia.

D. Myocarditis

■ **Description**

Condition of **myocardium affected by inflammatory or infectious process.** Myocarditis may be difficult or impossible to distinguish clinically from cardiomyopathy (see preceding sections). Some forms of cardiomyopathy may evolve from myocarditis.

■ **Symptoms**

Often **preceded by upper respiratory tract infection** (viral). Many cases mild and self-limited. In more severe cases, **fever, dyspnea, edema, chest pain.**

On exam, **tachycardia, CHF** (often biventricular), **gallops, cardiomegaly.**

■ **Diagnosis**

↑ESR   **History, exam. Chest x-ray** with cardiomegaly, CHF. Elevated sedimentation rate. Viral cultures and titers useful in some cases. Blood cultures (bacterial). Right ventricular endomyocardial biopsy may have a role.

■ **Pathology**

Viral—especially Coxsackie B, but also influenza, varicella, echo virus, infectious mononucleosis, Coxsackie A, measles, acquired immunodeficiency syndrome (HIV-2) and others
Bacterial diphtheria—streptococci or staphylococci as complication of endocarditis
Fungal
Giant cell myocarditis—cause unknown
Rickettsial—rare

V. PERICARDIAL DISEASES

A. Acute Pericarditis

■ Description

Inflammatory process involving pericardium, by spread either from myoepicardium or from adjacent structure.

■ Symptoms

Chest pain, often sharp and knifelike, central or left precordial, can radiate to shoulders or back. Often positional and with pleuritic component; however, may be asymptomatic.

■ Diagnosis

History. On exam, hallmark is three-component pericardial friction rub, but occasionally rub is not audible. No specific laboratory test, but often leukocytosis, elevated sedimentation rate. Acute and convalescent viral titers. The ECG with diffuse ST-T abnormality, typically with elevation of ST segment.

Echocardiography may show pericardial effusion. Important to establish etiologic diagnosis.

■ Pathology

Pericarditis can be caused by a wide variety of etiologies.

Infectious—includes viral, bacterial, fungal, parasitic, tuberculous. Most common infectious cause is Coxsackie type B virus.

Postcardiotomy and postmyocardial infarction—Dressler syndrome. Occur 2 to 12 weeks after cardiac insult, probably autoimmune basis.

Malignancy—invades pericardium by contiguous extension or metastasis.

Trauma

Radiation therapy

Systemic diseases—includes uremia, rheumatic fever, rheumatoid arthritis, myxedema, lupus erythematosus, scleroderma, periarteritis.

Drug related—procainamide, hydralazine, penicillin.

Idiopathic—cause unknown, probably the most common form in adults.

■ Treatment

Symptomatic and supportive. Aspirin, non-steroidal anti-inflammatory drugs (NSAIDs). Occasionally steroids are required.

Treat underlying disease.

B. Pericardial Effusion

■ Description

Accumulation of serous or serosanguinous fluid in pericardial space. Can be acute or chronic. Rapidity of fluid collection a major determinant of hemodynamic effect.

■ Symptoms

May be asymptomatic or have chest pain of pericarditis. Cardiac tamponade with hemodynamic collapse can occur.

■ Diagnosis

History, exam. May have pericardial friction rub or dullness at left lung base posteriorly due to compression of lung by pericardial sac (Ewart's sign). Chest x-ray with cardiomegaly. The ECG may show pattern of pericarditis, also electrical alternans; echocardiography documents presence and size of effusion.

■ Pathology

Most common causes are viral, idiopathic, tuberculous, and malignant pericarditis; however, any cause of pericarditis can cause pericardial effusion, and effusion may be the presenting sign of pericardial disease.

■ **Treatment**

Treat underlying disorder. Pericardiocentesis or surgical resection may be required for diagnosis or relief of tamponade.

C. Cardiac Tamponade (by Pericardial Effusion)

■ **Description**

Marked reduction of cardiac output due to interference with normal cardiac filling by the compressive effect of pericardial effusion. Rate of accumulation of pericardial fluid important. Rapid accumulation of fluid favors cardiac tamponade by relatively small volumes of pericardial fluid (as little as a few hundred milliliters).

■ **Symptoms**

Acutely ill. Dyspnea and hemodynamic collapse. If tamponade develops slowly, can mimic CHF.

■ **Diagnosis**

History, exam. Neck vein distention in setting of hypotension and pulsus paradoxicus. (↓ bp & pulse on inspiration)

[handwritten note: ↑ NVD on inspiration: Kussmaul's sign]

■ **Pathology**

Can occur with pericardial effusion of any cause, but most commonly associated with trauma, cardiac surgery, malignancy. Occasionally cardiac tamponade is due to pericardial effusion from viral or idiopathic pericarditis or following radiation therapy.

■ **Treatment**

Pericardiocentesis or surgical pericardiectomy without delay can be life saving.

Treat underlying disease after relief of cardiac tamponade.

D. Constrictive Pericarditis

■ **Description**

Chronic process of thickening of pericardium resulting in cardiac encasement.

■ **Symptoms**

Edema, ascites, hepatic congestion, weakness.

Exam shows signs of systemic venous congestion, especially neck vein distention. May have Kussmaul's sign and/or pericardial knock.

[handwritten note: ↳ NVD ↑ on inspiration]

■ **Diagnosis**

History, exam. The ECG is non-specific, but often shows low QRS voltage. Chest x-ray often with cardiomegaly, may show pericardial calcification. Echocardiography may show thickened pericardium. Cardiac catheterization confirms diagnosis by demonstration of characteristic hemodynamics ("dip and plateau" contour of ventricular diastolic pressure).

■ **Pathology**

Almost any cause of acute pericarditis can lead to pericardial constriction, but most commonly due to radiation therapy, virus, idiopathic process, collagen vascular disease, uremia, or malignancy.

Thickened non-compliant pericardial sac causes marked limitation to cardiac filling during ventricular diastole, resulting in systemic venous congestion and limitation of cardiac output reserve.

■ **Treatment**

Diuretic and salt restriction for mild cases, or cases with high surgical risk. Definitive management requires surgical pericardiectomy.

VI. VALVULAR HEART DISEASES

A. Acute Rheumatic Fever

■ Description

Inflammatory disease affecting skin, joints, heart, subcutaneous tissue, and central nervous system that develops following group A streptococcal pharyngitis. Common cause of valvular heart disease, but incidence declining in developed countries. Valvular sequelae include stenosis and/or regurgitation of aortic and/or mitral valves, less commonly affects right-sided heart valves.

■ Symptoms

Fever, malaise, polyarthritis, chorea, rash. Dyspnea from acute heart failure caused by valvular regurgitation and/or myocarditis. Acute pericarditis can occur. Many cases resolve without clinical sequelae. **Most common in children 5 to 15 years of age,** although can occur in any age group.

[handwritten: School age → children b/c they are most likely to get group A strep pharyngitis]

■ Diagnosis

History, exam. Many of the signs, symptoms, and laboratory findings of acute rheumatic fever (ARF) are non-specific, so the **modified Jones criteria** are often required for diagnosis: two major criteria, or one major and two minor criteria, and **evidence (usually serologic) of preceding streptococcal infection.**

1. Major Criteria

- ✓ Carditis—most common and most reliable sign
- ✓ Erythema marginatum
- ✓ Polyarthritis
- ✓ Chorea (Sydenham's)
- ✓ Subcutaneous nodules

2. Minor Criteria

- – Fever
- – Arthralgia
- – Prior documented ARF or pre-existing evidence of rheumatic heart disease
- – Prolonged PR interval on ECG
- – Elevated sedimentation rate or increased C-reactive protein

■ Pathology

Invasive infection with group A streptococcus probably elicits an antibody response with **cross-reactivity with host tissues (autoimmune mechanism).**

■ Treatment

Penicillin (but does not prevent subsequent heart disease), **bed rest, salicylates.** Corticosteroids if evidence of moderate or severe carditis. Diuretics, salt restriction if CHF develops. Sedatives for chorea. Cardiac surgery rarely required for severe valvular regurgitation during acute phase of illness.

■ Prevention

Prevention of **initial attack** of ARF by adequate and prompt antibiotic therapy for streptococcal pharyngitis. *at least 10d. of rx*

Prevention of **recurrent attack** of ARF by long-term prophylaxis against recurrent group A streptococcal infection.

B. Mitral Stenosis *— Diastolic rumble*

■ Description

[handwritten diagram: S₁ S₂ opening snap]

Narrowing of the mitral valve orifice by fusion following inflammation of anterior and posterior mitral leaflets and variable degree of fusion and shortening of chordae tendineae. Causes obstruction to LV inflow from the left atrium. May coexist with mitral regurgitation.

■ Symptoms

Dyspnea, often precipitated by **atrial fibrillation. Fatigue.** Left atrial thrombi can cause **systemic embolization.** In advanced cases, right heart failure with edema, hepatic congestion.

On exam, **loud S1, opening snap** in early diastole, **low-pitched diastolic murmur** ("rumble") at LV apex. May have **pulmonary congestion.** If RV failure, edema and neck vein distention.

■ Diagnosis

History, exam. Acute pulmonary edema with new onset AF may be presenting symptom of previously clinically silent MS. With left atrial enlargement or AF, ECG may have RVH. **Chest x-ray** with **left atrial enlargement,** pulmonary venous hypertension. **Doppler echocardiography** extremely helpful.

■ Pathology

Almost always a **sequel of rheumatic fever** (months to decades after acute attack). Rarely, congenital or due to mitral annular calcification. Atrial myxoma can mimic hemodynamic abnormality of mitral stenosis (MS). **Increase in left atrial pressure** causes pulmonary congestion, left atrial enlargement, atrial arrhythmias.

■ Treatment

Diuretic. Salt restriction. Control of atrial fibrillation, mitral valve surgery or percutaneous valvulotomy for patients with significant symptoms on medical therapy.

Bacterial endocarditis prophylaxis. Anticoagulation.

C. Mitral Regurgitation – holosystolic or crescendo systolic murmur radiating to axilla

■ Description

Reflux of blood from the **left ventricle** into the **left atrium** during ventricular systole through the mitral valve orifice. If regurgitation severe, causes **left ventricular volume overload** and pulmonary con-

gestion. May be acute or chronic, and may coexist with mitral stenosis.

■ Symptoms

Will vary markedly from **asymptomatic to severely compromised due to CHF,** depending on degree and acuteness of MR, left ventricular function, and associated arrhythmias. Systemic embolization may occur in setting of atrial fibrillation.

On exam, **holosystolic or crescendo (MVP) systolic murmur,** loudest at LV apex. May have S3 (chronic MR) or S4 (acute MR). Pulmonary congestion in severe cases.

■ Diagnosis

History, exam. Chest x-ray positive for cardiomegaly. The ECG often shows LVH, left atrial abnormality. **Doppler echocardiography** very useful to assess mechanism of MR.

■ Pathology

Mechanism of mitral regurgitation (MR) can involve **dysfunction of any portion of the mitral valve apparatus:** annulus, leaflets, chordae tendineae, papillary muscles, or adjacent left ventricular wall. Pathologic processes with potential to affect one or more valve components are multiple and include **rheumatic fever, endocarditis, acute myocardial infarction, mitral valve prolapse syndrome, Marfan syndrome, congenital lesions, trauma, mitral annular dilatation,** or **calcification.**

■ Treatment

Salt restriction, diuretic, vasodilators if CHF present. Control of arrhythmias. Anticoagulation in some cases. Severe MR often requires cardiac surgery (valve replacement or repair). Bacterial endocarditis prophylaxis.

D. Aortic Stenosis – *harsh systolic murmur*

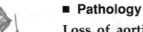

S_1 S_2

■ **Description**

Obstruction to blood flow from the left ventricle into the aorta at the level of the aortic valve. May coexist with aortic regurgitation.

■ **Symptoms**

Angina pectoris, congestive heart failure, syncope.

On exam, **crescendo decrescendo mid- or late-peaking harsh systolic murmur** in aortic area radiating to the neck. **Carotid upstroke diminished and late.** The S2 is absent or diminished.

■ **Diagnosis**

History, exam. ECG with LVH. **Chest x-ray** with cardiomegaly, CHF in some cases. **Doppler echocardiography** very helpful.

■ **Pathology**

need to rx by symptomatic or early rx → ↑ symptoms Much worse prognosis even ē valve replacement

Failure of the aortic valve orifice to open fully during ventricular systole may be caused by marked **thickening and calcification** of the aortic valve leaflets (as in calcific AS), **commissural fusion from inflammation** (as in AS after rheumatic fever), or may be **congenital in origin** (unicuspid or bicuspid AS).

■ **Treatment**

Surgical aortic valve replacement for symptomatic AS. Bacterial endocarditis prophylaxis.

E. Aortic Regurgitation – *diastolic murmur*

S_1 S_2

■ **Description**

Reflux of blood from the aorta into the left ventricle in ventricular diastole due to **incompetent aortic valve.** Can take acute or chronic form. May coexist with aortic stenosis.

■ **Pathology**

Loss of aortic valve competence can be caused by developmental abnormality, destruction of aortic leaflets, or by loss of support of aortic leaflets due to aortic root disease. Etiologic factors may be **endocarditis, congenital** (including bicuspid aortic valve), **trauma, inflammation** (rheumatic fever), **ascending aortic aneurysm, aortitis** (ankylosing spondylitis, syphilis, Reiter syndrome).

■ **Symptoms**

Dyspnea. Fatigue. Palpitations. Syncope and angina uncommon. If severe, CHF. Asymptomatic in mild cases.

On exam, **decrescendo diastolic murmur** loudest at left sternal border or aortic area, **cardiomegaly, S3 gallop.**

■ **Diagnosis**

History, exam. The ECG with LVH. Chest x-ray with cardiomegaly, possible CHF, aortic root dilatation often found. **Doppler echocardiography.**

■ **Treatment**

Salt restriction, diuretics, vasodilators if CHF present. **Aortic valve replacement** in advanced cases. Bacterial endocarditis prophylaxis.

F. Endocarditis

■ **Description**

Infection of endocardium, usually valvular but may involve mural endocardium or prosthetic heart valve. Subacute and acute forms, depending on organism involved. **Abnormal heart valves** and **congenital heart lesions** most often affected, but may occur in the normal heart.

■ Symptoms

Fever. Malaise. Anemia, weight loss, emboli, renal failure, metastatic abscess, arthritis, CHF.

On exam, elevated temperature, evidence of systemic (left heart involvement) or pulmonary (right heart involvement) embolization, cardiac murmurs (any regurgitant lesion), signs of CHF.

[handwritten: spiking fevers of unknown origin 2° periodic bacteremia]

■ Diagnosis

History, exam. High index of suspicion if pre-existing cardiac lesions or illicit intravenous drug use. **Blood cultures.** *(2x's)* **Doppler echocardiography.** Elevated sedimentation rate, rheumatoid factor.

■ Pathology

Most common causative organism is *Streptococcus viridans* (subacute course), but also caused by *Staphylococcus aureus* (acute course), *Staphylococcus epidermidis*, gram-negative bacteria, fungi, pneumococcus, gonococcus, and (rarely) spirochetes and rickettsiae. **Mitral valve most commonly involved,** followed by aortic and tricuspid. Pulmonic valve rarely affected by endocarditis.

[handwritten: → esp IVDA → esp tricuspid valve]

■ Treatment

Early treatment (often presumptive while blood culture results pending) **with appropriate bacteriocidal antibiotics.** Cardiac surgery for complications of severe CHF due to cardiac valve dysfunction, recurrent emboli, myocardial abscess.

G. Prosthetic Heart Valve

■ Description

Artificial device designed to be **surgically implanted** as a functional **replacement for a cardiac valve** that is severely malfunctioning. Valve repair is sometimes an alternative to replacement.

1. Prosthetic Valve Types

Mechanical prosthesis—designs include ball-in-cage (Starr Edwards) and tilting disc (St. Jude, Hall Medtronic, Bjork Shiley) models, are considered durable, but require chronic anticoagulation.

Bioprosthesis—designs (porcine or pericardial) generally do not require long-term anticoagulation, but valve deterioration a problem in younger patients.

2. Complications of Prosthetic Heart Valves

Endocarditis—(early or late after implantation), **embolization,** perivalvular **leak, mechanical failure, hemorrhagic complications** of anticoagulation.

VII. CONGENITAL HEART DISEASES

Present at birth, resulting from **abnormality of development.** Wide spectrum of clinical expression, depending on severity of defect. Cause unknown in most cases, but recognized contributing factors include chromosomal abnormalities (Down syndrome, Turner syndrome), older maternal age, maternal rubella infection in first trimester, maternal exposure to certain drugs (eg, anticoagulants). Prevention efforts involve adequate prenatal care, rubella immunization before conception, and genetic counseling in appropriate settings.

A. Ventricular Septal Defect

■ Description and Pathology

Most common congenital heart disease lesion. Persistent **opening in the upper portion of the ventricular septum** (membranous septum) with resultant **left-to-right shunt** at the ventricular level.

[handwritten: non cyanotic]

■ **Symptoms**

Harsh systolic murmur at left sternal border, radiates to right precordium. **Spontaneous closure 30 to 50% of cases.** If shunt small, may be asymptomatic. If shunt large, CHF and potential of pulmonary vascular disease with reversal of shunt and Eisenmenger syndrome.

the larger the hole, the smaller the murmur i.e. Grade II/VI murmur means smaller hole than Grade IV/VI

↳reversal of shunt

■ **Diagnosis**

History, exam. The ECG may show LVH. **Doppler echocardiography** should be diagnostic. **Chest x-ray with cardiomegaly** and increased pulmonary vasculature if shunt significant. Cardiac catheterization.

■ **Treatment**

For asymptomatic patient with **small ventricular septal defect (VSD), observation.** Bacterial endocarditis prophylaxis. **If shunt flow significant, surgical repair.**

Must have good follow-up!
Or if shunt doesn't close

B. Atrial Septal Defect

■ **Description and Pathology**

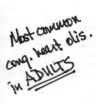

Most common cong. heart dis. in ADULTS

Persistent **opening in atrial septum,** most commonly in region of fossa ovalis [atrial septal defect (ASD of secundum septum)], but can also occur in lower portion of atrial septum (ASD of primum septum) or in sinus node region of the atrial septum (sinus venosus ASD). **Left-to-right shunt at the atrial level.** More common in females.

■ **Symptoms**

Fixed split S$_2$

Often asymptomatic as child or teenager. **Dyspnea, fatigue,** and **atrial arrhythmias** develop in early or middle adulthood, sometimes sooner. **Right heart failure** can occur. In some advanced cases, severe pulmonary hypertension and Eisenmenger syndrome can develop.

On exam, **fixed splitting of second heart sound, systolic ejection murmur** at

left upper sternal border, and **right ventricular enlargement.** If CHF has developed, neck vein distention and edema. Mitral regurgitation due to MVP (secundum ASD) or cleft in anterior mitral leaflet (primum ASD).

■ **Diagnosis**

History, but note that patient may be asymptomatic. **Exam.** The ECG almost always with **incomplete or complete right bundle branch block (RBBB),** and in addition usually has left axis deviation in cases of ASD of primum septum. **Chest x-ray** with cardiomegaly and **increased pulmonary vasculature. Doppler echocardiography** diagnostic in most cases. Cardiac catheterization.

■ **Treatment**

Observation for small shunt in asymptomatic patient. **Surgical repair for significant shunt.**

C. Patent Ductus Arteriosus

■ **Description and Pathology**

Arteriovenous fistula between aorta and left pulmonary artery due to failure of embryonic ductus to close after birth. **Left-to-right shunt** increases work on the left heart. Fistulous connection commonly inserts near origin of left subclavian artery. More common in births at high altitude, in births to mothers exposed to rubella in first trimester of pregnancy, in premature babies, and in females.

■ **Symptoms**

Hallmark is **continuous "machinery" murmur** at upper left sternal border. S2 may be paradoxically split. **Wide systemic pulse pressure with abnormally low diastolic pressure.** Left ventricular volume overload can lead to CHF.

■ **Diagnosis**

History, exam. The ECG with LVH. Chest x-ray with **cardiomegaly** and **increased pulmonary vasculature.** Cardiac catheterization.

■ **Treatment**

Surgical closure, optimal time 1 to 2 years of age. Bacterial endocarditis prophylaxis.

Can give Indomethacin to try to encourage closure (NSAIDS)

D. Coarctation of Aorta

■ **Description and Pathology**

Narrowing of aortic lumen, usually immediately **distal to origin of left subclavian artery** near insertion of ligamentum arteriosum. Associated with Turner syndrome. A common cause of **secondary hypertension.** More common in males.

■ **Symptoms**

Vary greatly from asymptomatic to severe **hypertension** resulting in **headache** or CHF, **intracranial hemorrhage,** lower extremity **claudication.** Aortic rupture a risk.

On exam, **upper extremity hypertension** with **reduced or absent lower extremity pulses, systolic ejection murmur** (may be continuous) anterior chest and upper back. May also have aortic regurgitation due to bicuspid aortic valve, which is associated with coarctation of aorta.

■ **Diagnosis**

History, exam. The ECG often with LVH. Chest x-ray may show cardiomegaly, **rib notching, dilated aorta,** and left subclavian artery. **Aortogram.**

■ **Treatment**

Surgical correction, optimally aged 4 to 8 years. Bacterial endocarditis prophylaxis.

E. Tetralogy of Fallot

■ **Description and Pathology**

Most common **cyanotic** congenital heart lesion older than 1 year of age. Consists of

1. **Ventricular septal defect** (usually large).
2. **Narrowing of right ventricular outflow tract** (usually infundibular). *pulm. stenosis*
3. **Overriding of aorta above VSD.**
4. **Right ventricular hypertrophy.**

About 25% of patients have a right-sided aortic arch. The result of this complex of abnormalities is a **right-to-left shunt** at the ventricular level.

■ **Symptoms**

Polycythemia, retardation of growth, exercise intolerance. Characteristic "**squat maneuver**" after exercise. *(↑ peripheral vasc. resis)*

On exam, **prominent right ventricular impulse, systolic ejection murmur** with **thrill** at left sternal border, single S2, **cyanosis, clubbing.**

■ **Diagnosis**

History, exam. **Chest x-ray** with **decreased pulmonary vasculature,** Doppler echocardiography, boot-shaped heart ("coeur en sabot"). The ECG with RVH. **Cardiac catheterization** confirms diagnosis and defines level and severity of RV outflow obstruction.

■ **Treatment**

Surgical correction, either palliative procedure followed by definitive operation at a later time, or initial total surgical correction. Bacterial endocarditis prophylaxis.

F. Endocardial Cushion Defect

■ Description and Pathology

Persistent opening in lower atrial and upper ventricular septa associated with developmental abnormalities of tricuspid and/or mitral valves, caused by failure of the endocardial cushions to fuse properly during development. Spectrum of defect ranges from ostium primum ASD only (usually with some abnormality of mitral valve) to a complete atrioventricular canal defect with a common ASD/VSD and a common atrioventricular valve. The complete defect is associated with Down syndrome.

■ Symptoms

Depends on severity and complexity of lesion. The complete endocardial cushion defect (common AV canal) usually presents in infancy with weight loss, CHF, recurrent pulmonary infections.

■ Diagnosis

History, exam. Doppler echocardiography establishes diagnosis and extent of defect. The ECG with **first-degree AV block, left axis deviation. Chest x-ray** with cardiomegaly, **increased pulmonary vasculature,** and CHF in severe forms.

■ Treatment

Depends on extent and complexity of defect. "Partial" or "incomplete" defects (ASD of primum septum) usually repaired as child or young adult. **Surgical repair** for some patients with complete defect. Bacterial endocarditis prophylaxis.

VIII. SYSTEMIC ARTERIAL HYPERTENSION

A. Primary (Essential, Idiopathic) Hypertension

■ Description

Accounts for about **90% of cases of hypertension,** usual onset 25 to 55 years of age. Many with family history of hypertension or atherosclerotic disease. Often found in patients with other cardiovascular risk factors. **More common in blacks** (20 to 30% of blacks).

■ Symptoms

Often asymptomatic. Headache. **Most common cause of LVH and CHF.** Risk factor for myocardial infarction, cerebrovascular accident, renal failure.

■ Diagnosis

Documentation of systemic arterial pressure > 140/90 mm Hg on at least three different occasions at rest, in the absence of identifiable secondary cause of hypertension. Measurement of blood pressure (BP) on each patient visit to a health care professional and mass screening programs are important for detection.

ECG may show LVH. Urinalysis, blood urea nitrogen (BUN), creatinine may reveal kidney dysfunction.

On exam S4 and loud S2 common.

■ Pathology

Cause not identified, but abnormalities have been implicated in central nervous system, renin angiotensin system, systemic vascular resistance, baroreceptor activity, aldosterone system. Probably multiple mechanisms.

■ Treatment

Weight control. Low-salt, low-animal-fat diet. **Diuretics, beta blockers, vasodilators, calcium channel blockers.** Noncompliance a major problem and is minimized by patient education about risks of disease and goals of treatment.

B. Secondary Hypertension

■ Description

Elevated systemic arterial pressure (see preceding diagnostic criteria) **associated with a documented condition known to cause hypertension.** Accounts for **8 to 10% of all cases of hypertension.** Can occur at any age, but suspect if patient < 25 years or > 60 years of age.

■ Symptoms

Similar to essential hypertension, except may have signs and symptoms related to specific cause of secondary hypertension.

■ Diagnosis

History and **exam,** with special attention to symptoms and signs of secondary causes.

Electrolytes, blood urea nitrogen (BUN), creatinine, calcium, urinalysis. Further specialized testing (eg, aortogram, renal arteriogram; urinary collection for catecholamines, vanillylmandelic acid (VMA); or 17-hydroxycorticosteroids) as dictated by clinical circumstances.

■ Pathology

Renal artery stenosis, renal parenchymal disease, coarctation of aorta, arteritis affecting kidneys, **endocrine disorders** (Cushing syndrome or disease, pheochromocytoma, hyperaldosteronism), hypercalcemia, drug induced (certain steroids, chronic licorice ingestion), brain tumor, or hematoma.

■ Treatment

Eliminate underlying secondary cause, if possible. **Surgical cure possible in many cases.** Antihypertensive therapy if surgical approach ineffective or impossible.

C. Accelerated (Malignant) Hypertension

■ Description

Abrupt worsening of systemic arterial hypertension with **diastolic pressure > 120 mm Hg** associated with neurologic dysfunction (severe headache, CVA, visual disturbances, papilledema, convulsions), **acute renal failure** (with or without chronic renal insufficiency), or **cardiac dysfunction** (acute MI, pulmonary edema).

■ Symptoms

Eyeground hemorrhages. May have focal or nonfocal CNS signs. If CHF present, pulmonary congestion and cardiac gallops.

■ Diagnosis

Diastolic arterial pressure > 120 mm Hg associated with acute and severe manifestations of cardiac, neurologic, or renal dysfunction.

The ECG with LVH, may show acute cardiac ischemia.

CRX may show cardiomegaly.

■ Pathology

Can occur in patient with either primary (essential) or secondary form of hypertension.

■ Treatment

Prompt control of blood pressure to moderate range. **Sodium nitroprusside, diazoxide, trimethaphan.** Hydralazine or nifedipine. Adjunctive use of beta blocker or diuretic, depending on circumstances. Switch to oral antihypertensive agents when stable.

D. Pre-eclampsia/Eclampsia

■ Description

Pre-eclampsia is a syndrome of **edema, proteinuria, and hypertension occurring** after 20th week of pregnancy or in early puerperium. Affects 10 to 20% of pregnancies, **most common in primigravidas, black women, previous hypertensives.** In severest form, pre-eclampsia progresses to CNS irritability and **convulsions (eclampsia).**

↑LFTs
↓platelets
blurry vision
HTN
proteinuria

■ Symptoms

Clinical continuum from mild pre-eclampsia to eclampsia with convulsions. Blood pressure increases may be abrupt. **Major cause of prematurity, fetal and maternal death.** Renal and hepatic dysfunction may occur in severe cases.

■ Diagnosis

History, exam. Laboratory testing for **proteinuria, renal and liver function.**

■ Pathology

Unknown, but may result from impaired uteroplacental blood flow caused by decreased prostaglandin E (PGE) synthesis.

■ Treatment

Bed rest, salt restriction. Methyldopa, hydralazine. Interruption of pregnancy, cesarean section, or induction of labor for severe cases. Intravenous (IV) magnesium sulfate for convulsions.

Definitive rx = delivery

IX. SYSTEMIC ARTERIAL HYPOTENSION WITH SHOCK AND CYANOSIS

A. Systemic Hypotension with Shock

■ Description

Hypotension is usually defined as <90 mm Hg systolic in adults. Shock is said to exist when hypotension is accompanied by signs and symptoms of **poor tissue perfusion.** Shock can exist with systemic arterial pressure above 90 mm Hg systolic in some cases.

■ Symptoms

Signs of poor tissue perfusion (altered mental status, cool extremities, oliguria, metabolic acidosis) associated with systemic arterial hypotension.

■ Diagnosis

History, exam. Neck vein distention and pulsus paradoxicus clues to possible cardiac tamponade.

■ Pathology

Normal systemic arterial pressure is maintained by an **interplay between cardiac output and SVR.** A decline in one factor that cannot be compensated for by an increase in the other will cause systemic hypotension. Furthermore, at Cardiac Index under approximately 2.0 L/min per meter squared of body surface area (BSA), peripheral perfusion will be inadequate, no matter how high the SVR.

Hypovolemia—causes systemic hypotension by reducing venous return to the heart, thereby reducing cardiac output. Hypovolemia can be absolute (eg, hemorrhage, dehydration) or can be relative (eg, anaphylactoid reaction, sepsis).

Cardiogenic—cause of systemic hypotension is due to an **inadequate output of the heart** under conditions of adequate venous return (ie, hypovolemia not present). Inadequate cardiac output under these conditions can be due to severe mechanical (valvular or pericardial) or myocardial (eg, cardiomyopathy, acute MI) dysfunction.

Severe pulmonary artery obstruction (eg, severe pulmonary embolism, severe pulmonary vasculature disease) can uncommonly be a cause of hypotension by causing restriction of left heart filling.

■ **Treatment**

Hypovolemic shock—**IV fluids** (crystalloid, blood products if appropriate), **treat underlying cause**. If pressors used, only temporary measure until intravascular volume restored.

Cardiogenic shock—**inotropic agents** (dobutamine, dopamine, amrinone), vasodilator. **Intraaortic balloon counterpulsation** in certain circumstances. Pericardiocentesis for cardiac tamponade.

Shock secondary to severe pulmonary arterial obstruction—diagnose and treat underlying cause.

B. Cyanosis

■ **Description**

Bluish discoloration of skin and mucous membranes.

■ **Symptoms**

Central cyanosis is apparent on skin and warm mucous membranes.

Peripheral cyanosis is apparent on skin in exposed areas, where vasoconstriction may be present, and may not be so visible on warm mucous membranes.

■ **Diagnosis**

History, exam.

■ **Pathology**

Due to an **excess (> 4 g %)** of reduced hemoglobin in capillary blood.

Central cyanosis—caused by abnormally high amount of reduced hemoglobin in arterial blood due to **right-to-left intracardiac shunt** (usually congenital heart disease) or to inability of **severely diseased lung parenchyma** to adequately oxygenate systemic venous blood.

Peripheral cyanosis—caused by excess removal of oxygen from normally saturated blood during **abnormally slow flow** through capillary bed during **shock** or **cold exposure**.

■ **Treatment**

Treat underlying condition.

X. ATHEROSCLEROSIS AND LIPOPROTEINS

■ **Description**

Focal pathologic process affecting the **large arteries** (coronary, aorta, femoral, iliac, carotid, renal, mesenteric) characterized by accumulation within the intima of lipids, blood and blood products, calcium, complex carbohydrates, and fibrous tissue.

As process advances the media is involved, which leads to **arterial narrowing, aneurysm, ulceration, and dilatation.**

■ **Symptoms**

Depends on arterial segment affected and the nature of the destructive atherosclerotic process on that segment:

Coronary artery disease—angina, myocardial infarction, sudden death.

Aortic aneurysm, rupture, obstruction with claudication, emboli.

Femoral and iliac obstruction with claudication, emboli, aneurysm.

Mesenteric obstruction with intestinal angina, infarction of bowel.

Renal obstruction with hypertension, renal insufficiency.

Carotid obstruction and ulceration, transient ischemic attack and stroke.

■ **Diagnosis**

History, exam. Cholesterol testing with lipoprotein fractionation in most patients with atherosclerotic disease. **Specific functional and anatomic testing** (stress testing, ultrasound, Doppler, angiography) guided by location and severity of atherosclerotic disease.

■ Pathology

Complex interactions between blood elements, lipids, and arterial wall.

Multiple hypotheses, but current data support following sequence of events:

Injury to arterial wall and endothelium by cigarette smoking, hypertension, shear forces at bifurcations, hypercholesterolemia(?), free radicals.

Platelet and macrophage interaction with arterial wall, smooth muscle cell proliferation, and lipid entry.

Impairment of normal lipid-clearance mechanism, which leads to accumulation of lipids within cells and interstitium of wall.

Function of artery compromised by destruction of media/intima and arterial wall integrity.

Lipoprotein macromolecular complexes formed by blood fats (cholesterol, triglycerides) and certain proteins to allow the fats to circulate in blood plasma. Without lipoproteins, blood fats would be insoluble in plasma.

Chylomicrons—originate in small intestine, carry dietary fat.

Very low-density lipoproteins (VLDL)—originate primarily in liver, carry triglycerides to periphery, also carry cholesterol.

Low-density lipoproteins (LDL)—the major source of plasma cholesterol, and the lipoprotein most strongly associated with atherosclerosis. Carries cholesterol into artery wall.

High-density lipoproteins (HDL)—felt to have a role in cholesterol removal. Levels are inversely correlated with risk of atherosclerosis in some, but not all, populations.

Apolipoproteins are lipoproteins in a **delipidated** state. Several alipoproteins have been described. **Apo A-I** appears to be strongly inversely correlated with risk of coronary atherosclerosis.

Certain **clinical risk factors** have been firmly established to be predictive of increased prevalence, earlier age of occurrence, and accelerated progression of atherosclerosis:

- Cigarette smoking
- Family history of atherosclerosis
- Hyperlipidemia
- Systemic hypertension
- Diabetes mellitus
- Male sex

■ Treatment

Medical therapy may be all that is required. **Surgical therapy** on affected arteries often possible and advisable for advanced cases. **Percutaneous angioplasty** appropriate for certain clinical situations (renal, peripheral, coronary disease). **Risk-factor modification.** Prevention efforts involve risk modification in individuals at risk for atherosclerosis starting early in life.

XI. PERIPHERAL ARTERY VASCULAR DISEASES

A. Occlusive Arterial Disease

■ Description

Narrowing or occlusion of **large- and medium-sized arteries** resulting in reduction or total disruption of flow of oxygenated blood. Associated with hypertension, hypercholesterolemia, cigarette smoking, male sex, diabetes mellitus.

■ Symptoms

Claudication of lower (or less commonly, upper) extremities distal to the point of occlusion. Pattern of claudication useful in predicting level of occlusion [buttock, thigh, sexual impotence in males (iliac); calf (femoral, popliteal)]. **Rest pain** and **ulceration** of skin can occur in advanced cases.

On exam, diminished arterial pulsations, vascular bruits, and consequence of poor arterial flow (sparse hair, ulceration) may be seen.

■ **Diagnosis**

History, exam. Noninvasive evaluation *Doppler (duplex) studies* includes measurement of ankle and brachial arterial pressures before and after exercise. Angiography confirms site of obstruction and evaluates distal arterial runoff.

■ **Pathology**

Atherosclerosis is most common cause of occlusive peripheral artery disease; however, inflammation or trauma can also be a cause of arterial occlusive disease. Embolism or acute thrombosis can result in sudden total occlusion of an artery and is usually a medical emergency.

■ **Treatment**

Reconstructive arterial surgery or percutaneous angioplasty for disabling symptoms or rest ischemia. Risk-factor modification. Avoid vasoconstricting drugs.

B. Giant Cell Arteritis (Temporal Arteritis)

■ **Description**

Systemic disorder with involvement of aorta and large branches (particularly carotid). Usually in patients older than 55 years of age. *usually ♀*

■ **Symptoms**

Fever, malaise, myalgia. Headache, scalp tenderness, jaw claudication, visual symptoms. Loss of vision may not be reversible.

■ **Diagnosis**

History, exam. Laboratory findings of elevated sedimentation rate, abnormal liver function tests, and anemia are nonspecific. Biopsy (often temporal artery) of involved artery.

■ **Pathology**

Segmental granulomatous inflammation of unknown cause resulting in necrosis of media and occlusion of arterial lumen.

■ **Treatment**

Corticosteroids, usually for months. Disease generally self-limited.

C. Polyarteritis

■ **Description**

Segmental vasculitis of small- to medium-sized arteries causing dysfunction in multiple organ systems. Patients usually in middle age.

■ **Symptoms**

Clinical pattern determined by which organ systems involved, but systemic hypertension with kidney involvement in vast majority. Acute myocardial infarction may occur. Congestive heart failure can be found, due either to acute MI or hypertension. Other symptoms may reflect involvement of skin, GI tract, spleen, CNS.

■ **Diagnosis**

History, exam. Multisystem involvement with biopsy evidence of active arteritis.

■ **Pathology**

Small- to medium-sized arteries affected by segmental necrotizing granulomatous inflammation (varies from media only to full thickness) of unknown cause.

■ **Treatment**

Corticosteroids. Other therapy as indicated for specific organ dysfunction (eg, acute MI).

D. Arteriovenous Fistula

■ **Description**

Abnormal **communication between artery and vein.**

■ **Symptoms**

Many asymptomatic, especially congenital AV fistulae, which tend to be smaller than acquired type. Venous and/or arterial insufficiency in extremity affected. CHF **due to high-output state.**

■ **Diagnosis**

History, exam. **Thrill and bruit** over fistula. Prompt decrease in pulse rate (Nicoladoni Branham sign) when fistula is occluded. **Angiography** demonstrates location and size of fistula.

■ **Pathology**

May be **acquired** as result of trauma (blunt or penetrating) or **congenital.** Sequelae of AV fistula can be local (increased venous pressure with swelling of extremity, or arterial insufficiency distal to the fistula) or systemic (high-output CHF, decreased diastolic BP), and will depend on size of fistula and site involved.

■ **Treatment**

Surgical excision or intra-arterial embolization in most acquired cases. Congenital forms are often followed conservatively.

XII. DISEASES OF VEINS AND PULMONARY EMBOLISM

A. Varicose Veins

■ **Description**

Dilated and tortuous veins of lower extremities. Most common vascular disease of the lower extremities.

■ **Symptoms**

Many asymptomatic. May cause **pain in legs,** superficial skin **ulceration, increased pigmentation.**

■ **Diagnosis**

Observation of varicose veins with patient standing.

■ **Pathology**

Usually a secondary condition as a sequel to deep vein thrombosis (causing chronic deep venous insufficiency), or resulting from obesity, pregnancy, ascites, right heart failure, prolonged standing.

Less commonly, a **primary condition** as a result of hereditary weakness of valves and walls of veins.

■ **Treatment**

Elastic support. May require sclerotherapy or **surgical treatment** (stripping).

B. Thrombophlebitis

■ **Description**

Occlusion of a vein by thrombus with variable amount of **inflammation** of vein wall. Can occur in superficial veins (varicose or non-varicose) or in deep venous system (iliofemoral, femoropopliteal, calf, axillary-subclavian). Predisposing factors include CHF, obesity, MI, trauma, postoperative state, malignancy, pregnancy, oral contraceptives.

■ **Symptoms**

Superficial thrombophlebitis—pain and erythema in affected area. May cause fever and swelling. Embolism rare.

Deep vein thrombophlebitis—pain, swelling, fever. May cause increased superficial venous pattern around site of deep obstruction. **Pulmonary embolism** is common.

■ **Diagnosis**

Superficial thrombophlebitis—exam, history. Laboratory findings non-specific.

Deep vein thrombophlebitis—exam, history (especially regarding predisposing conditions). **Impedance plethysmography and Doppler flow studies** very helpful in documenting thrombosis proximal to calf veins. May need **contrast venography**.

■ **Pathology**

Interaction of **hypercoagulability, venous stasis,** and **endothelial damage**.

■ **Treatment**

Superficial thrombophlebitis—warm moist packs, NSAIDs. In recurrent cases, anticoagulation, surgery.

Deep vein thrombophlebitis—full anticoagulating dose of **heparin IV** for 7 to 10 days followed by **oral anticoagulation** for 3 to 6 months. Prevention with low-dose subcutaneous heparin, warfarin, or calf-compression devices during period of high risk.

C. **Pulmonary Embolism and Infarction**

■ **Description**

Thrombus material that has moved from a peripheral vein through the venous system to lodge in a pulmonary artery or branch thereof. **Most pulmonary emboli from deep leg veins,** but some from pelvic veins, right heart chambers, arm veins. **Significant morbidity and mortality;** can be difficult to recognize clinically. Predisposing factors similar to those associated with deep vein thrombophlebitis.

■ **Symptoms**

Varies from minimal (even absent) to sudden cardiovascular collapse. **Dyspnea, chest pain** (sometimes crushing and substernal acutely, may develop pleuritic quality hours or days later). **Tachypnea.** May have **hypotension, cyanosis,** splinting on respiration, **pleural friction rub, fever,** tricuspid regurgitation.

■ **Diagnosis**

History and **exam,** but since often non-specific must have **high index of suspicion. Chest x-ray** may have pleural effusion, atelectasis, elevated hemidiaphragm. The ECG with sinus tachycardia, non-specific changes; acute RBBB supportive.

Ventilation and perfusion lung scanning very helpful if negative or high probability for pulmonary embolism. If results of ventilation-perfusion lung indeterminate or equivocal, **pulmonary angiography** may be required and is most sensitive and specific diagnostic test for pulmonary embolism. **Doppler flow** and **impedance plethysmography** or **venous contrast study** of lower extremities may be used in some circumstances, but neither can exclude presence of pulmonary emboli.

■ **Pathology**

Venous stasis, hypercoagulability, endothelial damage interact as in deep vein thrombophlebitis. Embolism obstructs pulmonary arterial bed, causes ventilation-perfusion mismatch, and can cause systemic hypotension in severe cases. **Hemorrhagic necrosis (infarction) of lung parenchyma** follows in a minority of cases.

■ **Treatment**

Intravenous heparin for 7 to 10 days followed by oral anticoagulation for 2 to 6 months. If recurrent pulmonary emboli on adequate anticoagulation, or if anticoagulation contraindicated, IVC interruption by surgical or percutaneous method.

(Greenfield Filter)

XIII. AORTIC ANEURYSMS

A. Dissecting Aneurysm of Aorta

■ Description

Rupture of blood into the media of the aortic wall followed by dissection in circumferential and longitudinal fashion. **Severe clinical consequences.** Usually presents acutely (but may be chronic). Associated with **hypertension, Marfan syndrome, pregnancy, coarctation of the aorta, trauma** (usually blunt). Men more commonly affected than women. **Peak incidence 35 to 70 years of age.**

■ Symptoms

Sharp, knifelike chest pain of sudden onset, often felt initially substernally (ascending aortic dissection) but may then radiate to neck and interscapular area as dissection progresses distally. **Acute aortic regurgitation,** acute MI, **hemopericardium with cardiac tamponade,** paraplegia (occlusion of spinal arteries); CVA can occur as a consequence of destruction by the plane of dissection.

Three basic anatomic patterns of aortic dissection have been described:

Type I—Dissection begins in proximal aorta and extends distally for variable distance.
Type II—Dissection limited to aortic arch.
Type III—Dissection begins distal to left subclavian artery and extends distally for variable distance.

■ Diagnosis

History, exam. May have unequal blood pressure in upper or lower extremities, acute aortic regurgitation, cardiac tamponade, congestive heart failure. **Aortog-**

raphy generally required for confirmation of diagnosis, but CT scan or transesophageal echocardiography may also be useful.

■ Pathology

Separation of elements of media layer of aortic wall by an **intramural hematoma,** which gains access to the media through a **tear in aortic intima.** Underlying condition in most cases appears to be cystic medial necrosis. The intramural hematoma may or may not exit into the true aortic lumen distally.

■ Treatment

Severe clinical consequences with grave outcome if not treated promptly. **Immediate control of blood pressure** (if hypertensive) with fast-acting parenteral agents, **beta blockers** to reduce shear forces in ascending aorta. **Emergency surgical treatment** of type I and II. Type III may be treated surgically, or may be followed medically in some cases if stable.

B. Aneurysm of the Thoracic Aorta (Non-dissecting)

■ Description

Significant **dilatation of one or more segments of thoracic aorta.** Most commonly involves ascending aorta from root to origin of innominate artery. May involve transverse arch segment alone. Aneurysm of the descending thoracic aorta may extend into the upper abdominal aorta (thoracoabdominal aortic aneurysm), and is often associated with significant hypertension.

■ Symptoms

Depends on location and severity. May be asymptomatic. Dilatation of aortic root may lead to loss of aortic valve support and **aortic regurgitation** and CHF. **Com-**

pression of adjacent structures can lead to symptoms of chest pain, hoarseness, dysphagia. With severely dilated aneurysms, **rupture** with fatal hemorrhage is a constant threat.

■ Diagnosis

History, exam. Dilatation of the aorta will be apparent on **chest x-ray. Aortography** is required for anatomic localization of aneurysm if surgery is contemplated.

■ Pathology

Atherosclerosis is the most common cause. **Cystic medial necrosis** may be seen in some aortic aneurysms, especially those of ascending aorta. Trauma, syphilis, aortitis less common causes. Marfan syndrome.

■ Treatment

Surgical resection with graft replacement for severe aneurysms, especially with significant aortic regurgitation, evidence of rupture or impending rupture, local compression syndrome.

C. Aneurysm of the Abdominal Aorta

■ Description

Most common site of aneurysm of aorta. Usually originates distal to the origin of the renal arteries. **Most common in males 50 to 70 years of age.**

■ Symptoms

Many asymptomatic, but may present with **abdominal or back pain** from expansion or with **hemodynamic collapse** from rupture with massive hemorrhage. May also have occlusive symptoms of lower extremity **claudication** or evidence of distal arterial embolization.

■ Diagnosis

History. Exam may show prominent **pulsatile abdominal mass.** Calcification in aneurysm on abdominal roentgenography. **Ultrasound. Aortography.**

■ Pathology

Atherosclerosis is most common cause. Thrombus within aneurysm may cause occlusion or embolism distally. Expansion with rupture and severe hemorrhage a serious threat to life.

■ Treatment

Elective **surgical resection** in most cases. Emergency surgical resection after rupture associated with increased mortality.

XIV. HEART TRANSPLANTATION

■ Description

Homograft cardiac orthotopic transplantation in carefully selected patients with life-threatening, severely symptomatic, and otherwise inoperable myocardial, valvular, coronary artery, or congenital heart disease. In some cardiac patients with severe pulmonary vascular disease (most commonly congenital heart patients), a heart-lung transplant is required.

Clinical Aspects of Post-Transplantation Care

Infection with a variety of organisms (often pulmonary in location) and rejection are major causes of morbidity and mortality after cardiac transplantation. Clinical signs of rejection (CHF, gallop rhythm, low QRS voltage on ECG) are insensitive, and the best method for evaluating acute rejection is **right ventricular endomyocardial biopsy.**

Graft coronary atherosclerosis, probably a form of chronic rejection, is a common problem. The transplanted cardiac patient will not experience angina because the transplanted heart is denervated.

Remember: NO Angina b/c heart is denervated!

XV. CARDIOPULMONARY ARREST

■ **Description**

Cessation of effective cardiac and/or pulmonary function resulting in hemodynamic collapse or severe cerebral dysfunction. Spontaneous cardiopulmonary arrest most often of cardiac etiology in adults (usually ventricular fibrillation due to coronary artery disease) and of pulmonary etiology in children.

■ **Symptoms**

Loss of consciousness (often abrupt) or severe lethargy. May be preceded by chest pain, palpitations, dyspnea. Must be distinguished from other causes of loss of consciousness or syncope (eg, neurologic, hemorrhagic, metabolic, toxic).

■ **Diagnosis**

Pulselessness (or ineffective very rapid or very slow pulse) in large artery of unresponsive victim.

■ **Treatment**

Basic Life Support (BLS).

A   Open airway.
B   Ventilate effectively—breathing.
C   Support circulation with external cardiac compression.

Assess effectiveness of BLS with evaluation of pupillary reactivity and palpation of pulsation in large artery. Continue until Advanced Cardiac Life Support available.

Advanced Cardiac Life Support (ACLS)

Maintain airway and adequate ventilation with adjunctive equipment (mask, endotracheal tube).

Arrhythmia recognition (ECG) and appropriate treatment (electrical and pharmacologic).

Intravenous access.

Often most important aspect of ACLS is prompt defibrillation for ventricular fibrillation (most common cause of cardiopulmonary arrest in adults).

BIBLIOGRAPHY

Brandenburg R, Fuster V, Guiliani E, et al. *Cardiology: Fundamentals and Practice.* Chicago, Ill: Year Book Medical Publishers, Inc; 1987.

Braunwald E. *Heart Disease.* 4th ed. Philadelphia, Pa: WB Saunders Co; 1992.

Dubin D. *Rapid Interpretation of EKG's.* Tampa, Fla: Cover Publishing Co; 1989.

Hurst J. *The Heart.* 7th ed. New York, NY: McGraw-Hill; 1990.

Perloff J. *The Clinical Recognition of Congenital Heart Disease.* 3rd ed. Philadelphia, Pa: WB Saunders Co; 1987.

Sokolow M, McIlroy M. *Clinical Cardiology.* Los Altos, Calif: Lange Medical Publications; 1986.

Young J, Gaor R, Olin J, et al. *Peripheral Vascular Diseases.* St. Louis, Mo: Mosby Co; 1991.

CHAPTER 2

Disorders of the Skin and Subcutaneous Tissue

JOEL S. GOLDBERG, DO

I. HEALTH AND HEALTH MAINTENANCE

A. Economic/Social Impact of Skin Disorders

■ **Description**

Consider ultimate cost in evaluation and treatment of sun-induced disorders. Consider financial and social/psychological impact (ie, acne).

B. Epidemiology and Prevention of Sun-Induced Skin Disorders

■ **Description**

Sun exposure results in pathologic skin changes termed actinic damage. Skin damage depends on multiple factors including individual skin sensitivity and current medications. Chronic sun exposure results in wrinkles and skin atrophy, and at some point precancerous and cancerous lesions (ie, malignant melanoma). Psoralens plus UVA (PUVA) has the **highest melanogenic potential.** Erythema and dyskeratotic cell potential is high with **ultraviolet B (UVB)** (290 to 320 nm). **Ultraviolet C (UVC) (1 to 290 nm) is absorbed by ozone layer.** Black light **(UVA) will go through glass, has a larger wavelength and causes aging and tanning; whereas UVB will not go through glass, has a shorter wavelength and causes sunburn.** Prevention of sun-induced lesions involves education, avoiding sun exposure, and/or use of sun blockers, especially with higher SPF (sun protective factor; 15 or more is excellent). **Para-aminobenzoic acid (PABA) protects against UVB.**

C. Epidemiology and Prevention of Contact Dermatitis and Drug Reactions

■ **Description**

Contact dermatitis is **epidermal inflammation** secondary to chemical compounds. It is noted to be **more common with fair skin,** and there may be a ge-netic tendency. **Drug reactions** may present as multiple types of skin eruptions. History and physical with attention to drug allergies is important, as is early discontinuation of the offending medication. **Common offending medications include penicillin, non-steroidal anti-inflammatory drugs (NSAIDs), and anticonvulsants. Any medication ingested may cause a skin reaction.**

D. Epidemiology and Prevention of Decubitus Ulcers

■ **Description**

Decubitus ulcers involve **skin necrosis** resulting **from excessive pressure.** The disorder is more common in individuals unable to move/react to this pressure (includes patients in coma, stroke/neurologic disorders). The key to **prevention** is **reduction** of **prolonged local pressure** via repositioning, therapy/ambulation if possible, or padding/pressure reduction via sheepskin, eggcrate, and air/water flow beds.

E. Epidemiology and Prevention of Dermatophytic Skin Disorders

■ **Description**

Fungal infection of keratinized tissue, via contact with an infected person, animal, or fomites. Increased frequency of fungal infections is noted in tropical conditions, with poor hygiene, with sweating and skin irritation, and immunological deficits. Control/moderation of these factors for prevention.

II. INFECTIONS

A. Herpes Simplex

■ **Description**

A **DNA virus** of type 1 (non-genital), and type 2 (genital) variety.

■ Symptoms

Fever and local tenderness. Primary infection of **type 1 most often presents as gingivostomatitis** with erosions and adenopathy. Reactivated infection of type 1 mostly presents as cold sores. **Type 2 (fever blisters—herpes labialis)** has high incidence of **systemic symptoms**, fever, and malaise, and presents with genital papules, vesicles, and erosions.

■ Diagnosis

Vesicle fluid virus culture, skin biopsy, history, and physical. **Tzanck preparation.**

■ Pathology

A prevalent sexually transmitted disease, herpes simplex virus (HSV) is transmitted by direct contact, via mucosal surface to surface.

■ Treatment

Acyclovir.

Additional Information. Herpetic whitlow is finger infection of HSV, a risk for physicians and dentists (wear gloves!).

B. Herpes Zoster

■ Description

Shingles is **recrudescence of latent infection of zoster/varicella virus.** Noted to be in boundary defined by a dermatome. Eruption is **most often unilateral** and indicates partial immunity.

■ Symptoms

Eruption of localized, painful, grouped vesicles, which is most often unilateral. Burning and paresthesias in the affected dermatome may be noted, as well as prodrome of fever and dermatome pain.

■ Diagnosis

Typical presentation in individual dermatome. Viral culture may be performed, along with cytologic smear or serologic studies. Tzanck smear **positive for balloon cells.**

Must have ⊕ varicella exposure!

■ Pathology

Dorsal nerve root latent virus reactivation.

■ Treatment

Acyclovir. Postherpetic neuralgia treated with capsaicin cream (Zostrix).

C. Varicella

■ Description

Zoster-varicella virus infection. Also called **chickenpox in childhood, confers 99% immunity.**

■ Symptoms

Itchy rash, fever. Presents as crops of vesicles centered in pink spots.

■ Diagnosis

Clinical picture is characteristic. Onset of papules, vesicles, and pustules, located on the thorax and face, prior to spread to the extremities. Typical lesions have a vesicle in the center of an erythematous spot. **Lesions in all stages of development are noted.** Positive **Tzanck** cytology showing giant and multinucleated giant cells.

■ Pathology

Varicella-zoster virus (a herpesvirus). **Incubation of 2 to 3 weeks**, with **transmission** possible **1 day prior to the rash to 6 to 7 days later.** Transmission via respiratory microdroplets as well as direct contact.

■ **Treatment**

Acyclovir is now used.

Additional Information. Dissemination may take place in individuals with immunologic disorders. High-risk patients [human immunodeficiency virus (HIV) positive, leukemia, etc.], may receive VZIG (varicella zoster immune globulin) as preventive immunization, even up to 3 days after exposure. **Complications** include **pneumonia** and **encephalitis.**

Now give kids VZIG

D. Cellulitis

■ **Description**

Subcutaneous and **dermal infection.**

■ **Symptoms**

Local area of **erythema, tenderness, warmth,** and **edema.**

■ **Diagnosis**

History and physical exam, may attempt culture.

■ **Pathology**

Bacterial skin infection, in **adults beta-hemolytic strep common. Skin break** allows germ entry.

■ **Treatment**

Heat, elevation, antibiotics.

Additional Information. **Erysipelas is strep infection, more superficial than cellulitis.** *Sharply demarcated, often of face*

E. Erythrasma

■ **Description**

Bacterial skin infection.

■ **Symptoms**

Red rash, sharp border, groin, axilla, beneath breasts.

■ **Diagnosis**

History and physical exam. **Glows under Wood's light, KOH prep.**

■ **Pathology**

Corynebacterium.

■ **Treatment**

Erythromycin.

F. Erysipeloid

■ **Description**

Cellulitis.

■ **Symptoms**

Red painful plaque.

■ **Diagnosis**

History and physical exam.

■ **Pathology**

Erysipelothrix (gram-positive rod). From touching dead animal material (fish, meat, etc).

■ **Treatment**

Penicillin.

G. Impetigo

■ **Description**

Bacterial skin infection.

■ **Symptoms**

Yellow crusty nose/mouth/facial lesions.
Honeycolored crusts

■ **Diagnosis**

Clinical, culture.

■ **Pathology**

Staphylococcus aureus, group A beta-hemolytic strep.

■ **Treatment**

Mupirocin (Bactroban) ointment, systemic antibiotics.

H. **Carbuncle**

■ **Description**

Abscess, deeper than boil. Several furuncles together.

■ **Symptoms**

Enlarging nodule drains, then ruptures; may have several draining points.

■ **Diagnosis**

History and physical exam. **Several draining points.**

■ **Pathology**

Abscess in area of hair follicles.

■ **Treatment**

Incise and drain, antibiotics for systemic signs, moist heat. **Furuncle is one nodule, secondary to staph.**

I. **Abscess**

■ **Description**

Local pus collection.

■ **Symptoms**

Tender swelling, fluctuant.

■ **Diagnosis**

Exam.

■ **Pathology**

Staph common cause.

■ **Treatment**

Incision and drainage, antibiotics for systemic symptoms.

J. **Gangrene**

■ **Description**

Tissue necrosis.

■ **Symptoms**

Similar to those of cellulitis but **bullae, crepitus** (from gas of anaerobic germ metabolism), pain.

■ **Diagnosis**

Suspect with poor antibiotic response, pain, and pus.

■ **Pathology**

Bacteria produce tissue necrosis. **Most often in extremities.**

■ **Treatment**

Surgical evaluation, cultures, and antibiotics.

K. **Dermatophytoses, Tinea Pedis, Tinea Capitis**

■ **Description**

Keratinized skin infection by fungi.

■ **Symptoms**

Tinea capitis may present as broken or hairless patch. **Tinea pedis** may present as toe-web scaling, cracking, or vesicles.

■ **Diagnosis**

History and physical exam, fungal culture, KOH preparation.

■ **Pathology**

Tinea capitis commonly due to *Trichophyton tonsurans,* and *Microsporum audouinii.* **Tinea pedis** may be due to *T. rubrum.*

■ **Treatment**

Topical antifungal for tinea corporis (body); tinea capitis and pedis may require systemic therapy.

L. Rubella

■ **Description**

Also termed **3-day measles,** or **German measles.**

■ **Symptoms**

Spreading macules and papules, face downward to trunk, **in 1 day,** fading by day 3. **Postauricular node enlargement.**

■ **Diagnosis**

History and physical exam. Serology to confirm if necessary.

■ **Pathology**

Rubella virus infection.

■ **Treatment**

None. **Prevention important as first-trimester infection may cause fetal anomaly. Prevent by immunization.**

M. Measles

■ **Description**

Rubeola.

■ **Symptoms**

Cough, coryza, fever, conjunctivitis, Koplik's spots.

■ **Diagnosis**

History and physical exam. Photophobia, malaise, macules and papules, may coalesce. May detect by serology. **Rash spreads over several days.**

■ **Pathology**

Measles virus. Respiratory transmission. Incubation 10 to 15 days.

■ **Treatment**

None. **Prevent by immunization. Complications include pneumonia and encephalitis.**

N. Roseola

■ **Description**

Also called exanthem subitum.

■ **Symptoms**

High fever 4 to 5 days and **rash after fever drops.** Occurs in first few years of life, with incubation of 5 days to 2 weeks. Rash of macules and papules, may be light pink in color. "lacey" rash

■ **Diagnosis**

History and physical exam.

■ **Pathology**

Viral. HHV 6

■ **Treatment**

None.

O. Erythema Infectiosum

- **Description**

Also called **fifth disease.**

- **Symptoms**

"Slapped cheek" rash, reticulate pattern rash, mild fever.

Child appears well

- **Diagnosis**

History and physical exam.

- **Pathology**

Parvovirus. B19

- **Treatment**

None.

P. Pilonidal Cyst

- **Description**

Sacral midline cyst.

- **Symptoms**

Swelling, tender, erythematous midline sacral mass.

- **Diagnosis**

History and physical exam.

- **Pathology**

Congenital, epidermal tissue beneath the skin surface.

- **Treatment**

Surgical removal, antibiotics.

Q. Viral Warts

1. *Common wart*—cauliflower shaped (caused by papillomavirus)

2. *Verrucae planae*—flat wart (faces and hands of children)

3. *Plantar wart*—back of foot

- **Description**

Hyperkeratotic growths.

- **Symptoms**

One or multiple verrucae of typical appearance.

- **Diagnosis**

Exam.

- **Pathology**

Human papillomavirus.

- **Treatment**

Freezing, acid, surgical removal.

R. Rocky Mountain Spotted Fever

- **Description**

Rickettsial, febrile disorder.

- **Symptoms**

Fever, headache, myalgia. Rash at about day four.

- **Diagnosis**

Evolving pink to dark red rash, starts on wrists and ankles. History and physical exam. Serologic testing for confirmation later.

- **Pathology**

Dermacentor andersoni **tick bite,** resulting in *Rickettsia rickettsii* transmission. Incubation 1 day to 2 weeks.

- **Treatment**

Tetracycline. If pregnant, give chloramphenicol. Complications include disseminated intravascular coagulation (DIC), shock and renal failure; **there may be no history of bite or rash in some cases.**

S. Lyme Disease

- **Description**

Tick-borne infection.

- **Symptoms**

Rash (erythema, *Chronicum* migrans), CNS, cardiac and joint symptoms. Fever, lethargy, headache.

- **Diagnosis**

History and physical exam, lyme serology enzyme-linked immunosorbent assay (ELISA), with confirmation by Western blot.

- **Pathology**

Borrelia burgdorferi, **via deer tick** *(Ixodes dammini).*

- **Treatment**

Doxycycline, amoxicillin.

T. Sexually Transmitted Diseases (Human Immunodeficiency Virus)

- **Description**

Human immunodeficiency virus (HIV).

- **Symptoms**

Kaposi's sarcoma, mollusca contagiosum, **oral hairy leukoplakia,** fungal infections, herpes zoster, oral thrush.

- **Diagnosis**

ELISA HIV testing with Western blot confirmation.

- **Pathology**

Acquired cell-mediated immunity defect. Decreased T4:T8 ratio.

- **Treatment**

Consult current literature.

Additional Information. **Oral hairy leukoplakia** is **white tongue plaque, due to Epstein–Barr virus (EBV), will not rub off,** no treatment.

Thrush can be rubbed off and **may respond to antifungal.**

Kaposi's sarcoma: purple/red macules and nodules, diagnosis by biopsy. Treat with radiation, chemotherapy, check current literature.

III. ALLERGIC DERMATITIS

A. Atopic Dermatitis

- **Description**

Epidermal and dermal **inflammation.**

- **Symptoms**

Itching.

- **Diagnosis**

History and physical exam. Family/personal history of atopy. **Xerosis (dry skin).**

- **Pathology**

Hypersensitivity reaction, type 1, with unknown etiology.

- **Treatment**

Topical steroids, skin hydration.

Additional Information. **May have allergy/ asthma history. Positive association with cataracts, and keratoconus.** Worse with itching and with stress.

B. Contact Dermatitis and Photodermatitis

■ **Description**

Dermal and epidermal inflammation secondary to toxin/chemical/foreign element exposure.

■ **Symptoms**

Itchy area of erythema, in exposed area (under watch, necklace, etc).

■ **Diagnosis**

History and physical exam. Itching.

■ **Pathology**

Type 4 delayed, cell-mediated, hypersensitivity reaction.

■ **Treatment**

Remove cause, topical corticosteroids, systemic steroids if severe.

Photodermatitis is light-induced, may show clear border between light-exposed and light-protected areas.

C. Cutaneous Drug Reactions

■ **Description**

Skin eruption resulting from medication (oral or topical).

■ **Symptoms**

May present as almost any type of dermatitis.

■ **Diagnosis**

History and physical exam.

■ **Pathology**

Types 1, 2, 3, and 4 hypersensitivity reactions.

■ **Treatment**

Stop suspected medication, systemic corticosteroids, antihistamines.

Additional Information. **Exanthematous rash is most common drug rash.** (Mono patient given amoxicillin.)

Fixed drug eruption will **present as lesion that will recur in same spot with same drug exposure.**

IV. PSORIASIS AND SEBORRHEIC DERMATITIS

A. Psoriasis

■ **Description**

Hereditary scaling dermatitis.

■ **Symptoms**

Chronic scaling plaques, knees, elbows, nails. Itching, and may have systemic symptoms. **Red plaques and silver-white scale.** Guttate psoriasis: multiple small papules.

■ **Diagnosis**

History and physical exam. Biopsy.

■ **Pathology**

Excess epidermal cell production.

■ **Treatment**

Topical corticosteroids. Phototherapy with PUVA, chemotherapy. Tar products.

Additional Information.

> **Koebner's sign**—trauma resulting in dermatitis.
>
> **Auspitz sign**—multiple bleeding points after scale removal.

B. Seborrheic Dermatitis

■ **Description**

Chronic scaling dermatitis.

■ **Symptoms**

Scales with or without erythema, common about nose, eyes, external ear canal (active sebaceous gland areas).

■ **Diagnosis**

History and physical exam.

■ **Pathology**

Etiology uncertain.

■ **Treatment**

Topical corticosteroids, tar shampoo.

Additional Information. **Leiner's disease: generalized infantile seborrheic dermatitis, rule out histiocytosis x.** Seborrheic dermatitis is most frequent cause of malar dermatitis. Seborrheic dermatitis on infant scale is "cradle cap."

V. BULLOUS DISORDERS

A. Bullous Impetigo

■ **Description**

Children's staph dermatitis.

■ **Symptoms**

Vesicles and bullae.

■ **Diagnosis**

History and physical exam.

■ **Pathology**

Exotoxin-producing staphylococcus.

■ **Treatment**

Antibiotics.

Additional Information. **Staphylococcal "scalded-skin" syndrome if excess toxin release in immunodeficient children or adults.**

B. Bullous Pemphigoid

■ **Description**

A type of bullous dermatitis.

■ **Symptoms**

Bullous eruption in elderly.

■ **Diagnosis**

History and physical exam, large tense blisters. **No Nikolsky sign** (skin not fragile). Confirm by biopsy.

■ **Pathology**

Autoimmune.

■ **Treatment**

Prednisone.

C. Dermatitis Herpetiformis

■ **Description**

Autoimmune bullous dermatitis.

■ **Symptoms**

Symmetrical vesicles on knees, shoulders, scalp. **No Nikolsky sign.**

■ **Diagnosis**

Physical exam, biopsy.

■ **Pathology**

Autoimmune vesicular disorder.

■ **Treatment**

Gluten-free diet, dapsone.

D. **Herpes Gestationis**

■ **Description**

Second- and third-trimester bullous disorder.

■ **Symptoms**

Tense, symmetrical blisters, itchy.

■ **Diagnosis**

History and physical exam, skin biopsy.

■ **Pathology**

Autoimmune.

■ **Treatment**

Prednisone, dapsone.

Additional Information. **Pemphigus—autoimmune disorder, flaccid blisters.**

VI. PRURITIC DERMATOSES

A. **Pruritus Ani**

■ **Description**

Anal area itching.

■ **Symptoms**

As the preceding section. May have minimal erythema, or severe excoriations from itching.

■ **Diagnosis**

History and physical exam.

■ **Pathology**

Etiology in soaps, itching, diet(?), irritating toilet tissue.

■ **Treatment**

Avoid etiologic factor, and treat primary cause if evident (pinworms, psoriasis, etc). Stop itch–scratch pattern. Sitz bath, topical corticosteroids, antihistamines.

B. **Factitial Dermatitis**

■ **Description**

Self-inflicted dermatitis.

■ **Symptoms**

Many types of dermatitis possible.

■ **Diagnosis**

History and physical exam, may have bizarre pattern, patient denies causing the rash, but may have clear psychological problems. **No rash in non-reachable areas (midback, "butterfly sign").**

■ **Pathology**

Rash produced by the patient.

■ **Treatment**

Psychiatric evaluation.

Neurotic excoriations: compulsive scratching. May also be termed lichen simplex chronicus.

Additional Information. **Rule out scabies, xerosis, uremia, Hodgkin's, and endocrine disorders** in chronic itching.

VII. ACNE VULGARIS

■ **Description**

Common acne.

■ **Symptoms**

Comedones, nodules, papules, pustules, and cysts.

■ **Diagnosis**

History and physical exam.

■ **Pathology**

Follicle plugging and inflammation, resulting from multiple factors including bacteria and androgenic influence.
    Bacteria: *Propionibacterium acne.*

■ **Treatment**

Benzoyl peroxide, topical and oral antibiotics, topical retinoids, isotretinoin (Accutane).

VIII. DECUBITUS ULCERS

■ **Description**

Bedsores. Skin/tissue necrosis.

■ **Symptoms**

Erythema, skin breakdown, open sores.

■ **Diagnosis**

History and physical exam.

■ **Pathology**

Pressure necrosis, and **ischemia.** Begins as blanchable erythema, then non-blanchable, then superficial to deep ulceration. Dry gangrene with tissue death may follow.

■ **Treatment**

Prevent by avoiding prolonged pressure in high-risk patients. Treatment options include iodine, antiseptic cream, occlusive dressing (Duoderm), debridement.

IX. STASIS DERMATITIS

■ **Description**

Chronic lower extremity dermatitis.

■ **Symptoms**

Pigmentation, erythema, and **edema.**

■ **Diagnosis**

Symptoms plus itching and petechiae.

■ **Pathology**

May result from phlebitis or venous insufficiency.

■ **Treatment**

Alleviate venous insufficiency. Support stockings, elevate legs, treat infection.

Additional Information. Stasis dermatitis may lead to stasis ulcer formation. Reduce edema, and treat infection.

X. URTICARIAL DISORDERS

■ **Description**

Urticaria are hives. Angioedema is urticaria of deeper dermal depth.

■ **Symptoms**

Fleeting itchy papules and swellings (wheals).

■ Diagnosis

History and physical exam.

■ Pathology

Vast etiology including <u>allergy</u> (drugs, chemicals, bites, etc), <u>hereditary</u>, <u>heat/cold</u>, <u>solar</u>, <u>and pressure</u>. May include both <u>type 1 hypersensitivity and type 3 reactions</u>. Increased <u>mast cells</u>, <u>dermal edema</u>, and <u>vascular fluid transudation</u>.

■ Treatment

<u>Eliminate offending agent, antihistamines</u>.

Additional Information. **Hereditary angioedema: autosomal dominant, C1 esterase inhibitor deficiency, subcutaneous and submucosal edema.**

 Dermographism: <u>scratching results in urticaria</u>.

XI. NEOPLASMS

The three most common skin cancers:

 1. Basal cell carcinoma
 2. Squamous cell carcinoma
 3. Malignancy melanoma

A. Squamous Cell Carcinoma

■ Description

<u>Skin and mucous membrane cancer</u>. <u>One percent per year metastasizes</u>.

■ Symptoms

<u>Indurated papule or nodule</u>, may be in <u>sun-exposed areas</u>.

■ Diagnosis

History and physical exam. Biopsy.

■ Pathology

Induced by the sun, radiation, chemicals.

■ Treatment

<u>Surgical or radiation</u>.

Additional Information

 Bowen's disease—<u>enlarging single lesion of CA *in situ*</u>. **May be arsenic-induced.**

 Erythroplasia of Queyrat—Bowen's on <u>the penis</u>, also *in situ* carcinoma.

B. Malignant Melanoma

■ Description

<u>Skin cancer</u> with <u>atypical melanocytes</u>. Some are <u>sun-related</u>. <u>Fifty percent have a 5-year death prognosis</u>.

■ Symptoms

May demonstrate **variegation of color, asymmetry, and irregular border**. May be <u>over 6 mm in size</u>.

■ Diagnosis

See symptoms; also skin biopsy by **total excision.**

■ Pathology

Atypical melanocytes, evolve in the epidermis. Metastasizes to the liver.

■ Treatment

<u>Surgical. Wide excision and metastatic work-up</u>.

Additional Information. **Most melanoma is superficial spreading type. Prognosis by Clark staging 1 to 5. Other types are nodular and lentigo.**

prognosis det. by depth of invasion

XII. ACTINIC KERATOSIS AND BASAL CELL CARCINOMA

A. Actinic Keratosis

■ **Description**

Also called **solar keratosis.**

■ **Symptoms**

Hyperkeratotic coarse scale, hard to remove.

■ **Diagnosis**

History and physical exam, biopsy.

■ **Pathology**

Sun-induced **keratinocyte damage.**

■ **Treatment**

Fluorouracil (5-FU), excision, cryosurgery.

Additional Information. **Most frequent premalignant skin lesion: actinic keratosis. On lips it is termed actinic cheilitis.**

B. Basal Cell Carcinoma

■ **Description**

As noted under Symptoms.

■ **Symptoms**

Pearly nodule, rolled border (rodent ulcer). Nodular is most common type. May also be pigmented, morpheaform, superficial, and infiltrative.

■ **Diagnosis**

History and physical exam, biopsy.

■ **Pathology**

Multiplication of atypical basal cells. Ninety percent occur in sun-exposed areas.

■ **Treatment**

Surgery, cryosurgery.

Additional Information. **Most common skin cancer: basal cell.**

XIII. PIGMENTED NEVI

A. Blue Nevus

■ **Description**

Benign papule or nodule.

■ **Symptoms**

Black/blue round nodule.

■ **Diagnosis**

History and physical exam, biopsy.

■ **Pathology**

Clumped melanin-producing **melanocytes.**

■ **Treatment**

Excise if desired.

B. Capillary Hemangioma

■ **Description**

Birthmark, **Strawberry nevus.**

■ **Symptoms**

Red/purple hemangioma.

■ **Diagnosis**

Clinical.

■ **Pathology**

Endothelial cell growth.

■ **Treatment**

Elective cosmetic removal or cryosurgery. May regress.

C. **Cavernous Hemangioma**

■ **Description**

Vascular anomaly.

■ **Symptoms**

Swelling, may have purple color.

■ **Diagnosis**

Clinical.

■ **Pathology**

Dilated vessels.

■ **Treatment**

Hope for regression, surgical treatment.

Additional Information

> **Kasabach–Merritt syndrome**—hemangiomas and thrombocytopenia.
> **Senile angioma**—cherry angioma, benign.
> **Venous lake**—benign purple nodule in elderly.
> **Spider angioma**—found normally, also in pregnancy, and liver disease.
> **Port-wine stain—congenital extensive purple lesion, will not regress.**
> **Sturge–Weber syndrome**—port-wine stain, brain calcifications and leptomeningeal angiomatosis, seizures.

XIV. CUTANEOUS MANIFESTATIONS OF SYSTEMIC DISEASE

A. **Behçet's Syndrome**

■ **Description**

Syndrome of recurrent **aphthous ulcers, genital ulcers, skin and eye lesions.**

■ **Symptoms**

As described. **Painful ulcers, erythema nodosum.** Arthritis, inflammatory bowel disease.

■ **Diagnosis**

History and physical exam.

■ **Pathology**

Immune complex in blood, with no known etiology. **Leukocytoclastic vasculitis.**

■ **Treatment**

Chlorambucil, oral antibiotic suspensions.

B. **Dermatomyositis**

■ **Description**

Multisystem disorder, consisting of striated muscle inflammation.

■ **Symptoms**

Heliotrope rash (eyelid erythema), **Gottron's sign** (purple papules on knees, knuckles), **proximal muscle weakness.**

■ **Diagnosis**

History and physical exam, elevated creatine phosphokinase (CPK), skin/muscle biopsy, abnormal electromyogram (EMG), typical rash.

■ **Pathology**

Muscle inflammation, abnormal CPK and muscle biopsy.

■ **Treatment**

Prednisone, rule out possible associated malignancy.

C. **Erythema Multiforme**

■ **Description**

Self-limited syndrome of targetlike skin lesions.

■ **Symptoms**

Fever, lethargy, **target lesions**, affect palms and soles, mucous membranes.

■ **Diagnosis**

History and physical exam. Skin biopsy.

■ **Pathology**

May be drug reaction, from infection (HSV infection), toxins, or other diseases. Perivascular infiltrate and dermal edema.

■ **Treatment**

Corticosteroids.

D. **Erythema Nodosum**

■ **Description**

Inflammatory disorder of subcutaneous tissue. Immunologic.

■ **Symptoms**

Lower extremity inflammatory nodules. May be tender.

■ **Diagnosis**

History and physical exam, skin biopsy.

■ **Pathology**

Panniculus inflammation. May present from infections, as Chron's disease, chronic ulcerative colitis, sarcoid, streptococcal or mycoplasma. Also drug exposure to sulfas or oral contraceptives.

■ **Treatment**

Supportive, NSAIDs, corticosteroids.

Additional Information. **Lofgren syndrome** —fever, erythema nodosum, possible sarcoid.

E. **Livedo Reticularis**

■ **Description**

Mottled skin color pattern.

■ **Symptoms**

As described, blotchy cyanosis.

■ **Diagnosis**

History and physical exam.

■ **Pathology**

Arteriole vasospasm. May exist with infection, vasculitis, or hematologic conditions. May be drug-induced.

■ **Treatment**

Avoid cold exposure, treat coexisting medical conditions.

F. **Lupus Erythematosus**

■ **Description**

Autoimmune disease involving vasculature and connective tissue.

■ **Symptoms**

Skin changes include malar erythema (butterfly rash), vasculitis, Raynaud's phenomenon, alopecia, and others. **Fatigue and fever**.

■ **Diagnosis**

History and physical exam, skin biopsy, serum autoantibody testing (ANA, double-stranded DNA).

■ **Pathology**

Epidermal basal cell destruction.

■ **Treatment**

Avoid sun exposure, topical cortico-steroids, antimalarials, systemic cortico-steroids.

G. **Amyloidosis**

■ **Description**

Extracellular amyloid deposition.

■ **Symptoms**

Macroglossia, waxy papules/nodules on face. Carpal tunnel syndrome.

■ **Diagnosis**

Exam, biopsy.

■ **Pathology**

Amyloid deposition in dermis and around vascular walls. **Congo red stain is used.**

■ **Treatment**

Prednisone(?), colchicine(?). Rule out multiple myeloma.

H. **Scleroderma**

■ **Description**

Multisystem disease, also called **progressive systemic sclerosis.**

■ **Symptoms**

Raynaud's, **dysphagia, masklike face,** thin lips, tight skin.

■ **Diagnosis**

History and physical exam, skin biopsy.

■ **Pathology**

Unknown etiology. Excessive collagen deposition, and endothelial cell damage.

■ **Treatment**

Symptomatic. **CREST syndrome: calcinosis, Raynaud's, esophageal dysfunction, sclerodactyly, telangiectasia.**

I. **Tuberous Sclerosis**

■ **Description**

Multisystem genetic disorder.

■ **Symptoms**

Retinal phakomas, cerebral tubers, sebaceous adenomas. Ash-leaf hypopigmented macules. _Seizures_

■ **Diagnosis**

History and physical exam, biopsy.

■ **Pathology**

Autosomal dominant. Dermal fibrosis.

■ **Treatment**

None. Control seizures. Supportive measures.

J. **Necrobiosis Lipoidica Diabeticorum**

■ **Description**

Chronic skin disorder, most cases associated with diabetes.

■ **Symptoms**

Yellow plaques, usually legs and ankles.

■ **Diagnosis**

History and physical exam, biopsy.

■ **Pathology**

Granulomatous reaction, and necrobiosis.

■ **Treatment**

Topical and intralesional corticosteroids.

K. Porphyria Cutanea Tarda (PCT)

■ **Description**

Heme pathway defect disorder.

■ **Symptoms**

Vesicles on the back of hands, fragile skin.

■ **Diagnosis**

Urine will fluoresce orange/red under Wood's light; hyperpigmentation. Blood/urine/stool studies for porphyrins, biopsy.

■ **Pathology**

Autosomal dominant; may be induced by chemicals, drugs, alcohol.

■ **Treatment**

Stop alcohol use, chloroquine. **Phlebotomy.**

Additional Information. **PCT is most common porphyria, association with heavy drinking, diabetes. No abdominal crises in PCT. Abdominal/neurologic symptoms** are found in variegate porphyria, acute intermittent, and hereditary coproporphyria.

L. Acanthosis Nigricans

■ **Description**

See Symptoms.

■ **Symptoms**

Black velvetlike axillary/neck patch.

■ **Diagnosis**

Clinical.

■ **Pathology**

May associate with malignancy, endocrine disease, obesity, or be familial.

■ **Treatment**

Rule out coexisting pathology.

M. Peutz–Jeghers Syndrome

■ **Description**

Familial polyposis.

■ **Symptoms**

Pigmented macules on lips and oral mucosa. Lentigines, pigmentation. Gastrointestinal (GI) polyps.

■ **Diagnosis**

History and physical exam, biopsy. **Melena, GI system complaints.**

■ **Pathology**

Extra melanin. **Autosomal dominant. Hamartomas are GI lesions.**

■ **Treatment**

None, monitor for GI malignancy. Surgery (GI tract lesions).

N. Thrombocytopenic Purpura

■ **Description**

Purpura and decreased platelets.

■ **Symptoms**

Sudden onset of **petechiae** and **ecchymosis**. Legs and mucous membranes typically.

■ **Diagnosis**

History and physical exam. Purpura will not blanch nor is it palpable. Coagulation studies.

■ **Pathology**

Decreased platelets. May follow infection in children.

■ **Treatment**

Prednisone, splenectomy(?).

O. **Disseminated Intravascular Coagulation**

■ **Description**

Bleeding disorder with many possible etiologies.

■ **Symptoms**

Cutaneous hemorrhage and ecchymosis.

■ **Diagnosis**

History and physical exam, **low plasma fibrinogen** and **elevated fibrin split products.** Elevated PT, PTT. Skin biopsy.

■ **Pathology**

Endothelial surface injury and tissue injury resulting in coagulation activation. (Crush injury, shock, sepsis, malignancy, abruptio placenta, eclampsia, vasculitis, hyperthermia, etc.)

■ **Treatment**

Treat primary cause, heparin, control coagulation abnormality.

XV. **NAIL SIGNS AND DISEASE**

A. **Onycholysis**

■ **Description**

Nail lifting off nail bed, **hyperthyroidism, psoriasis, injury.**

B. **Terry's Nails**

■ **Description**

Proximal two thirds of nail is white, **congestive heart failure (CHF), low albumin, cirrhosis.**

C. **Splinter Hemorrhages**

■ **Description**

Trauma, SBE.

D. **Beau's Lines**

■ **Description**

Horizontal nail depression, **nail growth cessation from stress.**

E. **Clubbed Fingers**

■ **Description**

Cardiopulmonary disease, cancer, or normal trait.

F. **Muehrcke's Nails**

■ **Description**

Two horizontal white stripes, **low albumin/nephrotic syndrome.**

G. **Yellow Nails**

■ **Description**

Lung disease, cancer.

H. **Half-and-Half Nails**

■ **Description**

Normal proximal half, distal brown, chronic renal failure.

XVI. OTHER NEWBORN AND INHERITED DISORDERS

A. **Erythema Toxicum Neonatorum**

■ **Description**

Newborn macule and pustule dermatitis; self-limited.

B. **Port-Wine Stain**

■ **Description**

Termed nevus flammeus; often facial and unilateral red lesion; treatment is usually inadequate and the argon laser is used.

C. **Café au Lait Spots**

■ **Description**

Pigmented macule; typical of neurofibromatosis.

D. **Mongolian Spot**

■ **Description**

Blue discoloration near sacral area; no clinical significance or treatment.

E. **Miliaria**

■ **Description**

Dermatitis secondary to sweat gland/duct blockage; avoid heat, and ensure cool room/patient to treat.

F. **Ataxia–Telangiectasia**

Telangiectases, and ataxia, bronchiectasis; autosomal recessive.

XVII. PRINCIPLES OF MANAGEMENT

A. **Acute and Infectious Disorders**

■ **Description**

Perform history and physical examination along with appropriate testing to determine diagnosis. Instruct patient on both therapy involved and future preventive measures. Advise isolation in contagious disorders when indicated.

B. **Chronic Dermatologic Disorders**

■ **Description**

Therapy includes not only current treatment plan, but patient education in nature of the disorder and chronicity. The need for continued therapy along with social and psychological implications should be discussed.

Additional Information. General treatment tools include antihistamines for itch, moisturizers for itch and lubrication, corticosteroids, antibiotics, antifungals, and antivirals.

If the lesion is wet, use soaks. If the lesion is dry, use an ointment.

Anti-itch compounds include menthol and phenol, Aveeno baths. Wet dressing might use Burrow's solution, or boric acid solution.

BIBLIOGRAPHY

Arndt K. *Manual of Dermatologic Therapeutics.* 4th ed. Boston, Mass: Little, Brown and Company; 1989.

Daniel CR III. *Pigmentation Abnormalities of the Nails. Pigmentation Disorders, Dermatologic Clinics,* Vol. 6. Philadelphia, Pa: WB Saunders; 1988.

Fitzpatrick TB. *Dermatology in Internal Medicine.* 4th ed., Vols. 1 and 2. New York: McGraw-Hill, Inc; 1993.

Fitzpatrick TB. *Synopsis of Clinical Dermatology, Common and Serious Disorders.* 2nd ed. New York: McGraw-Hill, Inc; 1992.

Maddin S. *Current Dermatologic Therapy.* Philadelphia, Pa: WB Saunders; 1982.

Roenigk HH Jr. *Office Dermatology.* Baltimore, Md: Williams and Wilkins; 1981.

Rook A. *Practical Management of the Dermatologic Patient.* Philadelphia, Pa: JB Lippincott; 1986.

Sams WM Jr. *Principles and Practice of Dermatology.* New York: Churchill Livingstone; 1990.

Sauer GC. *Manual of Skin Diseases.* 6th ed. Philadelphia, Pa: JB Lippincott; 1991.

Shelly WB. *Advanced Dermatologic Therapy.* Philadelphia, Pa: WB Saunders; 1987.

CHAPTER 3

Endocrine and Metabolic Disorders

JOEL S. GOLDBERG, DO

I. HEALTH AND HEALTH MAINTENANCE

A. Hyperlipidemia

■ **Description**

Impact includes an elevated **risk of atherosclerotic disease** and other disorders (**pancreatitis**, tendinous xanthoma). **Screening** should be performed on all adult patients, and in younger individuals where there is increased family risk. **Prevention** of morbidity and mortality includes adequate treatment and follow-up, along with education (including the benefits of diet and exercise).

B. Diabetes Mellitus

■ **Description**

Impact includes US incidence of about 3%, and resulting complications (**nephropathy, neuropathy, retinopathy,** cataracts, etc). **Screening** is useful, especially in **high-risk** cases, by fasting blood glucose, or glucose tolerance test. **Prevention** of morbidity and mortality includes adequate education (value of diet and exercise), and treatment (prevent ketosis and abnormal blood glucose values/fluctuations). Early detection and treatment of complications may reduce potential severity (retinopathy-photocoagulation). In addition, coexisting medical conditions need to be treated (hypertension, hyperlipidemia).

C. Addisonian Crisis

■ **Description**

Prevention of **morbidity** and **mortality** includes **early recognition** and management of high-risk patients (Addison patients with stress: infection, surgery, trauma, glucocorticoids). Recognition includes both physician alertness and patient education. **Preventive therapy** includes additional glucocorticoid doses during patient stress and emergency bracelet use.

D. Neonatal Hypothyroidism

■ **Description**

Prevention of **morbidity** and **mortality** secondary to neonatal hypothyroidism (**cretinism**) includes **screening** for **family history** (and medications ingested by the mother), and **routine newborn L-thyroxine sodium (T_4), and thyroid-stimulating hormone (TSH) studies.**

E. Acquired Hypothyroidism

■ **Description**

Prevention of **morbidity** and **mortality** secondary to acquired hypothyroidism includes early detection by screening and judicious use and monitoring of medications (lithium, iodinated prescriptions), and contrast dye. Check for thyroid antibodies.

II. MECHANISMS OF DISEASE AND DIAGNOSIS

A. Thyroid Disorders

1. Thyroid Tests

Free T_4—(FT$_4$), active circulating T_4, not altered by illness or binding disorders.

T_4RIA—changes with thyroxine-binding disorders.

T_3RU—excess thyroxine binding (estrogen use) results in T_3RU decrease, T_4 elevated. Reduced binding states (malnutrition) results in T_3RU increased, T_4 decreased.

FTI equals T_4 T_3RU.

gold standard for hyperthyroid *TSH*—supersensitive assay.

Thyroid antibodies.

2. Thyroid Nodule

■ **Description**

Solitary thyroid lesion.

■ Symptoms

May be asymptomatic, or exhibit thyroid dysfunction—hot nodule.

■ Diagnosis

History and physical exam (25% chance of cancer if history of irradiation), needle aspiration or thyroid scan (most malignant nodules are non-functioning, cold), ultrasound and surgical removal.

■ Pathology

Most common benign lesion: follicular adenoma. Most common malignant nodule: papillary cancer. History of irradiation: very important to ask. Increased chance of malignancy if young.

■ Treatment

Cyst: aspirate/follow. Carcinoma: surgical/radioiodine.

3. Thyroid Carcinoma

■ Description

Thyroid gland cancer.

■ Symptoms

Asymptomatic—may be adenopathy present.

Anaplastic type—may have **hoarseness, rapid-growing mass.**

■ Diagnosis

History and physical exam, work-up as per previous Thyroid Nodule section.

■ Pathology

Papillary most often. Very slow growing. Thyroid carcinoma (CA) is

more common in the young; **in older patients, follicular CA more common;** anaplastic, older patient, very malignant; medullary CA with amyloid (MEN I & II).

↳ *must have it for MEN II*

■ Treatment

Excision (extent of surgery depending on extent of disease), **suppressive thyroid therapy preop,** and 6 weeks **postop** (levothyroxine), **radioiodine.**

Additional Information. **Marker for medullary cancer is calcitonin level. Thyroid lymphoma: use x-ray therapy. Largest percentage of thyroid cancer death is due to anaplastic CA. Risk of leukemia with increasing 131-I use.**

4. Acquired Hypothyroidism

■ Description

Juvenile hypothyroidism and **adult hypothyroidism.**

■ Symptoms

May be **asymptomatic, myxedema** of tissue, cold intolerance, dry skin, lateral **eyebrow thinning,** constipation, lethargy.

■ Diagnosis

Elevated TSH, low T_4, anemia.

■ Pathology

Secondary to **surgical removal, thyroiditis,** or **unknown etiology.** Other causes include medication (amiodarone), postpartum necrosis of pituitary (Sheehan's), (autoimmune—most common).

■ Treatment

Levothyroxine.

Additional Information. **Myxedema may result in an enlarged heart/heart failure.**

5. Congenital Hypothyroidism

■ **Description**

Cretinism.

■ **Symptoms**

Dry skin, lethargy, umbilical hernia, slow teething/sexual development.

Constipation

■ **Diagnosis**

History and physical exam, **elevated TSH, low T$_4$, bone stippling** and delayed maturation.

■ **Pathology**

Thyroid absent, or ineffective hormone secreted due to enzyme deficiency (familial goiter).

■ **Treatment**

Levothyroxine (synthetic L-thyroxine).

Additional Information. **Pendred syndrome: congenital goiter and deafness.**

6. Thyroiditis

■ **Description**

Thyroid gland inflammation.

■ **Symptoms**

Acute suppurative—thyroid pain/erythema/dysphagia, and fever. —s/p URI

de Quervain's—lethargy, pain, fever, malaise, may be asymptomatic. -s/p URI

Hashimoto's—goiter.

Riedel's—tracheal compression/sclerosing fibrosis.

■ **Diagnosis**

History and physical exam, thyroid scan, lab (thyroid peroxidase autoantibodies—autoimmune), **elevated T$_4$** and T$_3$RU, in de Quervain's, may be hypothyroid with Hashimoto's. **de Quervain's: elevated sed rate,** biopsy.

■ **Pathology**

Acute—(de Quervain's: subacute/viral; suppurative: infection)

Chronic—(autoimmune/**Hashimoto's,** Riedel's, suppurative and nonsuppurative).

■ **Treatment**

Suppurative: antibiotics. de Quervain's: aspirin, prednisone. **Autoimmune: thyroxine. Reidel's: thyroxine.**

Additional Information. **Hashimoto's thyroiditis is the most common thyroiditis. Etiology: autoimmune.** Elevated antibody titers present. **Reidel's is the most uncommon type.**

7. Thyrotoxicosis

■ **Description**

Effects of elevated thyroid hormone levels, **hyperthyroidism.**

■ **Symptoms**

lid lag, exophthalmos ↗

Graves' disease: goiter, **ophthalmopathy, pre-tibial myxedema,** tachycardia, diarrhea, tremor, weight loss, heat intolerance. ~~lid lag~~

If not Graves: no ophthalmopathy or pre-tibial myxedema

■ **Diagnosis**

History and physical exam, elevated T$_3$, T$_4$, and thyroid-stimulating immunoglobulins (TSI, found in Graves).

TSH low

Sick euthyroid: low thyroid hormones   ↓ thyroid fnctn in pregnancy

thyroid ok   ↓ FT$_4$, ↓ FT$_3$ RIA
pt is sick—rx
illness   TSH neo high

■ **Pathology**

Thyroid overactivity. **Diffuse toxic goiter (Graves' disease)** most common, autoimmune. Other disorders include toxic adenoma (Plummer's disease), thyrotoxicosis factitia (hormone ingestion), subacute thyroiditis, ovarian struma/hydatidiform mole.

■ **Treatment**

Antithyroid medication, radioactive iodine, subtotal thyroidectomy.

Additional Information. Other symptoms include onycholysis, bruit, high-output failure, thin hair, and confusion.

8. *Thyroid Storm*

■ **Description**

Severe thyrotoxicosis. sudden

■ **Symptoms**

Very high fever, delirium, tachycardia. , HTN

■ **Diagnosis**

Clinical, elevated T_4 and T_3-RIA and TSH suppressed.

■ **Pathology**

Severe thyrotoxicosis, may be postop, or after infection/stress.

■ **Treatment**

Control etiology, antithyroid medication (propylthiouracil—methimazole, iodine, beta blocker, glucocorticoids).

9. *Goiter*

■ **Description**

Thyroid enlargement.

■ **Symptoms**

May be asymptomatic, or compressive symptoms secondary to gland size.

■ **Diagnosis**

History and physical exam, T_4 normal, TSH may be normal or slightly elevated, ultrasound examination. No autoimmune antibodies present.

■ **Pathology**

Inadequate iodine or **excessive iodine.** Lithium use, familial goiter.

■ **Treatment**   to suppress thyroid? cause hypoplasia
Levothyroxine. If inadequate iodine in iodine deficiency countries, give iodine. Surgery (rare).

B. **Diabetes Mellitus**

1. *Type 1*

■ **Description**

Insulin-dependent diabetes mellitus (IDDM). Insulin deficiency, with **elevated plasma glucagon.**

■ **Symptoms**

Polyuria, polyphagia, polydipsia, hyperglycemia, urine/blood ketones.

■ **Diagnosis**   → rarely do GTT anymore
Two or more **fasting glucose levels over 140.** May have **islet cell antibodies** and **human leukocyte antigen (HLA) present.**
sometimes follows viral syndrome - usually child or adolescent
■ **Pathology**

No insulin production by pancreatic β cells under stimuli. A result of **genetic predisposition to pancreatic immune and/or environmental injury.**

Human leukocyte antigen markers common.

■ Treatment

Diet (monitor carbohydrates and be consistent with snacks/timing of meals), **exogenous insulin.**

Additional Information. **Regular insulin: rapid onset, peak 1 to 3 hours, lasts 5 to 7 hours.**

NPH/Lente—(30% semilente, 70% ultralente) onset in 2 hours, peak 8 to 12 hours, lasts 18 to 24 hours. NPH (70/30) human insulin.
Ultralente—onset 4 to 5 hours, peak 8 to 14 hours, lasts 25 to 36 hours. Somogyi effect—nocturnal hypoglycemia causes elevated morning glucose (reduce insulin dose to treat). Dawn phenomenon—early morning hyperglycemia (etiology in reduced insulin effectiveness at that time).

2. Type 2

■ Description
Non-insulin-dependent.

■ Symptoms
Polyuria, polydipsia, blurry vision. **May be asymptomatic,** skin/vaginal infections noted, large infant size.

■ Diagnosis

Two or more **fasting glucose levels over 140.** Also, two or more **glucose levels over 200 on glucose tolerance test** (during the first 2 hours, and at 2 hours).

■ Pathology

Etiology unknown. **No ketoacidosis, but tissues not responsive to insulin**

secreted, and pancreas poorly responsive to elevated glucose levels.
assoc. c̄ obesity & HTN

■ Treatment

Diet (restrict calories to reach ideal body weight), **oral hypoglycemics, weight control, exercise.**

Additional Information. **Glycosylated hemoglobin (HbA$_{1C}$) elevation** indicates **hyperglycemia over prior 2 to 3 months.**

3. Ketoacidosis

■ Description

Diabetic patient with acidosis and ketosis.

■ Symptoms

Lethargy, nausea/vomiting, polyuria, abdominal pain, confusion, **Kussmaul's** respiration, dehydration, fruity breath.
takes hours to happen

■ Diagnosis

History and physical exam, **elevated glucose** (400 to 600 mg/dL), ketonuria/ketonemia, low pH on arterial blood gas (ABG), **metabolic acidosis** with **increased anion gap.**
hyperkalemia b/c K⁺ can't enter cells

■ Pathology

May result from infection/illness/not taking insulin, and is associated with lack of insulin.

■ Treatment

Insulin (continuous infusion 5 to 10 U/h or 0.1 U/kg/h), **correction of fluid/electrolyte abnormality. Use isotonic saline to start,** check glucose every hour, potassium every 2 hours. **Replace potassium as necessary** and monitor blood pressure (BP), electrocardiogram (ECG), and sodium.

risk of hypokalemia c̄ insulin Rx

Additional Information. **Most common severe complication: cerebral edema.**
Potassium will fall during treatment if not replaced.

4. Hyperosmolar Coma

■ **Description**

Extracellular hyperosmolality associated with hyperglycemia.

■ **Symptoms**

Severe dehydration, lethargy, confusion, coma.

takes days to happen (usually)

■ **Diagnosis**

History and physical exam, **very high glucose.**

■ **Pathology**

Elevated glucose without ketosis resulting in cellular fluid loss.

■ **Treatment**

Replace sodium, water (hypotonic saline), **give insulin** (lower doses required than in ketoacidosis).

5. Lactic Acidosis

■ **Description**

Excess lactic acid in the blood.

■ **Symptoms**

Coma, confusion, hyperventilation.

■ **Diagnosis**

high anion gap metabolicacidosis

Do NOT give lactated Ringers

History and physical exam [critically ill diabetic with complication(s)], **elevated plasma lactate, negative ketonuria, positive anion gap.**

■ **Pathology** *high exercise → liverdisease*

Overproduction or inadequate removal of lactic acid.

■ **Treatment**

Treat etiology, sodium bicarbonate, supportive.

6. Diabetes Mellitus Chronic Complications

■ **Description**

Renal—nephropathy (Kimmelstiel–Wilson lesions).
Neurologic—neuropathy (sensory: Charcot joint, motor-nerve palsy). *stocking/glove sensory loss*
Ophthalmic—retinopathy (non-proliferative, proliferative), cataracts (subcapsular, **senile most common**). *→ not diabetic*
Other—peripheral vascular disease, dermopathy, infection.

↑ risk MI, stroke

Additional Information. ***For patients with IDDM requiring major surgery:*** morning of surgery give **10 units regular insulin then insulin (regular) drip of 0.1 U/kg/hr.** Titrate up as needed.

C. Hypoglycemia, Pancreatic β-Cell Tumors

■ **Description**

Fasting hypoglycemia; **insulinoma.**

■ **Symptoms**

Lethargy, diplopia, headache, in AM or when fasting.

■ **Diagnosis**

History and physical exam, **typical hypoglycemic symptoms, blood glucose under 40 mg/dL, response to glucose.** Elevated serum insulin level during hypoglycemic episode. **Elevated proinsulin level,** and **lack of C peptide suppression.**

- **Pathology**

<u>Islets of Langerhans adenoma</u> most often; <u>usually benign.</u>

- **Treatment**

Surgical excision of tumor; preop give diazoxide (Proglycem). **Emergency therapy: give 50 mL 50% dextrose IV.**

Additional Information. **Other etiologies of hyperinsulinism** states include <u>sulfonylurea overdose</u>, <u>insulin overdose,</u> pentamidine use (hypoglycemia).

D. Parathyroid Disorders

1. *Hyperparathyroidism*

- **Description**

<u>Excess parathyroid hormone secretion.</u>

- **Symptoms**   *2° hypercalciuria*

Asymptomatic or **kidney stones,** bone pain/lesions (**osteitis fibrosa cystica**). Symptoms of elevated calcium (memory loss, depression, **proximal muscle weakness,** nausea, weight loss, polyuria).

- **Diagnosis**

↑PTH   **Elevated serum calcium,** and immunoassay for parathyroid hormone (**iPTH**). ✗Subperiosteal bone resorption on x-ray✗

- **Pathology**

Etiology unknown; **single chief cell adenoma most common.** Hyperplasia in MEN syndromes.

- **Treatment**

<u>Surgical resection.</u>

2. *Hypoparathyroidism*

- **Description**

Decreased parathyroid hormone amount or effect. <u>Thyroid surgery or genetic.</u>

- **Symptoms**

Symptoms of **hypocalcemia (positive Chvostek's and Trousseau's signs),** → bp cuff 3 min get tetany **circumoral paresthesia, tetany,** <u>cataracts,</u> intracranial calcifications, seizures.

- **Diagnosis**

History and physical exam, **hyperphosphatemia, hypocalcemia, normal renal function,** parathyroid hormone (<u>PTH</u>), and <u>urinary cyclic adenosine monophosphate (cAMP) level.</u>

- **Pathology**

Physiologic effects of <u>reduced calcium.</u>

- **Treatment**

Vitamin D and **calcium.** +/- PTH replacement

E. Pituitary and Hypothalamic Disorders

1. *Diabetes Insipidus*

- **Description**

Water-loss syndrome. <u>Nephrogenic:</u> kidney does not respond to vasopressin. <u>Neurogenic/central:</u> inadequate vasopressin. ↳ pituitary or hypothalamus

- **Symptoms**

<u>Polyuria, nocturia, thirst.</u> May crave ice.

■ Diagnosis

History and physical exam, routine urinalysis and labs, <u>urine specific gravity under 1.005, urine osmolality under 250,</u> water loss more than 3 L per day. *(Diabetes Mellitus does not get 3L of urine output!)*

Water-deprivation test—pitressin injection followed by plasma/urine osmolality studies.

Nephrogenic diabetes insipidus—cannot concentrate urine.

Primary polydipsia—no urine osmolality change (or minimum increase) **after injection.**

Central diabetes insipidus—<u>urine osmolality greater than plasma osmolality.</u>

(margin note: take out H₂O → r/o psychogenic polydipsia then give pitressin to get neuro vs nephro DI)

■ Pathology

Insufficient antidiuretic hormone (ADH), or lack of response to ADH, resulting from <u>pituitary injury, tumor, or other disorder</u> (tuberculosis, sarcoid, etc).

■ Treatment

<u>Antidiuretic hormone replacement (pitressin tannate, 1-deamino-8-D-arginine vasopressin [DDAVP]).</u>

(margin note: Chlorpropamide → causes SIADH given in nephrogenic diabetes insipidus H- thiazide)

2. Inappropriate ADH Secretion

■ Description

Syndrome of inappropriate secretion of antidiuretic hormone (SIADH).

■ Symptoms

Confusion, lethargy, seizures, coma.

(margin note: +/- edema)

■ Diagnosis

History and physical exam, **hyponatremia, serum hypo-osmolality, urine hyperosmolarity.**

(margin note: low/high)

■ Pathology

(margin note: small cell lung CA)

Associated with **malignant/non-malignant lung disease,** other tumors, <u>en</u>docrinopathy, <u>central nervous system (CNS) disease, drugs.</u>

■ Treatment

<u>Fluid restriction, demeclocycline,</u> hypertonic saline in emergency.

3. Panhypopituitarism

■ Description

<u>Reduced or lacking pituitary hormone secretion.</u> Affecting single or several hormones.

■ Symptoms

Lack of TSH: hypothyroid symptoms. Lack of ACTH: adrenocortical insufficiency symptoms (hypotension, nausea/vomiting, confusion). Lack of **gonadotropins:** impotence/amenorrhea. Evidence of lack of **prolactin and/or growth hormone.**

■ Diagnosis

<u>History and physical exam, thyroid functions, serum testosterone, endocrine stimulation testing.</u>

■ Pathology *Sheehan's syndrome*

Infarction, tumor, infection, trauma, and other causes.

■ Treatment

<u>Glucocorticoids, thyroid replacement, estrogen/testosterone replacement.</u>

4. Acromegaly

■ Description

Excessive **growth hormone** secretion.

■ **Symptoms**

As child—gigantism, delayed puberty.

As adult—enlarging hands/feet, coarse features, deep voice, wide teeth, large tongue, joint pain. *diaphoresis*

■ **Diagnosis**

History and physical exam, lab (serum growth hormone, somatomedin-C), glucose suppression test. → *elevated*

(glucose should ↓ ↑ growth hormone level)

■ **Pathology**

Excess growth hormone secretion by pituitary adenoma.

■ **Treatment**

Surgical (transsphenoidal), radiation, medication (bromocriptine) somatostatin *(octreotide)*

F.   Adrenal Disorders

1. Adrenocortical Insufficiency— Acute

■ **Description**

Abrupt lack of adrenocortical hormones.

low | high
high | low → *low*

■ **Symptoms**

Confusion, weakness, abdominal pain.

■ **Diagnosis**

History and physical exam, elevated potassium, low sodium! Low plasma cortisol.

■ **Pathology**

Trauma, infection, gland necrosis, glucocorticoid withdrawal (in steroid-dependent patient).

■ **Treatment**

Hydrocortisone sodium succinate 100 mg IV, then infusion, then taper.

Additional Information. Corticosteroid use complications: hypokalemia, peptic ulcer, hyperglycemia, hypertension (sodium retention), psychosis, infection.

Patient should be on a high-protein diet. Give potassium as necessary. Sudden discontinuance of corticosteroids may result in adrenal insufficiency, as noted previously.

2. Adrenocortical Insufficiency— Chronic

■ **Description**

Addison's disease. — *1° adrenal insufficiency need to lose 90% of adrenals*

■ **Symptoms**

Lethargy, skin pigmentation, hypotension, nausea/vomiting.

■ **Diagnosis**

History and physical exam, hyponatremia, hyperkalemia, low plasma cortisol, adrenocorticotropic hormone (ACTH) stimulation test.

■ **Pathology**   → *Addison's*

Most often autoimmune and history of long-term glucocorticoid use etiology. *also TB, sarcoid, metastatic lung CA*

■ **Treatment**

Usually both hydrocortisone (glucocorticoid), and fludrocortisone (mineralocorticoid) needed.

Additional Information. Primary adrenocortical insufficiency: elevated plasma ACTH. Secondary adrenocortical insufficiency: plasma ACTH normal or low.

3. Cushing Syndrome

■ **Description**

Glucocorticoid overabundance.

■ **Symptoms**

Centripetal **obesity, striae/bruising, hypertension, hirsutism,** weakness, osteoporosis.

moon facies, buffalo hump

■ **Diagnosis**

History and physical exam, **overnight dexamethasone suppression test, 24-hour urine for free cortisol,** elevated urine 17-hydroxysteroids, metyrapone stimulation test.

↑ high (met. alkylosis)   *high*

■ **Pathology**

Cushing's disease most common (usually pituitary adenoma), but Cushing syndrome may also result from adrenal tumor, or ectopic ACTH hypersecretion.   *↳ lung cancer*

■ **Treatment**

Surgery, radiation, medication.

Additional Information. **Cushing syndrome: moon face, buffalo hump appearance.**

4. Adrenogenital Syndrome

■ **Description**

Virilizing female disorder.

■ **Symptoms**

Hirsutism, amenorrhea, deep voice, acne, enlarged clitoris.

■ **Diagnosis**

History and physical exam, **high urinary 17-ketosteroids,** ultrasound, laparoscopy, high 17-hydroxyprogesterone.

■ **Pathology**

In child: usually due to congenital adrenal hyperplasia. **In adult:** ovarian disease (polycystic ovary), or adrenal disease.

■ **Treatment**

Surgical excision (if tumor), estrogen spironolactone (for polycystic ovary syndrome). For congenital adrenal hyperplasia, give glucocorticoid replacement.

Additional Information. **Congenital adrenal hyperplasia:** due to **11- or 21-β-hydroxylase deficiency.** Diagnosis by high levels of **11-deoxycortisol or 17-hydroxyprogesterone.**

5. Hyperaldosteronism

■ **Description**

Mineralocorticoid excess.

■ **Symptoms**

May be **asymptomatic** or show evidence of **hypokalemic symptoms,** weakness, hypertension.

high high high low

■ **Diagnosis**

History and physical exam, **sodium retention, hypokalemia, hypertension, low plasma renin, elevated plasma/urine aldosterone.**

■ **Pathology**

Aldosterone overproduction by zona glomerulosa, from adenoma (Conn syndrome) or hyperplasia.

■ **Treatment**

Adrenalectomy, give spironolactone preop.

Additional Information. Differential diagnosis between adenoma and hyper-

hypoaldosteronism: low   high   assoc. c̄ diabetes mellitus

plasia: after salty diet, AM plasma aldosterone over 20 ng/dL in adenoma; under 20 ng/dL in hyperplasia.

Pseudohyperaldosteronism: Liddle syndrome, (?)renal tubule defect results in hyperaldosteronism symptoms without excess aldosterone production.

Overindulgence in licorice may cause hyperaldosteronism-like picture, but aldosterone excess is absent. Treatment: switch to another junk food!

6. Pheochromocytoma

■ Description

Catecholamine-producing chromaffin cell tumor.

■ Symptoms

Episodes of headache, flushing, diaphoresis, diplopia, weight loss, hypertension. *(+) orthostatic ↓bp!*

■ Diagnosis

usually → mediastinal
10% extraadrenal
10% bilateral
10% malignant

History and physical exam, tachycardia, 24-hour urinary vanillylmandelic acid (VMA), or metanephrines, serum catecholamines. Urinary catecholamines may be elevated by Aldomet and other meds. MRI.

■ Pathology

Tumor, may be adrenal or elsewhere. May be familial (see additional information subsequently).

■ Treatment

Surgical excision, give phenoxybenzamine preop. *long-acting α blocker +/- β blocker while awaiting surgery*

Additional Information. Multiple endocrine neoplasia 2: pheochromocytoma, thyroid cancer, hyperparathyroidism. Multiple endocrine neoplasia

medullary carcinoma ←

3: pheochromocytoma, thyroid cancer, mucosal neuromas, no hyperparathyroidism. Hippel-Lindau: pheochromocytoma, CNS hemangioblastomas. *von* Recklinghausen's disease: pheochromocytoma, neurofibromas.

G. Ovarian Disorders

1. Turner Syndrome

■ Description

Ovarian agenesis.

■ Symptoms

Short stature, sexual infantilism, cardiac anomalies, webbed neck/shield chest, micrognathia.

■ Diagnosis

History and physical exam, 45,X chromosomal pattern, elevated follicle-stimulating hormone (FSH), luteinizing hormone (LH).

■ Pathology

45 X0 Chromosomal abnormality (only one X chromosome) 45 X0.

■ Treatment

Estrogen/progesterone growth hormone. *→ counselling*

Additional Information. Pituitary dwarf has low FSH.

2. True Hermaphroditism

■ Description
Ambiguous genitalia.

■ Symptoms

Ambiguous genitalia.

■ **Diagnosis**

History and physical exam, chromosome studies, <u>histologic evaluation of ovotestis tissue.</u>

■ **Pathology**

<u>Ovarian and testicular tissue present</u> (ovotestis).

true hermaphrodite meaning both ♂ & ♀

■ **Treatment**

Varies with age and genitalia development.

3. Polycystic Ovary Syndrome

■ **Description**

<u>Stein–Leventhal syndrome.</u>

■ **Symptoms**

<u>Amenorrhea, hirsutism, obesity, infertility.</u>

■ **Diagnosis**

<u>History and physical exam, ultrasound.</u>

■ **Pathology**

Etiology unknown. *— get multiple cysts on ovaries c̄ low estrogen, high testosterone*

■ **Treatment**

<u>Oral contraceptives, spironolactone.</u>

4. Premature Ovarian Failure

■ **Description**

<u>Younger than age 35.</u>

■ **Symptoms**

<u>Cessation of menses.</u> *— menopausal sx: hot flashes, mood swings, depression, night sweats, fatigue*

■ **Diagnosis**

History and physical exam (normal), serum **FSH and LH elevated.**

■ **Pathology**

<u>Autoimmune.</u>

■ **Treatment**

<u>Estrogen/progesterone.</u> *(like post menopause pt)*

5. Amenorrhea and Galactorrhea

may be Prolactinoma

■ **Description**

As the previous.

■ **Symptoms**

As the previous. If tumor, may have visual field cut or headache. *amenorrhea, galactorrhea*

■ **Diagnosis**

History and physical exam, <u>**prolactin level, MRI of head** with gadolinium.</u>

■ **Pathology**

Etiology in <u>**breast stimulation, medication, pituitary tumor.**</u>

■ **Treatment**

<u>Surgery and/or bromocriptine.</u>

H. Lipid Metabolism Disorders

1. General Information

Very low-density lipoprotein (VLDL) —predominantly **triglyceride carrier.**

Low-density lipoprotein (LDL)—predominantly **cholesterol carrier.**

Lipoproteins—combination of cholesterol, triglyceride, protein, and phospholipid.

<u>**Coronary heart disease (CHD) risk factors** include **elevated cholesterol, smoking, elevated BP, de-**</u>

creased high-density lipoprotein (HDL), diabetes, severe obesity, peripheral vascular disease, family history. Total cholesterol may be obtained in fasting or non-fasting state.

2. Hyperlipidemia

■ Description

Elevated blood lipoproteins (cholesterol and/or triglycerides).

■ Symptoms

Often asymptomatic. See following sections for common presentations.

■ Diagnosis

Lab evaluation (total serum cholesterol, HDL, LDL, triglycerides).

■ Pathology

Elevated lipids may result in atheroma formation. Isolated cholesterol increase due to LDL. Elevated triglycerides with some cholesterol increase is due to elevated VLDL and/or chylomicrons. If both cholesterol and triglycerides are high, usually increased VLDL and LDL is the etiology.

■ Treatment

See following sections.

3. Hypertriglyceridemia—Primary

■ Description

Elevated triglycerides; lipoprotein phenotype 4.

■ Symptoms

May be asymptomatic or pancreatitis, lipemia retinalis (white tint color to retina), xanthomas, hepatosplenomegaly.

■ Diagnosis

History and physical exam, very high serum triglyceride levels. Normal LDL cholesterol.

■ Pathology

May be familial trait.

■ Treatment

For impending pancreatitis, give nothing by mouth (NPO), and give IV glucose. Hypertriglyceridemia: diet (reduce fat, avoid alcohol).

Additional Information. Secondary hypertriglyceridemia may result in diabetes, nephrosis, alcohol abuse, hypothyroidism. Control primary disease, diet, medications minimally effective. Severe hypertriglyceridemia (over 1000), may be type 5 (excess chylomicrons and excess VLDL), or type 1 (only chylomicron excess). If diet fails try gemfibrozil and fish oil.

4. Hyperlipoproteinemia

■ Description

Broad beta disease, familial, phenotype 3, also termed dysbetalipoproteinemia.

■ Symptoms

Palmar and tuberous xanthomas, obesity, early atherosclerosis.

■ Diagnosis

History and physical exam, laboratory evaluation (elevated cholesterol and triglycerides).

■ Pathology

Genetic predisposition, with elevated beta-VLDL.

■ **Treatment**

Diet, clofibrate, nicotinic acid, gemfibrozil.

Additional Information. Combined cholesterol and triglyceride elevation is also noted in **familial combined hyperlipidemia, type 2-B,** with excess **VLDL and LDL,** and elevated coronary artery disease (CAD) risk. Try niacin or gemfibrozil, or lovastatin. **Nicotinic acid:** Niacin, for elevated **LDL/triglycerides,** elevates HDL; side effects: flushing (give aspirin to prevent).

5. *Primary Hypercholesterolemia*

■ **Description**

Familial hypercholesterolemia, **phenotype 2-A.**

■ **Symptoms**

Tendinous xanthomas (Achilles and patella common), **early CAD,** xanthelasma, corneal arcus.

■ **Diagnosis**

History and physical exam, lab evaluation, **clear serum.**

■ **Pathology**

Autosomal dominant, **increased LDL.**

■ **Treatment**

Diet (low fat, low cholesterol); medication (cholestyramine [Questran], nicotinic acid [Niacin], statins; quit smoking.   *LDL determines rx choice*

Additional Information. Secondary hypercholesterolemia is associated with hypothyroidism, anorexia nervosa, nephrosis, and cholestasis. Treat the primary disorder.

6. *Hypolipidemia*

■ **Description**

Tangier disease.

■ **Symptoms**

Large orange tonsils, neuropathy, splenomegaly.

■ **Diagnosis**

Low serum cholesterol, corneal opacities, cholesterol ester storage in multiple body areas.

■ **Pathology**

Deficiency of HDL, autosomal recessive.

■ **Treatment**

Supportive, gene therapy?

I. **Mineral Metabolism Disorders**

1. *Hemochromatosis*

■ **Description**

Disorder of iron excess.

■ **Symptoms**   *→ may have cirrhosis c̄ ascites*

Hepatomegaly, skin pigmentation, **cardiomegaly,** pancreatic disease.

■ **Diagnosis**

History and physical exam, abnormal liver function, elevated serum iron/ferritin, liver biopsy.

■ **Pathology**

Autosomal recessive.

■ **Treatment**

United States Medical Licensing Exam (USMLE) early diagnosis/treatment disorder. Phlebotomy, deferoxamine.

2. *Wilson's Disease*

■ **Description**

Hepatolenticular degeneration.

■ **Symptoms**

Kayser–Fleischer ring, neurologic (tremor), hepatic (cirrhosis).

■ **Diagnosis**

Low ceruplasmin, increased urinary copper.

■ **Pathology**

Autosomal recessive, excess copper deposits in liver, brain.

■ **Treatment**

USMLE early diagnosis/treatment disorder. Oral penicillamine.

J.   **Other Disorders**

1. *Klinefelter Syndrome*

■ **Description**

Hypogonadism disorder.

■ **Symptoms**

Gynecomastia, mental retardation, small testes.

■ **Diagnosis**

History and physical exam, chromosome analysis (usually 47,XXY), testicular biopsy.

■ **Pathology**

Seminiferous tubule dysgenesis.

■ **Treatment**

Testosterone I.M. or patch.

2. *Fabry's Disease*

■ **Description**

Metabolic inborn error disorder.

■ **Symptoms**

Renal failure, skin lesions as **telangiectasia**, and **angiokeratomas**, **pain/ fever episodes.**

■ **Diagnosis**

History and physical exam, **deficient** serum/tissue α-D-galactosidase A.

■ **Pathology**

Glycosphingolipid deposition in tissues (eyes, kidney, heart, CNS, etc).

■ **Treatment**

Supportive.

3. *Gaucher's Disease*

■ **Description**

Familial glucosyl ceramide lipidosis.

■ **Symptoms**

Lethargy, anemia, splenomegaly, bone/ joint pain, with or without CNS signs/ symptoms.

■ **Diagnosis**

History and physical exam, **Gaucher's cells in marrow.**

- **Pathology**

Excess glucocerebroside deposition.

- **Treatment**

Treat complications, gene therapy?

4. Obesity

- **Description**

Excess adipose tissue storage of triglyceride.

- **Symptoms**

Excessive weight.

- **Diagnosis**

History and physical exam, **weight 20% or more over average.**

- **Pathology**

Large adipocytes stuffed with triglycerides. **Number of adipocytes regulated in response to caloric intake as infant. Overweight baby becomes overweight adult.**

- **Treatment**

Reduce calories, exercise, investigational drugs.

Additional Information. **No true endocrine etiology for obesity.** Syndromes including obesity include **Prader–Willi** (mental retardation, hypogonadism), and Laurence–Moon–Biedl (nerve deafness, retinal pathology).

5. Gestational Diabetes

- **Description**

Pregnancy-associated diabetes.

- **Symptoms**

May be asymptomatic.

- **Diagnosis**

Fasting blood sugar. Glucose tolerance test at 24 to 28 weeks (give 50 g glucose, then check sugar hourly; over 140 to 150 mg/dL is abnormal.

- **Pathology**

May result in fetal macrosomia (large birth weight), intrauterine growth retardation (IUGR), congenital anomalies, elevated bilirubin, and neonatal hypoglycemia.

- **Treatment**

Diabetic diet, insulin.

6. Endocrine Disorders and Cancer

- **Description**

Carcinoma may produce chorionic gonadotropin, ACTH (lung most often), growth hormone, gastrin (Zollinger–Ellison), hypercalcemia from secretion of parathyroid-like compounds (lung most often), and others.

7. Carcinoid Syndrome

- **Description**

Serotonin-secreting, argentaffin cell tumor. *asymptomatic until get liver involvement*

- **Symptoms**

Diarrhea, flushing, bronchospasm, and heart valve lesions.

- **Diagnosis**

History and physical exam, **urinary 5-hydroxyindoleacetic acid (5-HIAA).**

■ **Pathology**

Tumors from enterochromaffin cells. Pulmonary and gastrointestinal (GI) tract sites common.

■ **Treatment**

Surgery, cyproheptadine.

8. Mastocytosis

■ **Description**

Mast cell disorder.

■ **Symptoms**

Flushing, vomiting, diarrhea, tachycardia, hypotension, syncope, in episodic attacks.

■ **Diagnosis**

History and physical exam, may have urticaria pigmentosa, histamine and histamine metabolite studies, skin/bone marrow biopsy. May show Darier's sign (stroking skin lesion results in elevated/erythematous reaction: dermographism).

■ **Pathology**

Release of mast cell mediators (heparin, histamine, enzymes). Cutaneous and systemic types.

■ **Treatment**

Epinephrine, antihistamines (block both H_1 and H_2 receptors), and antiprostaglandins.

BIBLIOGRAPHY

DeGroot LJ. *Endocrinology*, Vols. 1, 2, 3. Philadelphia, Pa: WB Saunders Co; 1989.

Ellenberg M. *Diabetes Mellitus, Theory and Practice*. New York: Medical Examination Publishing Company, Inc; 1983.

Felig P. *Endocrinology and Metabolism*. 3rd ed. New York: McGraw-Hill; 1995.

Greenspan FS. *Basic and Clinical Endocrinology*. 2nd ed. East Norwalk, Conn: Appleton-Century-Crofts; 1986.

Havel RJ. *Metabolic Control and Disease*. 8th ed. Philadelphia, Pa: WB Saunders; 1980.

Ingbar SH. *The Thyroid: A Fundamental and Clinical Text*. 6th ed. Philadelphia, Pa: JB Lippincott; 1992.

Layon JA. *Fluids and Electrolytes in Critical Care*. Philadelphia, Pa: JB Lippincott Company; 1988.

Scriver CR. *The Metabolic Basis of Inherited Disease*. 7th ed. New York: McGraw-Hill; 1994.

Speroff L. *Clinical Gynecologic Endocrinology and Infertility*. Baltimore, Md: Williams & Wilkins; 1989.

Styne DM. *Reproductive Endocrinology*. 2nd ed. Philadelphia, Pa: WB Saunders; 1986.

Thompson JS. *Genetics in Medicine*. Philadelphia, Pa: WB Saunders; 1986.

Wilson JD. *Textbook of Endocrinology*. 8th ed. Philadelphia, Pa: WB Saunders; 1992.

———————————— CHAPTER 4 ————————————

Gastroenterology

ARTHUR TUCH, MD

I. GASTROINTESTINAL BLEEDING

A. Acute Upper Gastrointestinal Bleeding

■ Description

Site of bleeding is esophagogastric (EG) junction (varices, esophagitis, Mallory–Weiss tears), **one third**; **stomach** (ulcers, gastritis), **one third**; and **pyloroduodenal region** (ulcers, duodenitis), **one third.**

■ Symptoms

Vomiting blood or melena.

■ Diagnosis

Esophagogastroduodenoscopy (EGD) identifies source in 95%. In ulcers, visible vessel in ulcer base indicates rebleed of 50%, and clean ulcer base, rebleed of 1%.

■ Pathology

Peptic disease, portal hypertension, shearing forces in Mallory–Weiss (MW).

■ Treatment

Mortality unchanged at 10% in past 40 years. H_2 blocker, correct coagulopathy if present, transfuse as needed, bicap may be helpful in ulcer disease. Varices: Pitressin and nitroglycerin (NTG) drip, sclerotherapy. Surgery may be needed if visible vessel in ulcer bed or if greater than 6 units required in 24 hours, or if 3 to 4 U/day in 3 days.

Rx cause

B. Acute Lower Gastrointestinal Bleeding

■ Description

Diverticulosis, angiodysplasia, neoplasm, colitis.

■ Symptoms

Bright red blood per rectum.

■ Diagnosis

Colonoscopy when bleeding stops. Angiography if bleeding persists.

■ Treatment

Replace blood, correct coagulation factors if needed. Vasopressin infusion at angiographic bleeding site.

Rx cause

II. INFLAMMATORY BOWEL DISEASE (IBD)

A. Ulcerative Colitis

■ Description

Chronic idiopathic inflammation. *Continous inflammation beginning @ rectum*

■ Symptoms

Small frequent bloody diarrheal stools often associated with **tenesmus.** Abdominal pain, fever, and leukocytosis. Fulminant colitis is associated with worsening systemic toxicity and may show colonic dilatation (transverse diameter > 5 cm).

■ Diagnosis

Rule out antibiotics and other drugs, stool for ova and parasites, culture and sensitivity (O&P, C&S), and *Clostridium difficile* toxin (*Escherichia coli* 0157:H7—culture negative hemorrhagic colitis, after raw beef or milk causes hemolytic anemia syndrome, 35% mortality in elderly). Histologic exam of mucosa. Colonoscopy and ileoscopy, barium enema if not megacolon, and small bowel series.

may get backwash ileitis

■ Pathology

Crypt abscesses and superficial ulceration compatible with diagnosis.

pseudopolyps

■ Treatment

acute flare up? {Azulfidine 4 g/day; folic acid 1 mg daily for 2 to 3 weeks.} Amebiasis should be excluded before beginning steroid therapy. Oral prednisone (30 to 60 mg daily) responds usually in 2 weeks, taper by 5 mg weekly. **Maintenance** prophylactic therapy: **sulfasalazine** 500 mg by mouth (PO) 4 times daily (qid) and **folate** 1 mg daily.

Surgery (colectomy) is curative

B. Crohn's Disease

■ Description

Chronic idiopathic inflammation.

Skip lesions, any part of GI tract, transmural

■ Symptoms

Small intestinal sites cause pain, bloating, diarrhea, weight loss, fever. Obstruction causes crampy abdominal pain followed by vomiting. Perianal disease (fistula, perianal abscess, fissures), fistulae (to the bladder, vagina, colon, skin, among loops of bowel), or abdominal masses due to abscesses.

■ Diagnosis

Skip lesions

Stomach or small bowel involvement, rectal sparing, fistulization. Deep fissures, ulcer, granulomas, or patchy distribution of colonic inflammation. Upper GI/small bowel, barium enema with flexible sigmoidoscopy versus colonoscopy.

■ Pathology

Transmural, "fat wrapping" on serosal surface, noncaseating granulomas.

■ Treatment

1. **Sulfasalazine:** 4 g/day, and if confined to the colon, 1 mg folic acid for 2 to 4 weeks, if sulfa allergic.
2. **Metronidazole:** 10 mg/kg daily. If no response in 4 weeks, then
3. **Prednisone:** 30 to 60 mg daily should be used instead (start with

Surgery is useless

prednisone if symptoms are severe). If patient responds to treatment 1 or 2, continue for 4 to 6 months; then stop if symptoms gone. No prophylactic therapy. Twenty percent of cases of IBD are neither specifically ulcerative colitis nor Crohn's disease. Sulfasalazine and prednisone appear safe in pregnancy and during lactation.

III. PEPTIC ULCER (DUODENAL AND GASTRIC ULCER)

■ Description

Peptic ulcers are defects in GI mucosa extending to the submucosa, into the muscle layers, and require acid and pepsin. The major complications of duodenal ulcers are bleeding, perforation, gastric outlet obstruction, and penetration into the pancreas.

■ Symptoms

Epigastric pain, dull ache relieved by food or antacids within about 15 minutes or radiation to the back, and often associated with heartburn.

Bleeding ulcers may be painless, but with hematemesis, melena, anemia, or hematochezia.

Gastric outlet obstruction may present with repeated vomiting and dehydration.

■ Diagnosis

Upper endoscopy, 90% in experienced hands (biopsy and brush of gastric ulcers to rule out cancer [CA]). Radiographic exam somewhat less accurate.

■ Pathology

Superficial erosion (see Description).

■ Treatment

Gastric ulcer: treat with H_2 blocker full dose for 8 to 12 weeks, and re-evaluate for com-

Rx: antibiotics! for H. pylori +/- H₂ blockers

plete healing. Ulcers greater than 1 cm often require 3 months or more for complete healing.

Duodenal ulcers heal faster. Treat with H_2 blocker full dose for 2 months, then consider maintenance therapy for prevention of recurrent ulcer, usually the same as acute treatment.

Prilosec (omeprazole) 20 mg every AM for duodenal ulcer for 2 months, especially helpful in reflux disease and Zollinger–Ellison syndrome.

Stop caustics: alcohol, non-steroidal anti-inflammatory drugs (NSAIDs), caffeine, nicotine.

IV. MOTOR DISORDERS OF THE GASTROINTESTINAL TRACT

A. Oropharyngeal Dysphagia

■ Description

Neuromuscular control of oral and oropharyngeal stage of **swallowing is impaired.** Skeletal muscle is primarily involved; 50% of nursing home patients in the United States have difficulty with eating and drinking.

■ Symptoms

Dysphagia.

■ Diagnosis

Barium video swallow with liquid to solid foods, neurological evaluation. Occasionally, esophageal manometry (ENT) evaluation.

■ Pathology

Cerebrovascular accident **(CVA) (most common),** Alzheimer's, bulbar and pseudobulbar palsy. Cranial nerve paralysis, myasthenia gravis, skeletal myopathies.

■ Treatment

Treat underlying condition where possible. If patient aspirates more than 10% of

barium test bolus and develops barium residue in oropharynx with sequential swallows, needs endoscopy or surgical gastrostomy.

B. Achalasia

■ Description

Achalasia is characterized by **increased basal pressure of the lower esophageal sphincter (LES),** incomplete LES relaxation after a normal swallow, and aperistalsis of the distal two thirds of the esophageal body.

■ Symptoms

Dysphagia for liquids then solids, chest pain, vomiting frequently without sour taste, nocturnal cough, pneumonia, lung abscess.

■ Diagnosis

Air fluid level near aortic arch with widened mediastinum on **chest x-ray. Barium swallow** may show dilated distal two thirds of the esophagus and smooth tapering at EG junction.

All patients with achalasia should have **upper endoscopy** to exclude tumors and to enter the stomach to differentiate the tonically contracted LES from a malignant stricture.

Esophageal manometry should be done and is the "gold standard" (see Description).

Computed tomography may be used to exclude extrinsic circumferential lesions simulating achalasia.

■ Pathology

Abnormalities are found in the dorsomotor nucleus of the vagus nerve and in the postganglionic neurons, which innervate the circular smooth muscle of the esophagus (Auerbach's plexus).

■ **Treatment**

Nifedipine 10 mg sublingually 1/2 hour before meals; if no help, then **pneumatic dilation**—transmural rupture of esophagus is an uncommon complication—if no help, then **surgical myotomy** (modified Heller's) with fundoplication, attempting to avoid esophageal stricture (20%) or Barrett's esophagus.

C. **Gastroesophageal Reflux Disease**

■ **Description**

Acid in an acid-sensitive esophagus. Dysphagia may develop due to benign stricture. Rare bleeding from erosive esophagitis.

■ **Symptoms**

Heartburn, occasionally chronic cough, nocturnal cough, choking, wheezing, laryngospasm, hoarseness, earache.

■ **Diagnosis**

Upper gastrointestinal endoscopy or (less sensitive) an air-contrast upper GI to exclude complications (eg, erosive esophagitis, benign peptic stricture, Barrett's esophagus, pill-induced esophageal injury, duodenal or gastric ulcer). If empiric medical treatment fails, then do acid perfusion, Bernstein test, continuous intraesophageal pH monitoring, or establish a relationship between symptoms and acid reflux.

■ **Pathology**

Hyperplasia of basal cells and prominent elongated papillae in squamous epithelium. Subtle histological changes occasionally having a normal gross appearance. Barrett's esophagus, columnar lined distal esophagus, as adaptive response to severe gastroesophageal reflux disease (GERD); rarely regresses despite control of reflux. Increased risk for adenocarcinoma. Esophagogastroduodenoscopy (EGD) every 2 to 3 years, more frequently if dysplasia.

■ **Treatment**

H_2 antagonist twice daily. Metaclopramide short term, less than full dose, complicated by 1 to 2% tardive dyskinesia, which is not always reversible. Omeprazole 20 mg in AM, not more than 8 to 12 weeks. Can be repeated occasionally for severe exacerbations (for severe medically resistant cases).

Surgical fundoplication, which may be effective for about 5 years; chewing gum, lozenges may be helpful by increasing salivary flow, which improves esophageal acid clearance.

D. **Scleroderma Esophagus**

■ **Description**

A patulous esophagus leads to reflux disease and dysphagia associated with Raynaud's phenomenon in 90% of cases.

■ **Symptoms**

Heartburn, dysphagia for liquids, then solids. (progressive dysphagia

■ **Diagnosis**

Air-filled esophagus on chest film. Prone view of esophagogram fails to empty. Esophageal manometry in advanced state includes decreased LES pressure, low amplitude or absent contractions in the smooth muscle esophagus, normal peristalsis in the striated muscle esophagus, and a normal upper esophageal sphincter (UES).

■ **Treatment**

See treatment for GERD. Surgery is unnecessary and probably contraindicated here because of the limited ability to empty the esophagus.

E. Gastroparesis

■ Description

Delayed gastric emptying without mechanical cause.

■ Symptoms

Nausea, vomiting, bloating, upper abdominal discomfort.

■ Diagnosis

Retained barium in stomach on UGI. Delayed nuclear medicine gastric emptying scan. Upper endoscopic exam within normal limits.

■ Pathology and Associated Conditions

Acute with intact vagi (blood sugar greater than 300 mg/dL, acute pancreatitis, trauma, abdominal surgery, porphyria, severe hypokalemia, or drugs [opiates, digitalis, ganglionic blockers, anticholinergic]). Chronic (most frequently caused by neuropathy [postvagotomy or diabetic] or myopathy [sclerodermal).

■ Treatment

Metaclopramide (a dopaminergic antagonist, 30% neurologic and psychiatric side effects). See GERD.

Domperidone (second generation; no CNS side effects).

Cisapride (increase endogenous release of acetylclodine), soon available.

Ondansitron (serotonin antagonist).

F. Constipation

■ Description

Symptomatic decrease in frequency of bowel movements and may also mean (to some patients) passage of dry stools, excessive straining, lower abdominal fullness, and a sense of incomplete evacuation.

■ Diagnosis

Rule out organic disease (endocrine pharmacologic, neurologic, and structural).

■ Treatment

Insoluble dietary bulk 15 g of crude fiber (eg, wheat bran [methylcellulose] or commercial psyllium products with 32 oz of water per day). Lactulose can be tolerated well for long periods. Occasionally mineral oil enemas can help relieve distal fecal impaction.

G. Diarrhea

■ Description

Twenty-four hour excretion weight or volume greater than 200 g/24 hours and greater than 10 g/kg in infants, and change in consistency—more liquid.

Not incontinence (the involuntary release of rectal contents).

■ Diagnosis

Osmotic diarrhea stool plasma osmolality = 290 mOsm/kg H_2O. Osm/(2 (NA + K) greater than 100 (Osm gap). Diarrhea should disappear when patient fasts.

H. Infectious Diarrhea

Certain systemic diseases are accompanied by diarrhea as a prominent symptom: graft-versus-host disease, hepatitis, legionellosis, listeriosis, Rocky Mountain spotted fever, psittacosis, otitis media in infants, and toxic shock syndrome. Conversely, certain enteric infections are accompanied by systemic symptoms that may be clues to their diagnoses. The hemolytic uremic syndrome can occur with shigellosis and enterohemorrhagic *E. coli*. Reiter syndrome can occur after infection with *Salmonella, Shigella, Campylobacter,* and *Yersinia*.

■ Treatment

The specific cause.

I. Antibiotic-Associated Diarrhea

■ Description

Any antibiotic (even 1 dose as long as 2 months before).

■ Diagnosis

Identifying *C. difficile toxin* in the stool. Finding characteristic **yellow adherent plaques on the colonic mucosa.** (pseudomembranes)

■ Treatment

Metronidazole (250 mg thrice daily [tid] costs less) **or vancomycin** (125 mg qid) are equally effective (80% response). Ten percent to 20% have recurrence within 1 month; retreat with same drug. With multiple recurrences, consideration should be given to bacitracin, rifampicin, prolonged therapy (1 month) with the initial antibiotic or adding cholestyramine 16 g daily tapered over 3 to 6 weeks.

V. COLORECTAL CANCER

■ Description

Cancer of colon is the most frequent neoplasm of the GI tract and is the second most common cause of cancer mortality in the United States. Early detection may lead to a substantial improvement in outcome.

■ Symptoms

Rectal bleeding, change in bowel habits.

■ Diagnosis

need to do DRE also

American Cancer Society recommends fecal occult blood testing of passed stool yearly after age 50 and flexible sigmoidoscopy every 3 to 5 years. Start earlier age with colonoscopy if genetic predisposition or prior disease.

The presence of heme in an asymptomatic person at risk is an indication for colonoscopy or flex sig and barium enema.

Colonoscopy is more sensitive, and a biopsy can be made; especially in high-risk patients whose first-degree relatives have colorectal cancer or who themselves have IBD, previous breast or genital CA, prior colonic adenomas, CA, or familial polyposis.

Finding even one adenoma should lead to total colonoscopy and polypectomy. Repeat colonoscopy in 1 to 2 years; if normal, can be followed by exams every 3 to 5 years.

■ Pathology

Ninety-five percent of malignancies of the colon and rectum are adenocarcinoma.

■ Treatment

The **only curative therapy is surgical resection of the primary tumor** and of the isolated hepatic metastases. Rule out synchronous lesions by doing full colonoscopy preop. Colonoscopy in 1 year to exclude recurrence and at 3 to 5 years to prevent the 8 to 10% incidence of second cancers, which occur within 10 years of the initial surgery.

VI. HEPATOBILIARY SYSTEM

A. Chronic Active Hepatitis

■ Description

Chronic active autoimmune hepatitis (CAAH) can present with striking increases in enzymes resembling viral hepatitis, but stigmata of chronic liver disease or marked elevations in gamma globulins may help identify it as chronic without evidence of other causes. The presence in serum of ANA or antismooth muscle antibodies strongly suggests autoimmune hepatitis.

■ Symptoms

Chronic hepatitis is suspected when physical examination reveals signs of chronic liver disease (eg, spider angiomata, ascites, and elevated serum glutamic-oxaloacetic transaminase (SGOT) or serum glutamate pyruvate transaminase (SGPT). Often the patient may have only increased fatigue and persistent elevated enzymes for 6 months or more.

■ Pathology

Piecemeal necrosis and bridging necrosis (fibrosis can lead to cirrhosis).

This disease is associated with three important patterns of autoantibodies in serum:

1. The first pattern characteristically has positive ANA, antismooth muscle antibody (ASMA) liver membrane autoantibodies.
2. The second pattern is associated with antibodies to a soluble liver antigen (antisoluble liver antigen [SLA]).
3. Positive sera for this are found in young women with hypergammaglobulinemia who respond well to immunosuppressive treatment.

Drugs producing a hepatitis that mimics chronic active autoimmune hepatitis (CAAH) are alpha-methyldopa and nitrofurantoin (especially women). Suspect Wilson's disease if hemolysis or neuropsychiatric signs noted, decreased serum ceruloplasmin, and Kayser–Fleischer rings on slit-lamp eye exam. Viral (B & C).

■ Treatment

Steroid therapy achieves symptomatic, clinical, and histological remission, but relapse occurs in 90% over 2 years, requiring long-term maintenance therapy leading to increases in life expectancy, but does not appear to stop progression to cirrhosis.

B. Complications of Cirrhosis

Cirrhosis is among the 10 most common causes of death in the United States, and the fourth most common (25 to 45%) in urban areas.

C. Ascites

■ Description

Fluid in peritoneal cavity.

■ Diagnosis

Ultrasound (US) or computed tomography (CT) more sensitive than physical exam.

Paracentesis 10 mL into blood culture bottles, acid-fast bacteria (AFB), fungal cultures, cytology, bilirubin, amylase, total protein, white blood cells (WBC) and differential, lactate dehydrogenase (LDH).

■ Pathology

All the factors in ascites mechanism and formation are not known.

■ Treatment

Sodium and fluid restriction and diuretics. Initially with spironolactone 50 to 400 mg/24 h; if no help in 3 to 4 days, start furosemide 40 mg daily. If no response, double daily up to 240 to 320 mg daily. Failure: other drugs, bumetanide, ethacrynic acid, or metolazone, watch for large diuresis; if no help, large-volume paracentesis if > 5 liters needed to give albumin 6 to 10 g/L of fluid removed. Can be done 1 to 3 times per month for life. Patient with intractable ascites who has bled from varices may benefit from intrahepatic shunting by a stent radiologically

Lactulose can cause diarrhea to remove ↑NH₃ & edema

placed through hepatic vein to the portal vein.

D. Spontaneous Bacterial Peritonitis

■ Description

Bacteria most likely reaches ascites through hematogenous spread; *E. coli* is most common pathogen. Mortality and recurrence is high even with antibiotics.

■ Symptoms

Fever, abdominal pain, encephalopathy in cirrhotic patient with ascites, but many patients may be asymptomatic.

■ Diagnosis

Greater than 250/mL WBC is reliable even if fluid is sterile, if symptoms are suggestive.

　Best ascites culture yields (> 80%) obtained by inoculation of 10 mL of ascites into each of three 100-mL blood culture bottles (aerobic, anaerobic, and micro-aerophilic) at the bedside. Protein usually less than 1 g/mL, greater than 10,000/mL, protein less than 2.5 with free air suggests ruptured viscus.

■ Treatment

Cefotaxime 2 g IV every 8 to 12 hours for 5 to 10 days. Repeat paracentesis in 49 hours after initiation of antibiotics; if ascitic fluid poly count not decreased by at least 50%, antibiotics should be changed and the problem re-evaluated.

E. Hepatic Encephalopathy

■ Description

Abnormal mental state and neuromuscular dysfunction **due to hepatic failure.**

■ Symptoms

Starting with **lethargy** and progressing to **stupor** or **coma** with dropping things and making mistakes as early signs.

■ Diagnosis

Can be spontaneous. Seek precipitating cause (eg, diuretics, hypokalemic alkalosis, hypovolemia, hyponatremia, azotemia, tranquilizer, sedative, analgesic drugs, infection, severe constipation, hypoxia, excessive dietary protein, and progressive liver damage).

■ Pathology

Pathogenesis not fully characterized.

■ Treatment

Protein restriction, lactulose 30 cc PO hourly until diarrhea, then every 6 hours. If PO not available, then 300 cc lactulose plus 700 cc tap water enema one to three times daily if deemed safe to give enemas. Treat underlying condition.

F. Liver Transplantation

■ Description

For end-stage liver disease, usually in postnecrotic cirrhosis, primary biliary cirrhosis (PBC), primary sclerosing cholangitis (PSC). Five-year survival from 55 to 85%. **Absolute contraindication:** active **sepsis** outside biliary tree, **metastatic hepatobiliary malignancy, advanced cardiopulmonary disease** and **AIDS.**

　Relative contraindications: active alcohol (ETOH)-induced liver disease (only 13 to 16% resume ETOH after), portal vein thrombosis, or previous portacaval shunt surgery. Clinically apparent hepatocellular carcinoma or cholangiocarcinoma, if HBsAg positive, liver disease and advanced chronic renal disease. In fulminant hepatic failure decide before stage IV coma (eg, drug-induced, hepatitis C viral hepatic failure, and fulminant Wilson's disease).

G. Viral Hepatitis

■ Description

Five viruses are clearly identified, and a sixth is suggestive epidemiologically (like non-B, non-C).

1. Hepatitis A

■ Description

The RNA virus: almost exclusive fecal–oral routes, usually early childhood. Rarely fulminant and fatal. Chronic A not described.

■ Symptoms

Easy fatigability, jaundice, anorexia, fever, but often not diagnosed because of mild anicteric disease.

■ Diagnosis

Immunoglobulin M (IgM) antihepatitis A virus (HAV) (+); immunoglobulin G (IgG) indicates previous infection with A. The SGPT greater than SGOT, greater than 1000, usually.

■ Treatment

Vaccines of killed and attenuated types produced, soon to be licensed.

2. Hepatitis B (HBV)

■ Description

DNA virus: transmitted perinatal, parenteral, and sexually, but not fecal–oral.

HBsAg is earliest marker, can be negative in fulminant hepatitis B. IgM anti-HBc will become rapidly positive and diagnostic.

HBsAg greater than 6 months = chronic B. HBeAg: whole virus replication (likely HBV-DNA is detectable in serum and is highly infective).

IgM anti-HBc AB titer can become low and persist in chronic hepatitis.

IgG anti-HBc with nL enzymes and no anti-HBs may have had viral B in the past, but failed to develop anti-HBs or lost it.

IgG anti-HBc found alone in a case may be associated with HBV detectable by polymerase chain reaction technique.

■ Symptoms

Flulike illness, jaundice in one third. Incubation a few weeks to 6 months. Ten percent to 20% (high) incidence of serum sickness—fever, arthralgia or arthritis, or skin rash, most frequently maculopapular or urticarial.

■ Diagnosis

IgM anti-HBc (see Description). SGPT greater than 1000.

■ Pathology

Cytotoxic T cells recognize hepatitis B core antigen receptors on liver cells. T cells attach to receptors, leading to cellular necrosis.

■ Treatment

Prevent with active (vaccine) and passive hepatitis B immunoglobulin (HBIG) immunization. Interferon alpha stops replications in chronic hepatitis. HBV-DNA and HBeAg disappear from serum. Patient is less infective in 35% of patients. In 10%, cure, HBsAg gone, and anti-HBs appeared.

3. Hepatitis D

Description

Unique RNA, requiring outer envelope of HBsAg for replication, co-infection, or superinfection (which is more likely to produce fulminant hepatic failure). **Prevalent among parenteral drug addicts, hemophiliacs, and homosexual men.**

■ Treatment

Interferon alpha treats D but relapses after therapy. Immunity to B prevents D.

4. Hepatitis C

■ Description

Anti-HCV defined this RNA viral infection. Makes up 85% of post-transfusion hepatitis, 70% of non-A, non-B.

5. Hepatitis E

■ Description

Transmitted by fecal–oral route—waterborne epidemics in especially India, Nepal, Pakistan, and Southeast Asia.

■ Symptoms

The disease is self-limited and does not evolve into chronic hepatitis, but has often been observed to be cholestatic, unique fulminant disease in pregnant women.

■ Treatment

Standard gamma globulin is ineffective and there are no active vaccines available.

H. Drug-Induced Liver Disease

■ Description

Acute hepatitis (INH), chronic active hepatitis (nitrofurantoin, alpha-methyldopa), cirrhosis (methotrexate), cholestasis (sulfonamides), fatty liver (corticosteroids), granuloma (allopurinol), benign and malignant neoplasms (estrogens), vascular lesions (vitamin A) and sclerosing cholangitis (5-fluorodeoxyuridine [5-FUDR]).

Anti-HCV: exposure to C in asymptomatic blood donors and in patients with chronic hepatitis. Screening blood donors for anti-HBc, increased alanine aminotransferase and HIV antibody has decreased incidence of post-transfusion hepatitis to anti-HCV; should reduce the incidence to less than 2%.

Anti-HCV: 0.5 to 1.4% blood donors in United States.

■ Diagnosis

Anti-HCV against a non-structural recombinant viral protein does not appear until several months after onset of the illness. More specific tests of acute infection will be forthcoming.

■ Pathology

Liver biopsy is not indicated in most patients with acute hepatitis, usually only when liver function tests (LFTs) abnormal for greater than 6 months.

Spotty necrosis of liver cells throughout the lobe, lymphocytes, and histocytes, bridging necrosis.

■ Treatment

Chronic hepatitis in 50%; cirrhosis in 20% in 1.5 to 2 years. Interferon alpha decreased enzymes to nL in 40%; 3 10^6 U subcutaneously three times weekly for 6 months. Enzymes do not increase before decrease, as in hepatitis B.

Fifty percent relapse in 6 months when treatment is stopped. Acetaminophen is suicide—greater than 15 g causes massive necrosis; generates toxic metabolites through P_{450} cytochrome. Cimetidine competes for oxidation by cytochrome P_{450}.

Alcohol increased P_{450} activity and toxic metabolites. Doses averaging 6 to 7 g/day (acetaminophen) taken by alcoholic has been associated with severe hepatotoxicity characterized by increased aspartate aminotransferase (AST) greater than 3000 to 10,000. The mortality in one series was 20%.

Antiarrhythmic amiodarone like alcoholic hepatitis (eg, stenosis, hepatocellular necrosis, and Mallory bodies).

Verapamil and captopril mixed hepatocellular cholestatic patterns; ketoconazole variable hepatocellular and in 40% cholestatic.

Methotrexate cirrhosis greater than 1.5 g total dose; low dose 7.5 mg/week for 2 years; not associated with bridging fibrosis or cirrhosis.

Most NSAIDs are found to be associated with some form of hepatotoxicity.

Total parenteral nutrition (TPN) associated with fragment cholestatic jaundice, much mixed origin but not characterized.

I. Primary Biliary Cirrhosis

■ Description

Autoimmune etiology characterized by antimitochondrial antibodies in the serum.

Anti-M2 is the major marker-specific mitochondrial antibodies against the inner mitochrondrial membrane.

■ Symptoms

Most common symptoms are insidious onset of **pruritus** and **fatigue,** early **hepatomegaly** and elevation of serum alkaline phosphatase before symptoms.

■ Pathology

Destruction intrahepatic bile ducts in the first stage with progression to macronodular cirrhosis in the final stage, with mononuclear infiltrate in the portal tracts and paucity of bile ducts.

■ Treatment

No specific effective treatment; ursodeoxycholic acid; methotrexate; transplantation in advanced stages.

VII. GALLSTONES

■ Description

Twenty percent with asymptomatic gallstones develop biliary colic, cholecystitis, or pancreatitis.

No indication for prophylactic cholecystectomy or non-surgical treatment in asymptomatic patient.

Cholecystectomy standard or laparoscopic cholecystectomy best therapy.

For symptomatic gallstones, if no major contraindications to surgery, operative mortality overall 1%. Lower for elective in 50-year-old, and as high as 10% in emergency situation in elderly.

■ Symptoms

Epigastric pain, which can be colicky, and advances to prolonged constant pain lasting more than 30 minutes, and usually moderately severe. May radiate to the midscapular area or to the top of the right scapula, the right shoulder, or neck.

assoc. NIV

■ Diagnosis

Kidney–ureter–bladder (KUB) studies.

Ultrasound (US)

Hepatobiliary scan (Disida)

Oral cholecystogram (OCG)(?)

■ **Treatment**

Laparoscopic cholecystectomy in qualified hands and appropriate cases is treatment of choice; second, open cholecystectomy (less frequently used).

1. Medical dissolution of cholesterol gallstones, especially with ursodeoxycholic acid.

2. Extracorporeal shock-wave lithotripsy (ESWL).

3. Endoscopic retrograde cholangiopancreatography (ERCP), sphincterotomy (where safe and feasible), and stone removal to remove common bile duct stones; subsequent cholecystectomy in selected cases.

4. Transhepatic techniques with radiologic guidance may be used as well.

VIII. MESENTERIC ISCHEMIA

■ **Description**

Strangulation obstruction of the small bowel—most common form of mesenteric ischemia. Splanchnic vasospasm: non-occlusive mesenteric ischemia.

■ **Symptoms**

Non-specific. *Pain far worse than expected from physical findings*

■ **Diagnosis**

Angiography is the standard. Leukocytosis, acidosis, abdominal pain and tenderness.

■ **Treatment**

Prompt laparotomy: re-establish arterial flow; assess bowel viability; resect frankly ischemic segments. Embolectomy or revascularization with second-look laparotomy 24 to 48 hours later to reveal intestine left *in situ*: 50 to 90% mortality from acute intestinal arterial occlusion.

IX. ACUTE PANCREATITIS

■ **Description**

Autodigestion producing inflammation, necrosis of pancreatic tissue, and peripancreatic fat.

Mortality is about 5 to 10%, **major causes are alcohol and biliary stone disease.**

■ **Symptoms**

Epigastric pain radiating to midback, better sitting up. Jaundice and fever are possible.

■ **Diagnosis**

Elevated serum amylase, swollen pancreas on CT scan. Elevated amylase also seen in perforated ulcer, mesenteric infarction, intestinal obstruction, pancreas, pseudocyst, and chronic pancreatitis; also in mumps parotitis, renal failure (if creatinine greater than 3, serum amylase can be 3 times normal on that basis), ovarian and oat cell tumor of lung, ruptured ectopic pregnancy, and macroamylasemia.

Lipase is slower to rise and fall and may also become elevated due to renal failure. *but still better than amylase (more sensitive)*

■ **Pathology**

See Description.

■ **Treatment**

Supportive care with nothing by mouth (NPO) versus analgesia, nasogastric tube if nausea and vomiting or ileus with abdominal distention (watch for poor prognostic signs: hypotension, serum calcium less than 8, PCO_2 less than 60, decreased Hgb) if hyperalimentation used, use H_2 blocker and avoid IV lipids. With severe gallstone pancreatitis, a gallstone impacted at duodenal ampulla may benefit from early ERCP with sphincterotomy and stone extraction, or if unsuccessful, surgical intervention, especially in the non-alcoholic with pancreatitis.

X. COMPLICATIONS OF ACUTE PANCREATITIS—PSEUDOCYST VERSUS ABSCESS

■ Description and Symptoms

Worsening of pain, nausea, and vomiting after initial improvement, with fever, increased WBC, and positive blood culture.

■ Diagnosis

Computed tomography of pancreas with Chiba aspiration, culture, and Gram stain.

■ Pathology

Phlegmonous mass, pseudocyst, or abscess.

■ Treatment

Antibiotics for proven abscess and possibly for phlegmon.

Surgical drainage of abscess reduces mortality from greater than 50% to 10 to 20%, if aspiration used for early diagnosis. For pancreatic pseudocysts that are symptomatic, expanding, or greater than 5 cm in size and unchanged in size for at least 6 weeks, interval surgical drainage into stomach or small intestine.

XI. PANCREATIC CANCER

■ Description

Fifth leading cause of cancer deaths in United States. **Five-year survival of 1%.**

■ Symptoms

Vague midabdominal pain, anorexia, and weight loss. Jaundice can occur in the absence of pain. Nausea and vomiting.

depression, bronze diabetes

■ Diagnosis

Ultrasound or CT. Chiba biopsy of mass. If negative, ERCP, since 90 to 95% of pancreatic cancers arise from the pancreatic duct system. Rare to do laparotomy for tissue diagnosis.

CA 19-9 and CA-50 in non-jaundiced patient has some validity and can be used as tumor marker after apparently curative surgery.

■ Pathology

Adenocarcinoma arising from ductular epithelium account for **three fourths** of pancreatic CA; 60 to 80% arise in the head; 10 to 20%, body; 5 to 7%, tail. At surgery, 85% have disseminated disease.

■ Treatment

Ten to 20% are candidates for attempted curative resection with small tumor in head of pancreas and no evident spread. Modified Whipple (pancreaticoduodenectomy) 5 to 10% mortality in the best centers. Endoscopic and percutaneous stent for biliary obstruction. Palliative gastric bypass and pain control.

XII. MALABSORPTION

■ Description

Abnormal labs, anemia, low serum iron, folate, vitamin C, vitamin B_{12}, calcium, phosphorus, magnesium, zinc, and other trace metals, elevated alkaline phosphatase (bone disease or cholestasis), or folate (blind-loop syndrome), and a prolonged protime.

■ Diagnosis

Steatorrhea (excess fat in stool): 100 g fat/diet/per day/times 3, after which stool is collected for another 3 days; greater than 7 g after 24 hours is abnormal. D-xylose, if abnormal, suggests small bowel disease. Normal value suggests focus on pancreatic disease: CT scan of the abdomen, serum amylase, gamma GT. If overgrowth considered, note response of malabsorption to antibiotic therapy.

■ Treatment

Treat underlying condition.

XIII. ESOPHAGEAL CANCER

■ Description

With squamous cell carcinoma, usually advanced in United States.

■ Symptoms

Dysphagia for solids.

■ Diagnosis

Endoscopic biopsy or cytology occasionally after initial barium swallow. Pathology, squamous cell carcinoma. → *usually. Risk factors = smoking, EtOH*

Adenoca – rarer – assoc. c̄ Barret's esophagus

■ Treatment

Five-year survival rate of only 5%. Resection if in lower, radiation in upper. Chemotherapy with cisplatin-containing combinations (50 to 60% response).

BIBLIOGRAPHY

McCarthy DM. MKSAP ix, Part B, Book 5, *Gastroenterology*. American College of Physicians, 1991.

Yamada T. Gastroenterology. In Kelley WN, ed. *Textbook of Internal Medicine*, 2nd ed. Philadelphia, Pa: JB Lippincott; 1992:390–669.

CHAPTER 5

Hematology

RICHARD J. GOLDMAN, MD

have hypersegmented → neutrophils, too

I. ANEMIA

A. General

1. Definition

Reduction in red cell mass. In women Hb < 12 g, Hct < 36%; in men < 14 g and < 42%.

2. Basic Measurements

Mean corpuscular volume (MCV): normal 80 to 100 cubic microns; separates anemias into microcytic, normocytic, macrocytic, but combined deficiencies may be normocytic. Use RDW (red cell distribution width) to assess anisocytosis.

   a. *Microcytic (< 80)*. Iron deficiency; thalassemia, chronic disease (usually normocytic).

   b. *Macrocytic (> 100)*. Megaloblastic anemias, chemotherapy, reticulocytosis, aplastic anemias, hypothyroidism. *(B12, folate deficiency)*

   c. *Pancytopenia.* Primary marrow disease, megaloblastic anemia, or hypersplenism.

   d. *Reticulocytes.* Since RBC survival is 120 days, reticulocyte count is about 1%; reticulocyte corrects for anemia severity and assesses marrow response.

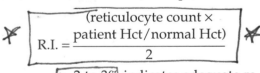

$$R.I. = \frac{\text{(reticulocyte count} \times \text{patient Hct/normal Hct)}}{2}$$

> 2 to 3% indicates adequate response; < 2 to 3% indicates hypoproliferative component

3. Red Cell Morphology

Rouleaux (myeloma); Burr cells (renal failure); tear drops and nucleated red cells (myelophthisic anemias); hypochromia and microcytosis (iron deficiency); targets (thalassemias, other hemoglobinopathies; obstructive jaundice); oval macrocytes (vitamin B_{12} or folate deficiency); basophilic stippling (lead poisoning); spherocytes (hereditary spherocytosis); schistocytes (microangiopathic hemolysis).

4. Value of Bone Marrow

   a. *Assess iron stores and presence of megaloblastic processes in combined deficiencies and chronic diseases and alcoholism.*

   b. *Look for primary blood dyscrasias (eg, leukemias) or invasion by metastatic tumor or infection. A core biopsy to evaluate cellularity or invasive processes.*

B. The Major Types of Anemia

1. Hypoproliferative

Marrow aplasias, anemia of chronic disease; drug causes include alkylating agents, chloramphenicol, phenytoin, benzene, gold.

2. Maturation Defects

Hypochromic anemias, megaloblastic; drug causes include alcohol, trimethoprim, triamterene, isoniazid (INH), lead.

3. Hyperproliferative

Hemorrhagic, hemolytic. *(hemoglobinopathics)*

4. Dilutional Anemias

Pregnancy.

C. Blood Loss (Acute and Chronic)

■ Description

Chronic is usually gastrointestinal (GI) or uterine.

■ Symptoms

Acute presents with signs of **hypoxia** and **hypovolemia**: weakness, hypotension, tachycardia. Significant hypovolemia (blood loss > 1000 cc) is manifest by postural signs. *Chronic* presents with fatigue, dyspnea, pallor.

■ Diagnosis

No significant drop in hematocrit initially. Increased white blood count (WBC), left shift; increased platelets and reticulocyte count (this leads to *increased* MCV acutely). Increased blood urea nitrogen (BUN) if GI bleeding. Hemoccult can detect 5 mL bleeding in 24 hours. Do three to six specimens.

■ Treatment

Correct hypovolemia. Whole blood as needed. **Look for source** of bleeding. Remember to check **coagulation tests.**

D. Iron Deficiency Anemia (IDA)

■ Description

The most common anemia; almost always due to **blood loss. In men** and **postmenopausal women** must be evaluated for **blood loss.** Common causes: GI bleeding; menstrual loss; pregnancy; diagnostic venipunctures; soft tissue bleeding after hip fracture/surgery.

■ Symptoms

Fatigue, palpitations, dizziness, dyspnea, headache. Angular stomatitis; glossitis. Thinning and flattening of nails, spoon-shaped nails (koilonychia) in advanced disease. Pica.

■ Diagnosis

Anisocytosis (increased RDW), decreased MCV, mean corpuscular hemoglobin (MCH), MCH concentration (MCHC). Central red cell pallor. Thrombocytosis. Low serum ferritin (< 12 γmg/dL). Decreased serum iron (< 60); increased total iron binding capacity (TIBC) (> 360).

Marrow not usually needed, but iron stores absent or severely reduced.

■ Treatment

Find the cause and treat. Iron daily for 6 to 12 months. Parenteral iron for special circumstances. Retics peak in 5 to 10 days; Hb rises over 1 to 2 months.

E. Nutritional Deficiencies: Pernicious, Other Megaloblastic Anemias

1. *General*

■ Description

A **macrocytic** nutritional anemia (with **pancytopenia)** due to impaired DNA synthesis. Etiology usually **cobalamin (vitamin B$_{12}$) or folate deficiency,** drugs.

■ Symptoms

Those of anemia; neurologic. *→ in B$_{12}$ deficiency*

■ Diagnosis

Macro-ovalocytic anemia, leukopenia, thrombocytopenia; increased bilirubin, iron, and iron saturation; decreased haptoglobin and uric acid. Increased MCV and RDW. **Hypersegmented** polys. **Increased** lactate dehydrogenase (LDH).

Marrow needed to rule out myelodysplastic syndrome, hematologic malignancy. **Nuclear-cytoplasmic asynchrony** (mature cytoplasm, immature nucleus). Marrow very cellular; increased mitotic figures; decreased M:E ratio (1:1); megaloblastic changes in erythrocytic and granulocytic series.

■ Pathology

Impaired DNA, but normal RNA synthesis leads to **ineffective erythropoiesis** and **hemolysis.**

2. Cobalamin (B₁₂) Deficiency

■ Description

Usually pernicious anemia, rarely dietary deficiency, gastrectomy, pancreatic disease, blind loop syndrome. Takes several years to develop.

↑in alcoholics

■ Symptoms

Symptoms of **anemia. Neurologic symptoms:** symmetric paresthesias in feet and fingers, disturbed vibratory sense and proprioception. Irritability, somnolence, "megaloblastic madness," abnormal taste, smell, vision, central scotomas.

■ Diagnosis

Decreased serum cobalamin. Responds within hours to cobalamin therapy. Folate usually increased. Increased serum and urine methylmalonic acid and homocysteine.

3. Pernicious Anemia

■ Description

A **gastric atrophy** condition, possibly autoimmune, leading to **decreased intrinsic factor** (IF) and cobalamin deficiency. Typically in older, fair-skinned, northern Europeans. Blocking and binding anti-IF antibodies.

■ Diagnosis

Achlorhydria after histamine stimulation. Decreased cobalamin absorption (**Schilling test** = decreased urinary excretion of [⁶⁵⁷Co]cyanocobalamin in 24 hours, corrected by oral hog IF).

■ Treatment

Cobalamin to replete the normal stores and to provide daily need for life. 500 to 1000 micrograms IM daily

for 2 weeks; two times per week for 4 more weeks; then **monthly for life.** Must also give iron if deficient. Folate given alone may worsen neurologic picture.

4. Folate Deficiency

■ Description

A usually dietary deficiency of folic acid. Folic acid is high in green vegetables, liver, kidney, yeast, mushrooms. Takes 4 months to become deficient. Causes include

Inadequate diet—as in alcoholism
Excessive cooking of foods
Malabsorption (sprue)
Phenytoin
Oral contraceptives
Pregnancy
Chronic hemolytic anemias
Metastatic cancer and leukemias

■ Diagnosis

Decreased serum folate; response to therapy; history of precipitating factors.

■ Treatment

Folic acid, 1 mg by mouth (PO) daily (4 to 5 weeks to replace stores).

F. Hemolytic Anemias: General

■ Description

Premature destruction of red cells due to **defective red cells,** or **noxious factors. Can be** intravascular or **extravascular** (more common)—cells sequestered by liver or spleen and destroyed.

■ Symptoms

Of anemia, jaundice, pallor, splenomegaly.

■ **Diagnosis**

Reticulocytosis, polychromatophilia, marrow hyperplasia; increased indirect bilirubin, LDH, free hemoglobin, urine hemosiderin and hemoglobin.

G. Hemolytic Anemias: Immune Hemolysis

1. General

Binding of antibodies and/or complement to RBC membrane. *Two types:* IgM—agglutinating ("complete") and work at colder temperatures; and IgG —non-agglutinating ("incomplete") and work at 37°C. The **direct Coombs'** (direct antiglobulin) test detects immunoproteins on the **membrane** and is (+) in nearly all immunohemolytic disorders. The **indirect Coombs'** (indirect antiglobulin) test detects **serum** antibodies.

2. Autoimmune Hemolytic Anemia (AIHA) Due to IgG Warm Antibodies

■ **Description**

The **AIHA is commonly secondary to underlying neoplastic or collagen vascular disease.**

■ **Symptoms**

Of hemolytic anemia and underlying disorder.

■ **Diagnosis**

Variable anemia, increased MCV, occasionally decreased WBCs and platelets. Spherocytosis, rouleaux formation, anisocytosis, reticulocytosis. (+) Direct Coombs'.

■ **Treatment**

Treat the underlying disorder. If mild, no treatment. If severe, **gluco-**

corticoids. If poor response consider **splenectomy, immunosuppressive drugs**, IV **gamma globulin, transfusion**. 75% obtain control with steroids and splenectomy.

3. Autoimmune Hemolytic Anemia Due to Cold-Reacting Antibodies

3–1. Cold-Agglutinin Disease

■ **Description**

IgM cold agglutinins are increased by **infection** (mycoplasma, Epstein–Barr, trypanasomiasis, malaria), but only rarely cause hemolysis. **Lymphomas** (especially large-cell lymphoma); idiopathic in some elderly.

■ **Symptoms**

Mild if from infection, worse if idiopathic or from lymphoma. Hemoglobinuria with severe chilling.

■ **Diagnosis**

Jaundice. Anticoagulated blood clumps. Warming to 37°C corrects. (+) **Cold agglutinin titer and direct Coombs'.**

■ **Treatment**

Treat underlying disorder. Avoid cold. Chlorambucil. Transfuse if necessary. Steroids/splenectomy no value.

3–2. Paroxysmal Cold Hemoglobinuria (Donath–Landsteiner Hemolytic Anemia)

Rare. Transient. Caused by **IgG** cold-reacting antibodies. In syphilis, infectious mononucleosis, measles, and mumps.

3–3. **Drugs Mechanisms**

a. Hapten type **drug binds to red cell (penicillin).**

b. Immune complex type complement-fixing antibodies against drug- protein complex on cell surface (sulfonamides, phenothiazines, quinine, quinidine).

c. **Alpha-methyldopa type** antibodies against altered cell membrane. (+) Direct Coombs (Alpha-methyldopa, levodopa, mefenamic acid). Treat by stopping drug.

3–4. **Paroxysmal Nocturnal Hemoglobinuria (PNH)**

■ **Description**

Rare acquired disorder with complement-mediated membrane damage. May develop **aplastic anemia** or **acute leukemia.**

■ **Symptoms**

Pallor, jaundice. **Veno-occlusive events.** Abdominal/back pain.

■ **Diagnosis**

Chronic hemolysis, **hemoglobinuria after periods of sleep,** mild pancytopenia. Increased LDH and decreased to absent haptoglobin. He-mosiderinuria. **Ham's test, sucrose hemolysis test** (more sensitive). Decreased to absent iron stores.

■ **Treatment**

Folic acid, iron, androgens, glucocorticoids, transfusions. Anticoagulation. Most die within 10 years, usually from thrombotic events, some with aplastic anemia or acute myeloblastic leukemia.

H. Hemolytic Anemias: Non-immune

1. **Glucose-6-Phosphate Dehydrogenase (G-6-PD) Deficiency**

■ **Description**

Enzyme deficiency leading to hemolysis. The G-6-PD deficiency decreases production of glutathione. Precipitating causes:

a. **Infection.**

b. **Drugs.** Including primaquine, atabrine; sulfonamides; nitrofurantoin (Furadantin), aspirin, acetophenetidin (phenacetin), sulfones (dapsone), naphthalene (mothballs), methylene blue, vitamin K, ascorbic acid.

c. **Fava beans.**

■ **Symptoms**

Acute intravascular hemolysis with jaundice 1 to 3 days after exposure. Abdominal and back pain. Symptoms of anemia. Occasional renal failure.

■ **Diagnosis**

Hemoglobinemia, hemoglobinuria, jaundice. Heinz bodies increased RBC methemoglobin. Can **assay enzyme levels; cyanide-ascorbate test.**

■ **Pathology**

Oxidation of hemoglobin produces **methemoglobin,** with characteristic Heinz bodies (denatured hemoglobin), which lead to red cell fragility and splenic "bites."

■ **Treatment**

Avoid offending agents.

2. **Hemoglobinopathies**

2–1. **General Structure**

Hemoglobin is **tetramer of globin polypeptide chains** (a pair of "α-like" and pair of "non-α" chains). Adult Hb is hemoglobin A ($\alpha_2 \beta_2$), and hemoglobin A_2 ($\alpha_2 \delta_2$). Fetal Hb is Hb F ($\alpha_2 G\gamma_2$) ($\alpha_2 A\gamma_2$).

■ Symptoms

Cyanosis, malaise, giddiness, altered mental state, loss of consciousness, coma, death.

■ Diagnosis

Cyanosis with normal PO_2. Blood chocolate brown. Symptoms occur if methemoglobin level > 30 to 50%.

■ Pathology

Usually inherited; may be acquired (toxin, neoplasms). Classification[1]

a. **Structural hemoglobinopathies**—mutated amino acid sequences, as in

   (1) **Abnormal polymerization** —(hemoglobin S) see the following.

   (2) **Reduced solubility**—(unstable hemoglobin).

   (3) **Altered oxygen affinity**— two types:

      (a) Increased oxygen affinity (eg, Hb Zurich).

      (b) Decreased oxygen affinity (eg, Hb Kansee).

   (4) **M hemoglobins—(methemoglobinemia).**

b. **Thalassemias**—see the following.

c. **Hereditary persistence of hemoglobin F.**

d. **Acquired hemoglobinopathies**—methemoglobinemia.

[1] Benz EJ Jr. Classification and basic pathophysiology of the hemoglobinopathies. In: Wyngaarden JB, Smith LH, Bennett JC, ed. *Cecil Textbook of Medicine.* 19th ed. Philadelphia, Penn: WB Saunders Co, 1992: Classification of Hemoglobinopathies: Table 136–2, p 878.

■ Description

Oxidation of hemoglobin from ferrous (Fe^{++}) to ferric (Fe^{+++}) state, which doesn't transport oxygen. May be due to:

a. **Globin mutation** leading to methemoglobin formation (M hemoglobin).

b. **Methemoglobin reductase deficiency** (very rare).

c. **"Toxic" oxidation to methemoglobinemia** by foreign substances (acetanilid, phenacetin, nitrites, aniline, and many others).

■ Treatment

M hemoglobin: no treatment. Reductase deficiencies: oral methylene blue (IV in emergency situations), ascorbic acid, or riboflavin.

2–2. Specific: Thalassemia Major (Cooley's Anemia)

Hypochromic, microcytic hemolytic anemia due to defective globin synthesis, leading to **unbalanced production** of α or β chains. Thalassemia trait protects from malaria. β-Thal more common in Mediterraneans, Africans, Asians. α-Thal more common in Asians.

■ Description

Defective β-globin synthesis. The α-globin precipitates and forms inclusions in red cells. Transfusions dependent.

■ Symptoms

Normal at birth, but by 6 to 9 months have severe anemia, poor growth, failure to thrive, hepatosplenomegaly, gross deformities, compression fractures.

■ Diagnosis

Hemoglobin 3 to 6 g. Severe microcytosis, hypochromia, cell fragmentation. Thalassemia trait in both parents. In patient, absent or low Hb A, large amount of Hb F, increased A_2 to 4 to 10%. Fetal DNA analysis from **chorionic villus biopsy** (early pregnancy), or amniotic fluid (later in pregnancy) allows option of therapeutic abortion.

■ Pathology

Ineffective erythropoiesis leads to severe anemia, hypercellular marrow, osteoporosis, compression fractures.

■ Treatment

Transfusion.
Splenectomy—(delay until 5 to 6 years old).
Iron chelation.
Vitamin C (to enhance iron excretion).

Hypertransfusion leads to **hemochromatosis.** Should receive Pneumovax and get penicillin prophylaxis.

2–3. Specific: Thalassemia Intermedia

■ Description

Milder disease with Hb >6 to 7 g, delayed organ damage from hemochromatosis, longer survival.

■ Treatment

Transfusion therapy recommended, but are **not transfusion dependent.** Splenectomy for hypersplenism.

2–4. Specific: Thalassemia Trait Description

Heterozygous α- or β-globin defect.

■ Symptoms

None.

■ Diagnosis

Mild hypochromic, microcytic anemia; rare splenomegaly. Increased A_2 hemoglobin (4 to 8%). **Must distinguish from iron deficiency.**

■ Treatment

None.

3. Sickle Cell Anemia

■ Description

Hemolytic anemia with red cells assuming characteristic **sickle cell (SC) shapes (drepanocytes)** due to abnormal β globin subunit of adult hemoglobin $β^s$ chain of Hb S ($α_2β^s_2$). Associated with other abnormal hemoglobins. People of African descent, but also in those around the Mediterranean, Saudi Arabians, Indians. May be malaria-protective. In United States, trait in 8 to 10% of blacks.

■ Pathology

Aggregation or polymerization of hemoglobin S molecules, leading to **gel state** when in the deoxy conformation (reversible, to a point), chronic hemolysis, tissue damage and **acute painful vaso-occlusive crises.**

■ Symptoms

Sickle cell trait. Asymptomatic. Not anemic. If anemia present, search for *other* causes.

Sickle cell anemia. **Chronic compensated hemolytic anemia.** Hb 6.5 to 10 g. Retics 10 to 25%. Mild jaundice. Increased indirect bilirubin. **Vaso-occlusive crisis** (pain in back, chest, extremities) precipitated by infection, dehydration, acidosis, hypoxia. If in vasculature, see cerebrovascular accident (CVA), seizures, pulmonary infarction, priapism. Occasional **hypoplastic or aplastic crisis,** especially with infection (parvovirus B$_{19}$). **Acute splenic sequestration crisis** (younger patients, or older with SC or SThal). **Megaloblastic crisis** due to folate deficiency. Aseptic necrosis of hip.

Sickle/β-thal and SC disease anemia less severe, less sickling. Fewer vaso-occlusive events.

Splenomegaly. More eye complications, aseptic necrosis of femoral head in SC.

■ **Diagnosis**

Screening: **sickle cell prep** (sodium metabisulfate) or **solubility test. Hemoglobin electrophoresis** for precise diagnosis (may need special electrophoresis).

■ **Treatment**

No specific therapy available. Supportive measures: large amount (2 to 3 times normal) of hypotonic and alkaline IV fluids. Analgesics. Antibiotics when appropriate. Oxygen. Exchange transfusion prior to general anesthesia for surgery to get Hb S < 50%. Do not transfuse for stable anemia (OK to leave at 6.5 to 7 g). Immunize with pneumococcal and *Haemophilus influenzae* vaccines.

Prevention. Genetic counseling. Prenatal diagnosis with fetal DNA analysis.

4. Spherocytosis (Example of Membrane Disorder): General

■ **Description**

Red cell membrane is composed of a bilayer of lipids, protein channels, and receptors that are responsible for membrane function.

5. Hereditary Spherocytosis

■ **Description**

Inherited hemolytic anemia with **increased osmotic fragility. Autosomal dominant** in 75%. Membrane instability.

■ **Symptoms**

Anemia, jaundice, splenomegaly. Hemolysis at all ages; worsened with some infections (mono) and intense physical activity. **Crises: hemolytic (mild). Aplastic (severe)**—frequently caused by human parvovirus. **Megaloblastic** (with pregnancy)—maintenance folic acid. Gallstones (bilirubin), gout, ankle ulcers.

■ **Diagnosis**

Reticulocytosis. Microspherocytosis. Incubated osmotic fragility test.

■ **Treatment**

Splenectomy for anemia or significant hemolysis; defer until age 6 to 7 because of sepsis potential. Pneumococcal vaccine.

6. Hereditary Elliptocytosis

■ **Description**

A spherocytosis variant with autosomal dominant inheritance and membrane skeleton defect. Several types exist.

7. Other Non-immune Hemolytic Disorders

1. **Hypersplenism**—excessive trapping and destroying of even normal (non-senescent) RBCs by an **enlarged spleen of any cause.** Poor correlation with spleen size.

■ **Treatment**

Splenectomy if transfusion dependent.

2. **Chemicals**—inorganic cations (arsenic, copper), organic substances (eg, chloroamine from water purification with alum and chlorine), amphotericin B. Toxins from *Clostridium welchii*, spiders, snake venom.

3. **Metabolic abnormalities**—spur cell hemolytic anemia: in severe liver disease with poor prognosis.

4. **Red cell parasites**
   a. **Malaria**—especially *Plasmodium falciparum*. A major cause of hemolysis worldwide. Splenomegaly.
   b. **Babesiosis.** Protozoans in red cells. Thrombocytopenia, disseminated intravascular coagulation (DIC). Deer tick vector. More common in northeastern United States.
   c. **Bartonellosis.** *Bartonella bacilliformis*. South America. Sand fly vector. Fever, chills, headache, musculoskeletal pain. Hemolysis. Responds to antibiotics.

5. **Trauma to red cells**
6. **March hemoglobinuria**—seen with marching, running, other repetitive contact (karate). See hemoglobinemia and hemoglobinuria.
7. **Fragmentational hemolysis**—due to cardiac or large vessel abnormality ("Waring Blender" syndrome).

■ **Description** *Hemolytic Anemia due to Intravascular hemolysis*

Usually **left side of heart** etiology; *mild* hemolysis from severe AS or AI, ruptured sinus of Valsalva, traumatic AV fistula, aortofemoral bypass surgery. More *severe* hemolysis from **prosthetic valves** (especially with aortic, artificial, metallic, defective, or poorly functioning valves).

■ **Diagnosis**

Increasing anemia. Slight reticulocytosis, schistocytes. Chronic urinary iron loss (hemosiderin) may lead to iron deficiency.

■ **Treatment**

Limit physical activity. Give iron. If transfusion requirement, **replace valve.**

8. **Microangiopathic hemolytic disorders.**

■ **Description**

Red cells are injured flowing through partially blocked channels. *Three main types:*

Disseminated intravascular coagulation (DIC)—thrombocytopenia, prolonged prothrombin time (PT), partial thromboplastin time (PTT), thrombin time. Increased fibrin degradation products (FDP). May be caused by gram-negative endotoxin-containing bacteria, amniotic fluid embolus, metastatic cancer.

Vascular lesions—cavernous hemangioma (Kasabach–Merritt syndrome), renal transplant undergoing rejection, malignant hypertension, eclampsia.

Thrombotic thrombocytopenic purpura (TTP) and **hemolytic-uremic syndrome** are characterized by hemolysis, thrombocytopenia, renal failure. See fever, jaundice, petechiae.

■ **Diagnosis**

Schistocytes, **helmet cells,** hemolysis, reticulocytosis, increased indirect bilirubin and LDH, decreased haptoglobin, hemosiderinuria.

■ **Treatment**

Treat the cause. Anticoagulation with heparin may help. Transfusion, platelet packs, cryoprecipitate. Plasmapheresis for TTP. High-dose gamma globulin.

I. Anemia Associated with Chronic Disease (ACD)

■ **Description**

A usually **normocytic, normochromic** anemia, but often hypochromic and occasionally microcytic, seen with **chronic infection, inflammatory disease,** or **cancer.**

■ **Symptoms**

Of anemia and the underlying disease.

■ **Diagnosis**

Decreased iron, transferrin, and transferrin saturation (but usually > 10%). Normal ferritin. Normal or increased marrow iron stores.

■ **Pathology**

Impaired iron utilization, shortened RBC lifespan, mild hemolysis. Leukocyte endogenous mediator (LEM) a possible humoral factor in ACD.

■ **Treatment**

Correct underlying problem. No benefit from iron therapy.

J. Anemia Associated with Chronic Renal Insufficiency

■ **Description**

Due to decreased erythropoietin production, but worsened by poor nutrition, blood loss, hemolysis.

■ **Diagnosis**

Hemoglobin 5 to 8 g. MCV normal. Burr cells.

■ **Treatment**

Recombinant human **erythropoietin.**

K. Aplastic Anemias; Pancytopenias

■ **Description**

Marrow failure, which may be due to

Aplastic process—(failure of stem cell to undergo differentiation

Myelophthisic process—(destruction of the marrow environment by invaders or inflammatory tissue). May see isolated deficiency (eg, pure red cell aplasia (PRCA), agranulocytosis, thrombocytopenia.

■ **Symptoms**

Bleeding (petechial, retinal), fatigue, pallor, bacterial infections.

■ **Diagnosis**

Cytopenia. Marrow replaced by fat. Ham test or sucrose hemolysis test (paroxysmal nocturnal hemoglobinuria); serum immunoglobulins (hypoglobulinemia); CT chest (thymoma). Must distinguish leukemia, myelofibrosis, other blood dyscrasia.

■ **Pathology**

Peripheral pancytopenia and marrow replaced with fat. Pathogenesis:

1. **Idiopathic** (50%).
2. **Dose-dependent, drug-related** (cytotoxic drugs, phenytoin, phenothiazines, chloramphenicol, thiouracil).
3. **Idiosyncratic, drug-related** (chloramphenicol).

4. **Environmental toxins** (solvents such as benzene; insecticides).

5. **Infections** (hepatitis, parvovirus).

6. **Preleukemia.**

■ **Treatment**

Options: Observation. Androgens. Bone marrow transplant. Antilymphocyte globulin. High-dose steroids. Immunosuppressive therapy. Red cell and platelet transfusions.

L. Anemia Associated with Intestinal Parasites, Especially in Children

1. Hookworm

■ **Description**

Hookworm disease is infection by *Necator americanus* ("New World hookworm"), *Ancylostoma duodenale* ("Old World hookworm"), or *A. ceylanicum* (Far East). Adults live in upper part of small intestine. Each adult extracts 0.2 mL blood daily.

■ **Symptoms**

Erythematous maculopapular rash, edema, severe pruritus (especially around toes). Cough, pneumonia, fever if severe pulmonary involvement.

■ **Diagnosis**

Iron-deficiency anemia, hypoalbuminemia. In young children may see severe anemia, cardiac insufficiency, and anasarca, retarded physical, mental, and sexual development. Hookworm eggs in fecal smear. Eosinophilia (as high as 70 to 80%).

■ **Treatment**

Antihelmintic agents: pyrantel pamoate; mebendazole. Iron replacement. Transfusion. Maintain good nutrition.

II. BLEEDING DISORDERS, COAGULOPATHIES, THROMBOCYTOPENIA

A. Mechanisms of Hemostasis

Normal hemostasis has three phases: vasoconstriction, platelet adhesion and aggregation, fibrin formation and stabilization; followed by clot destruction (fibrinolysis). Trauma → reflex constriction → platelet adhesion → release of tissue factor (TF) → activation of clotting cascade (TF-factor VIIa activates factor X ["extrinsic pathway"] and IX ["intrinsic pathway"]. Various platelet factors are released to further aggregation (adenosine diphosphate [ADP], prostaglandin G_2, thromboxane A_2).

Pathologic hemostasis is activated in response to abnormality in:

Vessel wall—(eg, atherosclerosis)

Platelets—(eg, myeloproliferative disorder)

Coagulation system—(eg, antithrombin III deficiency)

Diagnosis of bleeding disorders

History and **physical examination. Testing**—refer to specific disorders and see Algorithm to Evaluate Bleeding Disorders.[2]

B. Platelet Disorders

1. General

■ **Description**

Normal count 150,000 to 300,000 per mL. Normally 3 to 10 platelets seen per high power field (oil immersion). Megakaryocyte growth is stimulated by interleukin 6 (IL-6) and granulocyte and macrophage colony-stimulating factor (GM-CSF). Platelet circulation is 9 to 10 days. Spleen is usual site of destruction.

[2] Shuman M. Hemorrhagic disorders: abnormalities of platelet and vascular function. In: Wyngaarden JB, Smith LH, Bennett JC. *Cecil Textbook of Medicine.* 19th ed. Philadelphia, Pa.: WB Saunders Co; 1992. Algorithm for laboratory evaluation of bleeding disorders: Figure 154–4, p 991.

■ **Diagnosis**

Platelet function tests: **bleeding time reflects platelet and vascular components of coagulation;** is normal in coagulation factor deficiencies (except von Willebrand's disease). **Platelet aggregometry for congenital qualitative platelet disorders.**

2. *Qualitative and Quantitative*

Platelet deficiencies. General. Platelet count < 10,000, high risk for severe bleeding; < 20,000, may have sponta­neous bleeding; (?) > 100,000, no bleeding, even with major surgery. Decreased production. Aplastic anemia; marrow damage by drugs, chemicals, alcohol, and radiation, marrow replacement by leukemia, metastatic tumor, myelofibrosis; ineffective thrombopoiesis. Increased destruction.

Immune disorders; three mechanisms:

Autoantibodies against platelet membrane antigen

Immune complex binding to platelet Fc receptors

Lysis of platelets via complement fixation

a. Increased destruction: immune

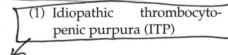

(1) Idiopathic thrombocytopenic purpura (ITP)

■ **Description**

Autoimmune bleeding disorder with antibodies to one's platelets. In children is **acute; seen after viral illness; 70% recover in 4 to 6 weeks.** In adult is more chronic; onset more gradual.

■ **Symptoms**

Petechiae, ecchymoses, epistaxis, menorrhagia.

■ **Diagnosis**

By exclusion of other disorders. Platelet antibody tests rarely helpful. Bone marrow exam is normal or shows increased megakaryocytes.

■ **Treatment**

Options: **observation, prednisone, intravenous gamma globulin, splenectomy, danazol, alkylating agents.**

(2) **Platelet antibodies in systemic disorders**

Cancer—lymphoproliferative disorders (chronic lymphocytic leukemia [CLL], lymphoma).

Systemic autoimmune disorders—systemic lupus erythematosus (SLE).

Viral illnesses—infectious mononucleosis, HIV, cytomegalovirus (CMV). HIV-thrombocytopenia may be multifactorial (treat with zidovudine [AZT], IV gamma globulin).

Drug-induced antibodies —many drugs involved, but common ones are quinine, quinidine, sulfa drugs, hydrochlorothiazide (HCTZ), phenytoin, methyldopa, heparin (3 to 5% of heparin users), digitalis derivatives.

b. **Increased destruction—non-immune disorders**

(1) **DIC.** See following sections

(2) **Thrombotic thrombocytopenic purpura (TTP)**

■ **Description**

Intravascular thrombotic disorder with thrombocytopenia.

■ Symptoms

Classically **wax and wane.** Severe **thrombocytopenia, microangiopathic hemolytic anemia, neurologic signs, fever,** mild **renal disease.**

■ Diagnosis

Acute thrombocytopenia, anemia, microangiopathic changes in red cells, minimal coagulation test abnormalities.

■ Pathology

Small vessels occluded by hyaline material (platelet thrombi).

■ Treatment

Large-volume **plasmapheresis** yields 70% cure rate. **Fresh frozen plasma. Glucocorticoids.** Red cell and platelet **transfusions.** Refractory disease: chemotherapy, splenectomy, cryosupernatant.

> **(3) Hemolytic-uremic syndrome (HUS)**

■ Description

Thrombocytopenic and hemolytic syndrome with **renal failure,** usually in infants and young children. Outcome: spontaneous recovery or severe chronic renal failure.

■ Diagnosis

Microangiopathic hemolytic anemia; mild to moderate thrombocytopenia; **prominent renal failure, severe hypertension,** no neurologic signs.

■ Pathology

Thrombosis and necrosis of intrarenal vessels.

■ Treatment

Correct hypovolemia, establish **diuresis, fresh frozen plasma, transfuse** as needed, **dialysis.**

#3 **c. Abnormalities of platelet function**

Acquired

1. **Drugs**
   - (a) Non-steroidal anti-inflammatory drugs (NSAIDs) (block platelet synthesis of prostaglandins).
   - (b) Penicillin.
2. **Renal failure**—usually mucocutaneous bleeding.
3. **Hepatic failure.**
4. **Paraproteinemias**—myeloma, macroglobulinemia. Treat with chemotherapy, plasmapheresis.

Hereditary

Von Willebrand's disease: see Disorders of Coagulation.

3. Thrombocytosis

Two types:

Essential. A myeloproliferative disorder (1 to 2 million platelets). Complications include thrombosis and/or bleeding. Also seen in agnogenic myeloid metaplasia, polycythemia vera, chronic myelocytic leukemia.

Reactive. In iron deficiency, hemorrhage, postsplenectomy, inflammatory bowel disease, leukemoid reactions. No specific treatment.

4. Platelet Transfusions

For surgery, bring platelets to > 50,000 (> 90,000 if in delicate area). Prefer single donor for each transfusion. On average, 1 unit raises count 10,000.

C. Vascular Disorders

1. Congenital

1–1. Hereditary Hemorrhagic Telangiectasia (Rendu–Osler–Weber Disease)

■ Description

The most common genetic cause of vascular bleeding; autosomal dominant.

■ Symptoms

Epistaxis; telangiectases on face, mucous membranes, GI tract; serious GI bleeding, cerebrovascular accident.

■ Treatment

Can treat some lesions surgically.

1–2. Congenital: Cavernous Hemangioma (Kasabach–Merritt Syndrome)

■ Diagnosis

Hemangioma with thrombocytopenia, mild DIC.

■ Treatment

Surgery, radiation, induced thrombosis; may involute spontaneously.

2. Acquired

2–1. Scurvy

Vitamin C deficiency. Lower extremity, perifollicular bleeding.

2–2. Purpura with Immunoglobulin Disorders

Cryoglobulinemia; benign hyperglobulinemia (Waldenström's purpura (may evolve into Sjögren's syndrome or SLE); amyloidosis (periorbital hemorrhages); Waldenström's macroglobulinemia and multiple myeloma; Henoch–Schönlein purpura (a childhood vasculitis with purpura, arthralgias, abdominal pain).

D. Disorders of Coagulation

1. General

Normal hemostasis requires interaction between blood vessels, platelets and monocytes, and blood coagulation proteins. This activates the **coagulation cascade,** as shown in the following figure.[3]

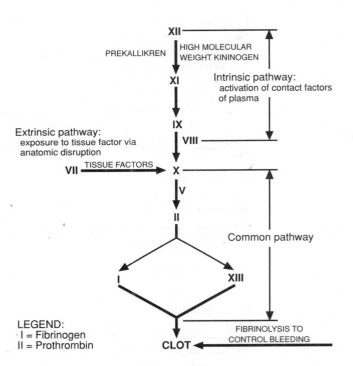

LEGEND:
I = Fibrinogen
II = Prothrombin

[3] Adapted from Mosher D. Disorders of blood coagulation. In: Wyngaarden JB, Smith LH, Bennett JC, eds. *Cecil Textbook of Medicine.* 19th ed. Philadelphia, Pa.: WB Saunders Co; 1992: Diagrams of interactions among coagulation factors: Figure 155–1, p 1001.

2. Evaluation of Coagulation Disorders

History—family history; response to trauma; menstrual history; response to meds (especially aspirin); joint problems.

Lab—complete blood count and morphology; **platelet count; bleeding time; prothrombin time** (PT) measures only **extrinsic** and common pathway; accelerated partial thromboplastin time (APTT) measures the **intrinsic and common pathway.** When doing PT and APTT, mixing of normal and abnormal plasma is used to distinguish **deficiencies** of clotting factors from presence of **inhibitors.** Fibrin clot solubility. Measuring specific coagulation factors.

3. Inherited Disorders of Blood Coagulation

Factor XI deficiency in Ashkenazi Jews. Treat with FFP.

Deficiencies of the extrinsic and common pathway (VII, X, V, II).

3–1. Hemophilia A (Factor VIII Deficiency)

■ Description

X-linked recessive inheritance. Of affected male: daughters will be carriers; sons will be normal. Of homozygous carrier female: 50% chance of producing a hemophiliac male or carrier daughter.

■ Symptoms

Level of factor VIII correlates with bleeding frequency. **Hematomas** in muscle or soft tissue (retroperitoneum). **Hemarthroses** (elbow, knee, ankle) may lead to crippling. Bleeding after surgery (must prep with factor VIII).

■ Diagnosis

Factor VIII level < 5% and usually < 1% of normal. History of joint and soft tissue bleeding. Must distinguish from factor IX deficiency (hemophilia B), von Willebrand's disease. Have normal PT, abnormal APTT (activated partial thromboplastin time). Can do factor VIII assay.

■ Treatment

Physical activity counseling. **Factor VIII (cryoprecipitate or lyophilized concentrate).** Analgesics. AIDS risk: whether or not positive HIV, still take care in exposure to patient's blood. Advise use of condoms for intercourse. Risk in maternal to newborn transmission of HIV.

3–2. Von Willebrand's Disease

■ Description

The **most common hereditary bleeding disorder**, due to deficient or abnormal von Willebrand's factor (vWf) and factor VIII-AHF. Autosomal dominant.

■ Symptoms

Variable. Usually superficial bleeding, epistaxis, easy bruising. Postop bleeding a major hazard; postdental extraction common. Menorrhagia.

■ Diagnosis

Low factor VIII-AHF (rarely < 5%, so bleeding generally mild); low level of immunoreactive vWf; long bleeding time. Abnormal platelet aggregation in response to ristocetin.

■ Treatment

Replacement with cryoprecipitate (but **not** with concentrate) similar to hemophilia A, to keep factor VIII in therapeutic range. Desmopressin (1-deamino-8-D-arginine vasopressin; DDAVP) is effective in stimulating vWf release.

3–3. Hemophilia B (Factor IX Deficiency; Christmas Disease)

■ Description

Similar to factor VIII deficiency with inheritance, with fewer symptoms, but with potential for severe bleeding.

■ Symptoms

As in factor VIII.

■ Diagnosis

Normal PT, prolonged APTT. Patient's plasma cannot correct prolonged APTT of known factor IX-deficient plasma.

■ Treatment

Options: **fresh-frozen plasma (FFP). Factor IX concentrate.**

3–4. Factor VII

Rare, mild.

■ Diagnosis

Inability to correct **abnormal PT** with factor VII-deficient plasma.

■ Treatment

Plasma (can also use factor IX concentrate to avoid volume overload).

3–5. Factor X

Rare. Both PT and APTT are prolonged. Mild to moderate bleeding.

■ Treatment

Plasma.

3–6. Factor V

Autosomal recessive. Variable course.

■ Treatment

Plasma (fresh or FFP).

3–7. Factor II (prothrombin)

Rare, recessive disorder.

■ Treatment

FFP.

3–8. Vitamin K-dependent Factors

Inherited; no liver disease, malabsorption or coumarin drugs present.

■ Treatment

Vitamin K.

4. Acquired Abnormalities of Blood Coagulation

a. Heparin. **Heparin** is a universally used anticoagulant for thromboembolic conditions. Regulate heparin anticoagulation with APTT, aiming for 1.5 to 2 (2-2.5) times control. Minimize bleeding complications by giving drug by continuous infusion, regular checking of APTT, avoidance of use in patients with bleeding diathesis or occult bleeding site, avoidance of aspirin or IM injection.

■ Treatment

Counteract with Protamine. Discontinue heparin.

b. Therapeutic fibrinolysis (thrombolysis). Streptokinase, urokinase, alteplase (tissue plasminogen activator, rt-PA) are used in treating deep-vein thrombosis, pulmonary embolus, acute myocardial infarction, peripheral arterial thromboembolism. May cause hemorrhage. Minimize bleeding complications by selecting appropriate patients, avoidance if bleeding disorder, recent GI or genitourinary (GU) bleed, severe hypertension, history of CVA, recent head trauma, major surgery or invasive procedure in last 2 weeks, or pregnant.

■ Treatment

Pressure. Discontinue drug. FFP.

c. Vitamin K deficiency and coumarin anticoagulants. Normally adequate vitamin K in diet (green leafy vegetables). May be deficient in malabsorption states, bile-salt deficient states, poor dietary intake, and with use of antibiotics.

■ Diagnosis

Increased PT.

> *Vitamin K deficiency of newborn*—routinely give vitamin K (1 mg IM at delivery) to avoid hemorrhagic disease of the newborn.
>
> *Malabsorption syndromes*—vitamin K deficiency seen with impaired fat absorption (adult celiac disease, regional enteritis, cholestyramine or neomycin use, biliary tract obstruction).

■ Treatment

Daily PO vitamin K_1.

> *Antibiotics in debilitated patients* —prevent with vitamin K_1.
>
> *Coumarin anticoagulants*—therapeutic level of PT usually 1.5 control (ie, 17 to 19 seconds). More bleeding seen at 2 control. Requirement can change with diet (vitamin K intake) and drugs that affect warfarin. Avoid aspirin.

■ Treatment

With FFP, vitamin K. Avoid coumarin in pregnancy between 6th and 12th week and after the 38th week.

> *Liver disease*—since the liver makes fibrinogen, plasminogen, vitamin K-dependent proteins, and anti-thrombin, bleeding is common with liver disease.

■ Diagnosis

Hypofibrinogenemia; acquired dysfibrinogenemia; increased fibrinolysis; DIC.

■ Treatment

Normalize the PT, fibrinogen concentration, platelet count prior to high-risk procedures (give vitamin K, platelets, FFP). No treatment of DIC unless clinically *SIGNIFICANT BLEEDING*.

d. **Renal disease.** Prolonged bleeding time. Platelet function abnormal; platelet count occasionally low.

■ Treatment

Correcting the anemia, cryoprecipitate.

e. Factor VIII inhibitors.

Commonly seen in factor VIII deficiency (hemophilia A).

■ **Treatment**

Factor VIII concentrate or cryoprecipitate.

  f. **Lupus-type inhibitors**
  g. **Disseminated intravascular coagulation (DIC), hypofibrinogenemia**

Clinical types:

Compensated DIC—ongoing **thrombosis** and **fibrinolysis** is traumatized or inflamed tissues in chronic serious diseases. Normal PT, platelets, **increased fibrinogen.** No bleeding seen.

■ **Treatment**

May require long-term heparin (Trousseau syndrome of "migratory" arterial and/or venous thrombosis; underlying neoplasm).

Defibrination syndrome—massive release of tissue factor causing depletion of fibrinogen, other factors, leading to thrombosis and/or bleeding, low platelets and fibrinogen, increased FDP, increased PT. Seen with shock, sepsis (Waterhouse–Friderichsen syndrome in meningococcemia), cancer, burns, obstetric complications.

■ **Treatment**

Platelets, cryoprecipitate, FFP, possibly heparin if poor response to other measures; vitamin K.

Primary fibrinolysis—primary release of plasminogen activator. Seen in CA of prostate, acute promyelocytic leukemia, hemangiomas, snake venoms.

■ **Symptoms**
Diffuse bleeding.

■ **Diagnosis**

Decreased fibrinogen, increased FDP, increased PT.

■ **Treatment**

Cryoprecipitate, epsilon-aminocaproic acid (EACA).

Microangiopathic thrombocytopenia.

■ **Description**

Syndrome seen in sepsis, malignancy, immune complex disease, vasculitis, malignant hypertension, eclampsia.

■ **Diagnosis**

Low platelet count, fragmented RBCs, increased FDP, but PT and fibrinogen OK.

■ **Treatment**

With FFP, **plasma exchange.**

Snake bite—venom contains toxic proteins and enzymes that cause tissue injuries.

■ **Treatment**

Antivenom, platelets, plasma.

Hemolytic uremic syndrome—see Microangiopathic Hemolytic Disorders.

III. LEUKOPENIC DISORDERS, AGRANULOCYTOSIS

A. Neutropenia

■ **Description**

Normal WBC 5 to 10 10^9/L. Neutropenia = neutrophils $< 2.0 \ 10^9$ (in blacks < 1.5

10^9), but usually no clinical problems until $< 1.0 \times 10^9$, and especially if $< 0.5 \times 10^9$. Causes:

1. **Marrow failure**—(many are drug-induced)
2. **Marrow invasion**—by cancer, hematologic malignancy
3. **Maturation arrest**—in folate or B_{12} deficiency

■ Symptoms

Range from asymptomatic to signs of severe infection. Signs may be absent because WBCs mediate the inflammatory response.

■ Diagnosis

Must distinguish primary versus secondary neutropenia. Vacuolization suggests infection. Bandemia > 20% suggests good marrow. Need bone marrow exam (aspiration and biopsy).

■ Treatment

Determine the cause. Treatment options: antibiotics, glucocorticoids or azathioprine, recombinant human granulopoietic factors (GM-CSF: colony-stimulating factor, granulocyte and macrophage; and G-CSF: colony-stimulating factor, granulocyte), bone marrow transplant, neutrophil transfusions.

B. Lymphocytopenia

■ Description

Causes:

1. **Decreased production**—as in protein-calorie malnutrition, radiation, immunosuppressive agents, congenital lymphocytopenic immunodeficiency states, viruses (measles, polio, varicella-zoster, HIV [AIDS]).
2. **Shunting**—of lymphocytes from peripheral blood in some bacterial or viral infections, or with trauma.
3. **Increased lymphocyte destruction**—from antilymphocyte antibodies, or in thoracic duct fistula, protein-losing enteropathy, severe congestive heart failure (CHF).

■ Symptoms

Of the underlying condition.

■ Treatment

Treat underlying cause. Investigational treatments include marrow transplant, fetal liver, thymic epithelial cells.

IV. NEOPLASTIC DISORDERS

A. Plasma Cell Disorders

1. General

■ Description

Neoplastic or potentially neoplastic disorders with proliferation of **single clone of plasma cells of B-cell series** producing **monoclonal gammopathies, paraproteinemias, dysproteinemias, or immunoglobulinopathies** due to secretion of **monoclonal proteins**. Each monoclonal protein is composed of two heavy and two light chains. Heavy chains include G, A, M, D, E. The light chains include kappa (κ) and lambda (λ).

■ Diagnosis

Serum protein electrophoresis (SPEP) is good for screening, but **immunoelectrophoresis is needed for confirmation**. Do SPEP if multiple myeloma, macroglobulinemia, amyloidosis is suspected, and for unexplained weakness or fatigue, anemia, back pain, osteoporosis, osteolytic lesions or spontaneous fracture. **Must distinguish monoclonal (usually neoplastic) from polyclonal (usually reactive or inflammatory) gammopathy.** Do **serum viscometry** for high globulins or if patient has blurred vision, oronasal bleeding, or other symptoms suggesting hyperviscosity. Urine: need sulfosalicylic acid to screen for light chains in urine. Do urine immunoelectrophoresis or immunofixation rather than Bence Jones. **Be aware that one can have negative urine protein test and electrophoresis, but have positive immunoelectrophoresis or immunofixation.**

2. Monoclonal Gammopathy of Undetermined Significance (MGUS; Benign Monoclonal Gammopathy)

■ Description

M-protein in serum **without evidence of neoplasm.** Significance: 20% go on to develop myeloma, macroglobulinemia, or amyloidosis.

■ Diagnosis

M-protein < 3 gm; < 5% plasma cells in marrow; insignificant M-proteinuria; **no lytic lesions or anemia, no hypercalcemia or renal insufficiency;** stable M-protein and no other abnormalities. Must distinguish from myeloma. **Follow-up of evolution** may be the only way to distinguish.

■ Treatment
Follow.

3. Multiple Myeloma

■ Description

A neoplastic proliferation of **single clone of plasma cells producing a** **monoclonal immunoglobulin.** Etiology unknown.

■ Symptoms

Bone pain in back, chest; vertebral collapse. Weakness, fatigue; symptoms and signs of anemia, renal failure, hypercalcemia, amyloidosis.

■ Diagnosis

Normochromic, normocytic anemia. Elevated sed rate. **Monoclonal serum band in 80%;** hypogammaglobulinemia in 10%. No serum M-protein in 10%. **Urine: 80% have monoclonal protein** by immunoelectrophoresis or immunofixation. Overall, 99% have M-protein in serum or urine at time of diagnosis. Marrow: > 10% of all nucleated cells are plasma cells (range from 5 to 100%). May be focal. Plain x-rays show **lytic lesions,** osteoporosis, fractures. Either CT or MRI can be used as backup. Do not use bone scan.

■ Pathology

Renal involvement caused by "myeloma kidney," hypercalcemia, amyloidosis, hyperuricemia, acquired Fanconi syndrome, or light chain deposition. Radiculopathy in thoracic and lumbosacral areas. Serum β_2-microglobulin (β_2-M) level is the most reliable prognosticator in untreated patients. **Myeloma variants** include **smoldering myeloma** and **plasma cell leukemia.**

■ Treatment

Can defer treating minimal disease. Primary modes of treatment are **chemotherapy, irradiation,** and **analgesics** for pain control. Chemotherapy includes melphalan + prednisone, or M2 protocol (melphalan, cyclophosphamide, carmustine [BCNU], vincristine, prednisone).

Long-term chemotherapy may cause myelodysplastic syndrome or acute leukemia. Treat 1 to 2 years and stop if M-protein is stable in urine and serum, and no other evidence of disease. α-Interferon may be of value. *Refractory disease:* other chemotherapy combinations. *Special complications include:*

1. **Hypercalcemia**—hydration, prednisone; consider mithramycin, diphosphonates, calcitonin, increased physical activity.
2. **Renal failure**—furosemide; hemodialysis if symptomatic; plasmapheresis; allopurinol.

4. Waldenström's Macroglobulinemia (Primary Macroglobulinemia)

■ Description

Production of large **monoclonal** immunoglobulin M (IgM) protein by abnormal proliferation of lymphocytes or plasma cells.

■ Symptoms

Weakness, fatigue, bleeding, pallor; impaired vision, weight loss; **hepatosplenomegaly; lymphadenopathy;** neurologic symptoms (sensorimotor peripheral neuropathy); infection; CHF.

■ Diagnosis

Severe normocytic, normochromic anemia; γ-globulin spike (IgM type on immunoelectrophoresis). About 75% have κ light chains. Bone marrow biopsy shows hypercellular marrow, **infiltrated with lymphoid cells and plasma cells.**

■ Treatment

Treat if anemic, if constitutional symptoms, hyperviscosity problems, or significant hepatosplenomegaly or lymphadenopathy. Options: **chemotherapy** (chlorambucil [Leukeran]; M2 protocol; α-2 interferon). **Transfusions. Plasmapheresis** for hyperviscosity.

5. Hyperviscosity Syndrome

■ Description

Syndrome of increased serum viscosity seen in Waldenström's macroglobulinemia, and occasionally in multiple myeloma.

■ Symptoms

Occur if relative viscosity is > 4 centipoises (cp). Manifest by mucous membrane bleeding, retinal hemorrhages, papilledema, decreased vision, dizziness, headaches, coma, aggravation of CHF.

■ Treatment

Plasma exchange until patient asymptomatic.

6. Heavy-Chain Disease

■ Description

Due to monoclonal protein composed of only the heavy chain. There are gamma, alpha, and mu types.

1. **Gamma (g.5g-HCD)—lymphomalike illness. Results fair with CVP chemotherapy.**
2. **Alpha (a.5a-HCD)—the most common type. Common involvement of the GI tract. Poor prognosis.** Some response to chemotherapy.

3. <u>Mu</u> (m.5m-HCD)—<u>seen in chronic lymphocytic leukemia or lymphoma.</u> Bence Jones proteinuria in two thirds. Treat with steroids and alkylating agents.

B. Polycythemia Rubra Vera; Other Cythemias, Including Eosinophilias

1. General

Must differentiate **relative polycythemia** (decreased plasma volume) from **absolute polycythemia** (increased total red cell mass). Can distinguish absolute from relative by measuring red cell mass (with ^{51}Cr-labeled RBCs) and plasma volume (with ^{125}I-albumin). Normal red cell mass is 30 ± 3 mL/kg in men, 27 ± 2 mL/kg in women. Normal hematocrit up to 54% in men, 48% in women.

2. Relative Polycythemia (also called Spurious Polycythemia, Stress Polycythemia, Gaisbock Syndrome)

■ **Description**

Consider relative polycythemia after ruling out dehydration, the most common cause of polycythemia.

■ **Diagnosis**

Hypertensive, smoking, middle-aged male.

■ **Symptoms**

May have no symptoms; risk of increased incidence of thromboembolic events.

■ **Pathology**

Common factors are smoking and diuretics (in hypertensives).

■ **Treatment**

Discontinue smoking. May need phlebotomy.

3. Absolute Polycythemia

1. **May be secondary or autonomous**

a. **Secondary polycythemia.** Two types:

Physiologically appropriate response to tissue hypoxia. **Increased erythropoietin. Seen in:**

(1) High altitude. Diagnosis: increase AP diameter of chest, ruddy cyanosis, engorged capillaries of skin, mucus membranes.

(2) Cardiopulmonary disease. Right-to-left shunts, chronic obstructive pulmonary disease (COPD).

(3) Alveolar hypoventilation (eg, pickwickian syndrome).

(4) Abnormalities of oxygen-hemoglobin dissociation curve. High oxygen-affinity hemoglobinopathies; hereditary methemoglobinemias; carbon monoxide exposure (smoking, industrial exposure).

Physiologically inappropriate response to tissue hypoxemia:

(1) Neoplasms and non-neoplastic renal disease. Neoplastic includes renal and adrenal cancer, cerebellar hemangioblastoma, hepatocellular carcinoma; non-neoplastic includes renal cysts and hydronephrosis. Increased erythropoietin production.

(2) Drug-induced. Testosterone, adrenal corticosteroids.

■ **Symptoms**

Ruddy cyanosis, headache, tinnitus, fullness in head and neck, lightheadedness; increased thrombotic events; epistaxis; upper GI bleeding.

■ **Diagnosis**

Can do blood or urine erythropoietin and bone marrow colony growth tests to distinguish primary from secondary polycythemia.

■ **Treatment**

In "Inappropriate" group, phlebotomize to hematocrit < 50%; in "Appropriate" group, phlebotomy may do more harm, so aim for hematocrit < 60%.

b. **Polycythemia vera**

■ **Description**

Malignant proliferative disorder of **erythroid, myeloid, and megakaryocytic** elements of marrow leading to **increased red cell mass** and often to increased granulocytes and platelets in blood. Related to myeloproliferative disorders. If treated, median survival increased from 1 to 10 years. **Thrombosis** the major cause of death. Low or undetectable erythropoietin.

■ **Symptoms**

Headache, tinnitus, lightheadedness, vertigo, blurred vision. Thrombotic and hemorrhagic episodes (epistaxis, **easy bruising,** UGI bleeding). Increased incidence of peptic ulcer disease and pruritus. Severe pain in the feet. Bone tenderness.

■ **Diagnosis**

Splenomegaly in 75%. Hepatomegaly in 40%. Increased hemoglobin, hematocrit, red cell count. Hypochromic, microcytic cells. Low serum iron. Hematocrit is best guide to red cell mass (> 60% is very suggestive). **Increased red cell mass** (> 36 in men; > 32 in women). Increased WBCs, platelets, trending to higher levels and more immature forms later in disease. Increased numbers of basophils and eosinophils. **Increased leukocyte alkaline phosphatase, B_{12}** and lysozyme levels. **Normal O_2 saturation** (> 92%). Low or absent erythropoietin.

■ **Pathology**

Marrow: hyperplasia of all elements. Megakaryocytes in sheets or clumps. Absent marrow iron stores.

■ **Treatment**

Phlebotomize initially to hematocrit < 45%. May need **myelosuppression.** Current recommendations: if > 70 years old, treat with ^{32}P and phlebotomy; if < 70 years old, use phlebotomy; **hydroxyurea** if poor response. Problems with chlorambucil or busulfan include excessive myelosuppression and development of secondary malignancies.

c. **Eosinophilic syndromes**

(1) **Parasitic diseases**—especially multicellular helminthic parasites. Diagnosis: often three or more stool specimens needed to diagnose.

(2) **Other infections**—allergic bronchopulmonary aspergillosis, coccidioidomycosis. Eosinophils depressed by bacterial and viral infections.

Can get eosinophilia c̄ Chlamydia pneumonia

(3) **Allergic diseases**—allergic rhinitis, asthma, hypersensitivity drug reaction, drug-induced interstitial nephritis.

(4) **Myeloproliferative disease** —idiopathic hypereosinophilia syndrome. Treatment: steroids; chemotherapy.

(5) **Neoplastic diseases**—eosinophilic leukemia; chronic myelocytic leukemia; occasionally in Hodgkin's disease; some carcinomas.

(6) **Cutaneous diseases**—scabies, bullous pemphigoid, episodic angioedema with eosinophilia.

(7) **Pulmonary eosinophilias**— see Pulmonary section.

(8) **Gastrointestinal disease**— eosinophilic gastroenteritis; inflammatory bowel disease.

(9) **Immunologic disease**—hypersensitivity vasculitis; allergic granulomatous angiitis (Churg–Strauss syndrome); some immunodeficiency syndromes (Wiskott–Aldrich syndrome, graft-versus-host disease.

(10) **Other**—Dressler syndrome; chronic peritoneal dialysis; eosinphilia–myalgia syndrome secondary to contaminated L-tryptophan; Addison's disease; hypopituitarism.

C. Reactions to Transfusion of Blood Components

1. Acute Hemolytic Transfusion Reaction

■ Description

Reaction occurs within minutes or hours of exposure. Intravascular destruction caused by complement activation. Extravascular destruction caused by antibodies without complement activation.

■ Symptoms

Fever, chest pain, wheezing, back pain, hypotension, DIC, bleeding diathesis, renal impairment.

■ Treatment

Discontinue transfusion. Correct hypotension. Control bleeding. Prevent acute renal failure (use IV fluids, mannitol, diuretics to maintain output at 100 cc/h).

2. Febrile Non-hemolytic Transfusion Reaction

■ Description

Reaction occurs within minutes or hours of exposure. In 0.5% of transfusions.

■ Symptoms

Transient flushing, palpitations, tachycardia, cough, chest discomfort, neutropenia. Latent period of 15 to 60 minutes; then increased blood pressure, headache, chills, rigors.

■ Pathology

Cytotoxic or agglutinating antibodies from prior transfusion.

■ Treatment

Discontinue transfusion and test for hemolysis. Antipyretics.

3. Acute Lung Injury

■ Description

Infrequent.

■ Symptoms

Fever, chest pain, dyspnea, cyanosis, cough, blood-tinged sputum, hypoxemia. Resembles CHF, but noncardiogenic.

■ Pathology

Anti-HLA antibody.

■ Treatment

Respiratory support, mechanical ventilation, fluid replacement.

4. Allergic Reactions

■ Description

Urticaria and pruritus in 1 to 3%. Is reaction of donor protein and patient IgE. Is usually mild. Anaphylaxis very rare.

5. Hypervolemia

6. Bacterial sepsis—very rare

7. Delayed Reactions: Delayed Hemolytic Transfusion Reaction

■ Description

Reaction occurs days or years after exposure. Antibodies occur as anamnestic response. History of prior transfusion or pregnancy. Positive direct Coombs'.

1. **Graft-versus-host disease.**

■ Description

Reaction seen in immunocompromised patient or in patients getting treatment for lymphoma or leukemia, 4 to 30 days after transfusion.

■ Symptoms

Fever, erythema, diarrhea, liver function test (LFT) abnormalities, pancytopenia. **Mortality 90%.**

■ Pathology

T lymphocyte mediated.

■ Prevention

Pretransfusion irradiation of blood or components.

2. **Iron overload**—see Hemochromatosis.
3. **Post-transfusion purpura.**

■ Description

Thrombocytopenia 5 to 9 days after transfusion.

■ Pathology

Alloantibodies to platelet antigens.

■ Treatment

Steroids, plasma/blood exchange, IV gamma globulin.

4. Delayed reactions: transfusion-transmitted disease.

   a. Hepatitis. **Hepatitis C** (non-A, non-B) most common, but also see it with A and B. Illness 7 to 8 weeks after transfusion; 50% of hepatitis C patients develop chronic hepatitis; 10 to 20% of these get **cirrhosis or hepatocellular carcinoma.** Aim for **prevention** with donor screening.

   b. **Retroviral infection.** 3% of AIDS is from transfusion, 7-year latency. Aim for **prevention** with donor screening.

c. **Cytomegalovirus (CMV).** Infection not serious if immunocompetent. Bone marrow recipients may be more severely affected and die. New filters help prevent this.

V. HEMOCHROMATOSIS (IRON-STORAGE DISEASE)

■ Description

Primary ("idiopathic") hemochromatosis is a common autosomal recessive genetic disease in Europeans. Secondary hemochromatosis is seen in anemias with ineffective erythropoiesis, increased iron absorption, and multiple transfusions.

■ Symptoms

Hepatomegaly, splenomegaly, **skin pigmentation,** weakness, lethargy, **chronic abdominal pain,** arthralgia, loss of libido, impotence. Atrial tachyarrhythmias, dilated cardiomyopathy, and congestive heart failure. Insulin-dependent diabetes mellitus. Cancer of liver occurs late.

2° scarring !

■ Diagnosis

Requires presence of these symptoms and signs, family history, index of suspicion, and **demonstration of iron overload** (saturated iron-binding capacity [60 to 100%], and high plasma ferritin level [> 300 µg/L in male, and > 200 in female]). **Liver biopsy is diagnostic.**

■ Pathology

The excess iron stored as **hemosiderin** is damaging to the parenchymal tissue, and leads to **fibrosis and cirrhosis** (in liver) of the organ. Slate-gray skin. Testicular atrophy.

■ Treatment

Early detection so phlebotomies started early. Treat with weekly phlebotomy for 2 to 3 years to restore iron to normal in full-blown disease; then at 2- to 3-month intervals. Treatment increases 5-year survival from 18 to 92%. In secondary hemochromatosis, treat with desferrioxamine.

BIBLIOGRAPHY

Bagby GC Jr. Leukopenia. In: Wyngaarden JB, Smith LH, Bennett JC, eds. *Cecil Textbook of Medicine.* 19th ed. Philadelphia, Pa: WB Saunders Co; 1992. An algorithm for the evaluation of patients with neutropenia: Figure 140–5, p 912.

Brain MC, Carbone PP. *Current Therapy in Hematology-Oncology.* 4th ed. Philadelphia, Pa: BC Decker; 1992.

Berk PD. Erythrocytosis and polycythemia. In: Wyngaarden JB, Smith LH, Bennett JC, eds. *Cecil Textbook of Medicine.* 19th ed. Philadelphia, Pa: WB Saunders Co; 1992: Algorithm for evaluation of an elevated hematocrit: Figure 142–2, p 923.

Benz EJ Jr. Classification and basic pathophysiology of the hemoglobinopathies. In: Wyngaarden JB, Smith LH, Bennett JC, eds. *Cecil Textbook of Medicine.* 19th ed. Philadelphia, Pa: WB Saunders Co, 1992: Classification of Hemoglobinopathies: Table 136–2, p 878.

DeVita VT Jr, et al. *Cancer: Principles and Practices of Oncology.* Philadelphia, Pa: JB Lippincott; 1989.

Mosher D. Disorders of blood coagulation. In: Wyngaarden JB, Smith LH, Bennett JC, eds. *Cecil Textbook of Medicine.* 19th ed. Philadelphia, Pa: WB Saunders Co; 1992: Diagrams of interactions among coagulation factors: Figure 155–1, p 1001.

Mosher D. Disorders of blood coagulation. In: Wyngaarden JB, Smith LH, Bennett JC, eds. *Cecil Textbook of Medicine.* 19th ed. Philadelphia, Pa: WB Saunders Co; 1992: Drugs and conditions that influence response to warfarin: Table 155–2, p 1014.

Schein PS. *Decision Making in Oncology.* Toronto, Canada: BC Decker; 1989.

Shuman M. Hemorrhagic disorders: abnormalities of platelet and vascular function. In: Wyngaarden JB, Smith LH, Bennett JC, eds. *Cecil Textbook of Medicine.* 19th ed. Philadelphia, Pa: WB Saunders Co; 1992. Algorithm for laboratory evaluation of bleeding disorders: Figure 154–4, p 991.

Williams WJ, et al (eds). *Hematology.* 4th ed. New York: McGraw-Hill Inc; 1990.

Wilson JD, Braunwald E, Isselbacher KJ, et al. *Harrison's Principles of Internal Medicine.* 12th ed. New York: McGraw-Hill Inc; 1991.

Woodley M, Whelan A. *Manual of Medical Therapeutics.* 27th ed. Boston, Mass: Little, Brown and Co; 1992.

Wyngaarden JB, Smith LH, Bennett JC. *Cecil Textbook of Medicine.* 19th ed. Philadelphia, Pa: WB Saunders Co; 1992.

CHAPTER 6

Oncology

RICHARD J. GOLDMAN, MD

I. GENERAL

A. General Statistics

In 1988, 985,000 new cancer cases was diagnosed in the United States, with 494,000 deaths, 22% of all deaths. One third of all people will develop cancer. Lung cancer on the rise, steadily in both males and females (has passed breast cancer as the major cancer in females). Stomach cancer on the decline.

B. Etiologic Factors

Multiple steps and factors are now known to exist. Carcinogens and cocarcinogens are acting with genetic assistance. Implicated agents include:

Chemicals (eg, chemotherapy for other malignancies or after immunosuppressive treatment in transplants).
Viruses (eg, papillomavirus and cervical cancer [CA]; acquired immunodeficiency syndrome [AIDS] virus, and Kaposi's sarcoma).
Physical agents (ionizing radiation, ultraviolet light).
Diet (**high-fat, low-fiber** and **low-calcium diet** [colon]).
High alcohol (oral).
Cocarcinogens (tobacco products are the major public health hazard. One third of cancer in United States and Europe is related to tobacco products).
Genetic (via **oncogenes** [pieces of cellular DNA found in oncogenic retroviruses], **proto-oncogenes** [DNA sequences in normal cells related to oncogenes]). **Oncogenes:** human genome has set of genes (20 to 100 loci) called proto-oncogenes or cellular oncogenes. The first studies were from viruses causing animal tumors. Retroviruses (RNA genes are copied into RNA by reverse transcriptase into the host). Retroviral oncogenes are misplaced copies of cellular genes acquired by a process known as transduction. May be tumorogenic because their usual controls were lost, or there may have been mutations. At least 11 proto-oncogenes have been identified in humans.

C. Histology

Cancer (CA) cells: **large, irregular, more numerous nuclei** with **increased mitotic figures.** Necrosis and hemorrhage (outgrow vascular supply). "Tumor blush" in angiograms. Carcinomas: epithelial origin. Sarcomas: mesenchymatous origin. Carcinomas can be squamous or adenocarcinomas.

D. Cytogenetics

Most common is **band deletion** or **reciprocal translocation** between two chromosomes. **Aneuploidy, addition, deletion, translocation.** Example: Philadelphia chromosome (Ph^1) in chronic myelocytic leukemia.

E. Growth Kinetics

A particular "doubling time" is characteristic of particular tumors. Clinically detectable (1-cm) tumor has undergone 30 doublings to reach 10^9 cells. Ten further doublings will produce lethal 1 kg of tumor burden.

F. Predicting Outcome

1. Staging

The TNM system (tumor, node, metastases) is generally used, but is not always clinically useful (is good in head and neck, breast, lung).

2. Other Determinants of Prognosis

Biologic characteristics of the tumor; **host resistance; host-tumor interaction; toxic:therapeutic ratio; hormone receptors** (breast).

G. Tumor Markers

Beta subunit of human chorionic gonadotropin (HCG), (AFP), thyrocalcitonin, breast cyst antigen, serum acid phosphatase, monoclonal immunoglobulins, urinary lysozymes, carcinoembryonic antigen (CEA), lactate dehydrogenase (LDH).

H. Extent at Diagnosis

One third in situ or localized; one fourth regional spread; one third distant metastasis; the rest undetectable; 40 to 50% are curable at time of diagnosis.

II. DETECTION AND SCREENING

TABLE 6–1. SUMMARY OF AMERICAN CANCER SOCIETY RECOMMENDATIONS FOR THE EARLY DETECTION OF CANCER IN ASYMPTOMATIC PEOPLE[1]

Test or Procedure	Sex	Age	Frequency
Sigmoidoscopy, preferably flexible	M & F	50 and over	Every 3 to 5 years
Fecal occult blood test	M & F	50 and over	Every year
Digital rectal examination	M & F	40 and over	Every year
Pap test	F	All women who are or who have been sexually active, or have reached 18, should have annual Pap and pelvic. After 3 or more consecutive satisfactory exams, the Pap may be done less often, at discretion of physician.	
Pelvic exam	F	18 to 40	Every 1 to 3 years
		Over 40	Every year

Table 6–1. Continued

Test or Procedure	Sex	Age	Frequency
Endometrial tissue sample	F	At menopause, women at high risk*	
Breast self-exam	F	20 and over	Every month
Clinical breast exam	F	20 to 40	Every 3 years
		Over 40	Every year
Mammography	F	40 to 49	Every 1 to 2 years
		50 and over	Every year
Health counseling	M & F	Over 20	Every 3 years
Cancer checkup	M & F	Over 40	Every year

* History of infertility, obesity, failure to ovulate, abnormal uterine bleeding, or estrogen therapy. Screening mammography should begin by age 40. To include exam for cancers of thyroid, testicles, prostate, ovaries, lymph nodes, oral region, and skin.

[1] Levin B, Murphy GP. Revision in American Cancer Society recommendations for the early detection of colorectal cancer. *CA-A Cancer Journal for Clinicians.* 1992;42(5):296–299.

III. MANAGEMENT

A. General

Define therapeutic strategies, do periodic reassessment after diagnosis and staging, and share with patients and family. Consider physical, psychological, and social situation.

B. Therapy Modalities

1. Biological Response Modifiers: Modulation of Host Immune System Interferons

Especially good in **hairy cell leukemia, Kaposi's sarcoma.** Interleukin-2 (increases number of peripheral lymphocytes, increases killer cells, increases cytotoxic activity, produces LAK [lymphokine-activated killer] cells): effective in **renal cell CA, malignant melanoma.**

2. Chemotherapy

a. **Four phases:** induction, consolidation, maintenance, adjustment.

b. **Measuring responses:** complete (no measurable tumor) versus partial (50% reduction).

3. Surgery

The **primary therapeutic modality** for most early cancers.

C. Supportive Care

Antibiotics, transfusions, antiemetics, anxiolytics.

D. Nutritional Problems

Reasons for anorexia and hypercatabolism include anatomical, dysphagia, paraneoplastic syndromes, chemotherapy, depression, secretion of peptides. **Must improve nutrition** to permit use of chemotherapy (may require parenteral or tube feedings).

E. Hyperuricemia and Hyperuricosuria

In lymphatic leukemia and lymphomas. Treat with **allopurinol** and **hydration.**

F. Deconditioning, Hypercalcemia, Fractures

Keep mobile.

G. Psychosocial Issues

Supportive family, physician, and staff. **Maintain optimism.**

H. Pain Control

Liberal use of narcotics for severe generalized pain. **Radiotherapy.** Neurological procedures.

I. Hospice and Home Care

Much preferred over continued hospitalization or nursing home.

IV. EPIDEMIOLOGY AND PREVENTION

Great variation in incidence among countries, regions, and cultures within countries suggests environmental and genetic factors. Most causes result from multiple exposures and susceptibility states.

A. Major Factors

1. Tobacco

The main hazard in western countries. In **lung, larynx, mouth, pharynx, esophagus, bladder, pancreas, kidney,** and possibly **cervix.** Two packs per day leads to 20-fold increase in lung cancer rate. Passive smoking is also carcinogenic.

2. Alcohol

Multiplies the effect of tobacco in cancer of mouth, pharynx, esophagus, larynx. **Liver cancer** in cirrhotics. Not carcinogenic alone.

3. Solar Radiation

Skin cancer (squamous and basal cell; melanoma).

4. Ionizing Radiation

Accounts for 3% of all cancer. Mainly **breast, thyroid,** and **bone marrow.**

5. Occupational and Environmental Pollution Hazards

Less than 5%. Examples: Aromatic amines: bladder cancer. Arsenic: lung, skin, liver cancer. Asbestos: lung, pleura, peritoneal, gastrointestinal (GI) track tumors. Benzene: leukemia.

Mustard gas: lung, larynx, and sinus cancer. Vinyl chloride: liver cancer.

6. Medication

Synthetic estrogen—adenocarcinoma of **vagina** and **cervix** occurring several years later in daughters **exposed in utero. Conjugated estrogen** for menopausal symptoms: **endometrial cancer.**

Oral contraceptives—possible role in benign liver tumors, endometrial cancer (with sequential oral contraceptives), cervical, and breast. However, note **decreased risk** reported in endometrial and ovarian cancer with **combined oral contraceptive.**

Alkylating agents—acute non-lymphocytic leukemia. **Immunosuppressives** such as azathioprine and corticosteroids in transplant patients: histiocytic lymphoma.

7. Infectious Agents

Papillomavirus and **herpes virus** —**cervical cancer. Epstein–Barr** (EBV): nasopharyngeal and Burkitt's lymphoma.

Hepatitis-C—hepatocellular cancer. Human T-cell leukemia virus (HTLV-I): adult T-cell leukemia. Human immunodeficiency virus (HIV) (HTLV-III or LAV): AIDS syndrome. AIDS: Kaposi's sarcoma; non-Hodgkin's lymphoma.

8. Nutrition

Fat—colon and breast cancer.

Fat and caloric excess—endometrial cancer.

Decreased fiber—colon cancer. **Decreased vitamin A, beta-carotene and selenium:** lung cancer.

Decreased fruits and vegetables and vitamin C—stomach cancer.

Increased alcohol and poor nutrition—esophageal cancer.

Aflatoxin (from fungus *Aspergillus flavus*): liver cancer.

9. Genetic

Chinese nasopharyngeal cancer. Native Americans and **Hispanic** groups: gallbladder cancer. **Whites:** skin cancer. Autosomal dominant heredity: **retinoblastoma, polyposis coli.** Hereditary preneoplastic syndromes (neurofibromatosis leading to sarcomatous change, gliomas of brain and optic nerve, acoustic neuroma, meningioma, and acute leukemia).

B. Chemoprevention Trials Are Currently in Progress

Transretinoic acid (cervix); folic acid (cervix); wheat bran + calcium carbonate (colon); calcium (colon); beta-carotene (colon, lung, skin, oral cavity).

V. PARANEOPLASTIC SYNDROMES

A. General

Syndromes due to **remote or biologic effects of proteins or hormones secreted by tumor.** Often improve after treatment of tumor.

B. Syndromes

1. Wasting of Host (Tumor Cachexia)

Most common paraneoplastic syndrome. Possibly multifactorial.

■ Treatment

Treat the tumor; hyperalimentation if surgery planned or if hope of significant remission or cure with therapy.

2. Endocrine

2–1. Ectopic ACTH

■ Description

Cushing syndrome: about 50% from the lung. The agent may be POMC (proopiomelanocortin). Adrenal tumors produce cortisol, but not adrenocorticotropic hormone (ACTH).

■ Symptoms

Often subtle. Mild weakness, hypokalemia, psychosis, abnormal glucose tolerance curve.

■ Diagnosis

Extremely high plasma ACTH that **does not suppress with dexamethasone** (but does in Cushing's disease).

■ Treatment

Surgery; chemotherapy. Alternate therapy: metyrapone, aminoglutethimide, or ketoconazole.

2–2. Hypercalcemia

■ Description

Seen in solid tumors **(lung, kidney, ovary),** and hematological disease **(multiple myeloma and adult T-cell lymphoma).** Mechanisms include release of osteoclast-stimulating factor, increased renal calcium absorption.

■ Symptoms

Polyuria, constipation, lethargy, personality change.

■ Treatment

Mobilization. Saline infusion. Furosemide. Mithramycin (emergency). **Calcitonin** and **glucocorticoids** (short-term). **Biphosphonate** and **oral phosphate** (long-term).

2–3. Hypophosphatemia

Rare.

2–4. Chorionic Gonadotropin

Cleared rapidly from serum; little clinical effect; rarely see gynecomastia.

2–5. Hypoglycemia

Most commonly in mesotheliomas, hepatic carcinomas, adrenal cortical carcinomas. Due to factors with insulinlike activity.

2–6. Growth Hormone and Growth Hormone-Releasing Hormone (GHRH)

Acromegaly in bronchial carcinoid or pancreatic islet cell tumor.

2–7. Calcitonin

Little or no biologic effect in normal adults, so no symptoms. Good hormonal marker for medullary carcinoma of thyroid.

2–8. Vasopressin

Causes syndrome of inappropriate antidiuretic hormone (SIADH). Seen in carcinoma of the lung.

2–9. Erythropoietin

Benign and malignant **kidney conditions** (hypernephroma, renal cysts, hydronephrosis). Nonrenal conditions include hemangioblastomas, uterine fibromas, adrenal cortical neoplasms, ovarian neoplasms, hepatomas, pheochromocytomas.

3. Neurological

Subacute cerebellar degeneration, subacute motor neuropathy, sensory neuropathy, Eaton–Lambert syndrome, dermatomyositis.

4. Hematological

4–1. Erythrocytosis

From erythropoietin secretion, renal or liver tumors (see Endocrine section).

4–2. Leukemoid Reactions

From colony-stimulating factor (CSF) secretion. Also see granulocytosis (lung, gastric, pancreatic, brain, melanomas, lymphomas) or eosinophilia (lymphomas, Hodgkin's, GI carcinomas).

4–3. Anemia

Anemia of chronic disease common in most cancers. Autoimmune hemolytic anemia in B-cell lymphoproliferative neoplasms, and occasionally with ovarian and lung CA.

4–4. Microangiopathic Hemolytic Anemia

In stomach, breast, lung.

4–5. Granulocytopenia

Usually from chemotherapy, radiation therapy, infection, marrow involvement.

4–6. Idiopathic Thrombocytopenic Purpura (ITP)

Usually in lymphomas.

5. Thromboembolic Paraneoplastic Syndromes

■ **Description**

Hypercoagulable state. Three types:

a. Migratory thrombophlebitis (Trousseau's syndrome). Usually GI neoplasm, but also lung, breast, ovarian, prostate.

■ **Treatment**

Difficult; may require long-term heparin if warfarin doesn't work.

b. Disseminated intravascular coagulation (DIC). **May be common and subclinical.**

■ **Treatment**

Treat the tumor. May use heparin.

c. **Non-bacterial thrombotic endocarditis (NBTE, marantic endocarditis).** Usually mucin-secreting adenocarcinomas. May embolize.

■ **Treatment**

Treat the tumor.

6. Renal Paraneoplastic Syndromes

a. SIADH.
b. Nephrotic syndrome. Hodgkin's (lipoid nephrosis, minimal change glomerulopathy). Non-Hodgkin's lymphoma (immune complex).
c. **Myeloma and amyloid kidney.**
d. **Hypokalemia.** Myelogenous leukemia (lysozyme-related).

7. Dermatologic

Acanthosis nigricans, dermatomyositis, flushing in carcinoid, Gardner syndrome.

8. Gastrointestinal

Protein-losing enteropathy, malignant hepatopathy (Stauffer's syndrome).

9. Miscellaneous

Fever (lymphomas, hypernephromas). **Lactic acidosis** (acute leukemias, lymphomas). **Hypokalemia and hypertension** (lung, hypernephroma, Wilms'). **Hypertrophic pulmonary osteoarthropathy** (lung, mesothelioma, other metastases to lung). **Amyloidosis** (myeloma, lymphoma, carcinomas). **Systemic lupus** (lymphomas, leukemias, thymomas, testicular, lung, ovarian).

VI. TUMOR MARKERS

Usefulness: screening, early detection, assessing **tumor burden** and **prognosis,** assessing **response to therapy,** evaluating **early recurrence. Examples:**

Hormones—**beta subunit of human chorionic gonadotropin** (beta-HCG): testicular cancer, choriocarcinomas, hydatidiform mole. *Others:* Human placental lactogen, ACTH, vasopressin, calcitonin, gastrin-releasing peptide.

Oncofetal proteins—**alpha fetoprotein** (AFP): hepatoma and testicular cancer. The level has predictive value in follow-up.

Carcinoembryonic antigen (CEA)—GI tract, breast, lung, ovarian tumors. Increased by smoking and inflammatory processes, so should not be used for screening.

Immunoglobulins—myeloma and some other lymphoproliferative disorders; good for following response to treatment. Heavy chains and light chains in myeloma and Waldenström's macroglobulinemia.

Enzymes—L-Dopa decarboxylase: small-cell lung cancer. Creatine phosphokinase (CPK-BB): small-cell lung and prostate cancer. **Prostatic acid phosphatase:** one third of occult prostate and 75% of more advanced prostate cancer. **Lysozyme:** monocytic and myelomonocytic leukemias. **(Lactic dehydrogenase).**

Tumor antigens—CA 125: ovarian. CA 19-9: colon cancer and other epithelial tumors. β_2 **microglobulin** (a human leukocyte antigen [HLA] class I antigen): assessing response in myeloma therapy.

VII. SPECIFIC TYPES OF NEOPLASTIC DISORDERS

A. Blood and Blood-Forming Organs

1. Hodgkin's Disease

■ **Description**

Lymph node malignancy of unknown etiology; average age 32; male more than female.

■ **Symptoms**

Painless cervical or other **adenopathy.** Chest x-ray may show mediastinal mass, infiltrates, effusions. **Fever,** sometimes cyclic (Pel–Ebstein fever). **Night sweats. Pruritis.** Superior vena cava obstruction. Spinal cord compression. Hepatic and splenic enlargement. Infections (herpes zoster, cryptococcosis, *Pneumocystis carinii* pneumonia, toxoplasmosis). Immunologic abnormalities common.

■ **Diagnosis**

Use **CT of chest and abdomen, lymphangiography. Bilateral bone marrow biopsy** in all patients suspected of diffuse or bone disease.
Staging:

   I. Single lymph node or group.
   II. More than one node or group; same side of diaphragm.

III. Spleen and nodes; both sides of diaphragm.

IV. Liver or marrow.

■ Symptoms

Fever > 38.5; night sweats; 10% weight loss over 6 months.

■ Pathology

Anemia of chronic disease, but occasionally due to hypersplenism, marrow invasion, Coombs'-positive hemolytic anemia. Leukocytosis, eosinophilia. Pathognomonic **Reed–Sternberg giant cell** (large bilobed cell with prominent eosinophilic nucleoli).

■ Treatment

Biopsy first. Staging before treatment. **Staging laparotomy (with splenectomy)** is widely used, and may affect therapy. Treat with **radiotherapy:** 3600 to 4000 rads. Radiation alone initially in stages I and II. Stage IIIA: either radiation or chemotherapy. **Chemotherapy:** in advanced (IIIB and IV) disease. **Standard is MOPP program** (nitrogen mustard, vincristine [Oncovin], procarbazine, and prednisone), minimum of six cycles, produces complete remission in 70 to 80%; disease-free 10 to 20 years later in 50% of these. Greatly improved prognosis due to staging, radiotherapy, and chemotherapy advances.

2. Non-Hodgkin's Lymphoma

■ Description

The largest group of immune system neoplasms, characterized by monoclonal proliferation of B or T lymphocytes. Preceding immune dysfunction (eg, AIDS). Possible viral etiology in Burkitt's, adult T-cell leukemia.

■ Symptoms

Similar to Hodgkin's.

■ Diagnosis

Node pathology; B- and T-cell typing studies. Use CT of abdomen, pelvis, and chest. Immunoglobulins, bone scan, upper GI studies (UGI), bilateral bone marrow biopsies.

■ Pathology

Classifying systems: Rappaport Classification, Lukes and Collins, The NCI Working Formulation (1982). Usually at Stage III or IV at time of diagnosis.

■ Treatment

Depends on grade and stage. Modalities include multiagent **chemotherapy** (C-MOPP = cyclophosphamide, vincristine, procarbazine, prednisone), **whole-body irradiation,** or **combined chemo/irradiation.**

■ Special Problems

Superior vena cava obstruction: irradiate. Gastric lymphoma: resect. CNS disease: irradiate. Urate nephropathy: allopurinol to prevent.

3. Acute Leukemia in Children

3–1. Acute Lymphoblastic Leukemia

■ Description

Malignant proliferation of lymphoid precursors, with replacement of normal cells; 75% of the 2500 new acute leukemias.

■ Symptoms

Pallor, fatigue, bleeding, fever, bone pain, adenopathy, arthralgias, hepatosplenomegaly.

■ Diagnosis

Marrow **morphology, cytochemical staining, immunologic cell surface markers, cytogenetics.**

■ **Pathology**

Marrow infiltrated or replaced with lymphoblasts.

Treatment

Cure rate 65 to 70%. **Multiple-drug chemotherapy** (prednisone, vincristine, doxorubicin, methotrexate, asparaginase) + **intrathecal chemotherapy** (methotrexate or cytarabine) or **cranial irradiation.** Because of high cure rate, no marrow transplant with first remission, but is recommended after second remission.

3–2. Acute Myeloblastic Leukemia

■ **Description**

Malignant proliferation of myelocytic precursors, with replacement of normal cells; 15 to 20% of acute leukemias.

■ **Symptoms**

Similar. Usually sicker than patients with acute lymphocytic leukemia (ALL).

■ **Diagnosis**

Similar.

■ **Pathology**

Marrow infiltrated or replaced with myeloblasts.

■ **Treatment**

Intensive **chemotherapy** with daunorubicin and cytarabine, often with thioguanine or etoposide. **Intrathecal chemo** or **irradiation.** Produces 80% complete remission rate, 65% remain in continuous CR.

4. Acute Leukemia in Adults

■ **Description**

Malignant unregulated proliferation of immature myeloid or lymphoid precursors, with replacement of normal cells. Inciting agents include ionizing radiation, oncogenic viruses, genetic and congenital factors, chemical agents.

■ **Symptoms**

Anemia, hemorrhage, infection, leukemic infiltrates (bone pain, meningitis, mediastinal mass, chloromas), lymphadenopathy, splenomegaly.

■ **Diagnosis**

Anemia, abnormal blood counts, thrombocytopenia and abnormal bone marrow. Elevated serum and urine lysozyme in acute myeloblastic leukemia (AML). Must distinguish from infections, other cancers, drug effects.

■ **Pathology**

Bone marrow: **morphological, histochemical techniques, surface markers** (immunologic techniques), **cytoplasmic markers** (enzymes), chromosomal changes. 80% are acute myelogenous (ANLL, acute non-lymphocytic leukemia).

■ **Treatment**

First correct complications. Allopurinol. Then **aim for cure** (30%) with **chemotherapy.**

Acute myelogenous (ANLL, acute non-lymphocytic leukemia)—remission achieved in majority of patients older than 60 with one course of cytosine arabinoside (ara-C) and daunomycin or doxorubicin. Bone marrow transplant (patients younger than 45 with HLA-identical donors) for relapse after first remission. Cure rate 20% in adult AML.

Acute lymphoblastic (acute lymphocytic, ALL)—vincristine, prednisone, and a third drug, such as L-asparaginase, doxorubicin, or daunorubicin, gives 80% remission in adults. Need CNS prophylaxis (cranial irradiation plus intrathecal methotrexate), then maintenance or continuation therapy. For relapse, give systemic chemo and local irradiation. Bone marrow transplant (30% survival rate in autologous transplant).

5. "Myelodysplastic Syndromes" or "Preleukemia"

Characterized by normal to increased marrow cellularity and ineffective erythropoiesis. **Many develop AML** within 6 to 18 months. Consider bone marrow transplant.

6. Chronic Leukemic States

6–1. Chronic Myelogenous Leukemia

■ Description

Originates in primitive myeloid stem cell. Characteristic **Philadelphia (Ph[1]) chromosome.**

■ Symptoms

Fatigue, anorexia, weight loss, sense of abdominal fullness. Headaches, fever, sweats, bone pain. Hemorrhages, thromboses, fever.

■ Diagnosis

Splenomegaly. Leukocytosis with immature cells. **Thrombocytosis. Anemia** with marked leukocytosis. Markedly decreased leukocyte alkaline phosphatase. Elevated uric acid, LDH, vitamin B$_{12}$, urinary lysozyme. **Myelofibrosis.** Enters a **blastic** or **accelerated phase** (myeloblastic or lymphoblastic) after 3 years in 80%.

■ Pathology

Bone marrow aspiration reveals hypercellular marrow, increase in eosinophils, basophils, megakaryocytes. Diagnosis confirmed by Philadelphia chromosome.

■ Treatment

May just **follow if asymptomatic** and white blood cells (WBC) < 50,000. For advancing disease, **hydroxyurea** the main drug, though cyclophosphamide and busulfan also effective. Acute leukostatic or thrombotic complications require immediate chemotherapy, leukapheresis, or plateletpheresis. Good hydration and allopurinol. Splenic radiation to reduce spleen size and white count. Treatment of blastic phase very difficult.

6–2. Chronic Lymphocytic Leukemia

■ Description

25% of all leukemias. Monoclonal proliferation of long-lived, usually B **lymphocytes.** Unknown etiology. May be asymptomatic. High incidence of **second malignancies.**

■ Symptoms

Asymptomatic lymphocytosis. **Adenopathy, splenomegaly.** Malaise, fatigue, weight loss, anorexia, fever, night sweats, bacterial infections; herpes zoster is common.

■ Diagnosis

Lymphocytosis, with >50% of small lymphs with round nuclei in the marrow. May need to do cell marker studies.

■ Pathology

Lymphocytosis can be massive. Anemia, thrombocytopenia, neutropenia. Coombs'-positive **autoimmune hemolytic anemia** is common.

■ Treatment

Should **avoid vaccination for smallpox and other viral illness. Treat only if progressive** and symptomatic. Chlorambucil (Leukeran). Corticosteroids for acute symptoms, hemolytic anemia, thrombocytopenia. Local radiotherapy to splenomegaly or massive adenopathy.

6-3. Hairy Cell Leukemia (Leukemic Reticuloendotheliosis)

■ Description

A chronic **B-cell leukemia;** 2% of all leukemias.

■ Symptoms

Of marrow suppression and hypersplenism.

■ Diagnosis

Progressive splenic enlargement. Pancytopenia. **Hairy cells** in blood and marrow. May need marrow biopsy.

■ Pathology

Medium to large lymphocyte with hairy projections. Surface monoclonal immunoglobulin.

■ Treatment

May observe, as it is slowly progressive. **Splenectomy** for progressive cytopenias. α-INTER-FERON (the treatment of choice) and pentostatin (2-deoxycoformycin) highly effective when relapse after splenectomy.

6–4. Mycosis Fungoides

■ Description

A **cutaneous T-cell lymphoma.** The Sézary syndrome is the leukemic form of mycosis fungoides.

■ Symptoms

Skin eruption with **appearance of eczema or psoriasis.**

■ Diagnosis

Multiple biopsies necessary.

■ Pathology

Prolonged course, beginning with **non-specific lesions** (premycotic stage) that slowly evolve into **cutaneous plaques and patches** (mycotic stage), and then into **ulcerative nodules and tumors** (tumor stage). May involve lymph nodes and internal organs later.

■ Treatment

Combination **chemotherapy** as in Hodgkin's disease.

6–5. Polycythemia Rubra Vera

■ Description

A myeloproliferative disease with excessive production of erythroid, myeloid, and megakary-ocytic elements, leading to in-creased red cell mass, throm-boses, and hemorrhages.

■ Symptoms

Headache, lightheadedness, ver-tigo, blurred vision, tinnitus, thromboses, hemorrhages, peptic ulcer disease, pruritis, severe foot pain.

■ Diagnosis

Plethora, cyanosis, **splenomeg-aly** in 75%, hepatomegaly in 40%. **Increased red cell mass** as-sociated with increase in all ele-ments. Normal oxygen satura-tion.

■ Pathology

Hypochromic, microcytic cells, low serum iron. Hematocrit > 60%. **Leukocytosis to leuke-moid** picture. Increased leuko-cyte alkaline phosphatase. High lysozyme. High B_{12} (> 900). Often marked **thrombocytosis** (> 400,000). Increased indirect bilirubin, increased LDH, in-creased uric acid. Marrow hy-perplastic; panmyelosis; marked megakaryocytic hyperplasia. **Ab-sent iron stores.**

■ Treatment

Prolongs survival and prevents thrombotic and hemorrhagic events. **Phlebotomy** to Hct < 45%. **Myelosuppression** with radioactive phosphorus or hy-droxyurea. Increased long-term risk of second malignancies, es-pecially with chlorambucil use.

B. Nervous System and Special Sense

1. Primary Neoplasms of the Brain

■ Description

Most common cancer in children. "Benign" brain tumors can be lethal. **Cerebral edema** is a major cause of morbidity.

■ Symptoms

Headache (morning), mental changes, generalized convulsions, papilledema (25%), vomiting, vasomotor/auto-nomic, hormonal changes.

■ Diagnosis

Use CT and magnetic resonance imag-ing (MRI) of head. Must distinguish from benign intracranial hypertension (non-focal), stroke (acute event), sub-dural hematoma, Alzheimer's.

■ Pathology

Types:

1. **Neuroectodermal** are the most common. These include **astrocy-toma** (more benign), **glioblas-toma multiforme** (more malig-nant).
2. **Mesodermal meningioma** (be-nign, though grow very large).
3. **Pituitary adenoma** and **cranio-pharyngioma.**
4. **Pineal** (produce endocrinopa-thies).
5. **Metastatic.**
6. **Vascular** arteriovenous malfor-mations (AVM), hemangioblas-tomas.

■ Treatment

Surgery for **cure** in meningioma, be-nign cerebellar tumors, or acoustic schwannomas. **Radiation** for malignant tumors. *Medical therapy:* **steroids** relieve edema; **anticonvulsants; chemotherapy.** *Metastatic tumor:* irradiation and steroids yield marked improvement in two thirds to three fourths.

2. Metastases to the Brain

■ Description

Most CNS tumors are metastatic. Brain metastases are from **lung** and **breast;** melanoma has high propensity to spread to brain.

■ Symptoms

Neurologic symptoms, seizures, headaches, motor weakness.

■ Diagnosis

Use **MRI, CT with contrast.** Distinguish from seizure, meningeal carcinomatosis, paraneoplastic syndrome. May need gadolinium MRI or repeat CT in 4 to 6 weeks to make diagnosis.

■ Treatment

Depends on primary and the extent of disease. Options include

1. **For solitary lesions, surgery and steroids.**
2. **For multiple metastases, irradiation (chemotherapy** for small-cell lung CA and testicular).

3. Leptomeningeal metastases

■ Description

About 8% of cancer patients develop meningeal spread. Most common are **Hodgkin's, leukemia, melanoma,** adenocarcinoma of **breast, lung,** and **GI tract.**

■ Symptoms

Headaches, altered mentation, cranial nerve defects, lumbosacral radiculopathies, seizures.

■ Diagnosis

Lumbar puncture (LP); (5 to 100 cells, increased protein, decreased glucose). **Positive cytology** (repeat LPs may be needed) to confirm diagnosis. The MRI, CT usually normal, but with contrast see diffuse enhancement.

■ Treatment

Cranial irradiation; intrathecal chemotherapy.

4. Acoustic Neuroma

■ Description

Schwannomas of eighth nerve.

■ Symptoms

Hearing loss, tinnitus, less often vertigo.

■ Diagnosis

Brainstem auditory-evoked responses (BAERs); CT or MRI with contrast.

■ Pathology

Composed of myelin-forming Schwann cells that cover the acoustic nerve fibers. Slow-growing masses that compress normal tissue.

■ Treatment

Microsurgery or **radiosurgery** yields 85 to 95% control rate.

5. Retinoblastoma

An **autosomal dominant hereditary** tumor of the retina. The most common intraocular tumor of children.

C. Circulatory System (Kaposi's Sarcoma; Kaposi's Hemorrhagic Sarcoma)

■ **Description**

Seen after **immunosuppressive therapy** and **HIV infection** (50% of homosexual men with AIDS).

■ **Symptoms**

Hemorrhagic **nodules** with violaceous, dark brown lesions. Before AIDS epidemic, was primarily on lower extremities. With AIDS, see **mucocutaneous and lymph node involvement.**

■ **Diagnosis**

Clinical picture; biopsy.

■ **Pathology**

Proliferation of mixed cell population, including endothelium; vascular appearance.

■ **Treatment**

α-**Interferon** yields 30 to 40% response rate, as does **vinblastine** and **doxorubicin.** Radiation helpful in localized lesions.

D. Respiratory System

1. Carcinoma of the Nasopharynx

■ **Description**

Risk factors include **alcohol, cigarettes.**

■ **Symptoms**

Pharyngitis, lymphoid hypertrophy, voice change, conductive hearing loss, dysphagia, odynophagia, halitosis, weight loss.

■ **Diagnosis**

Endoscopy, biopsy.

■ **Pathology**

Most common is **squamous cell.** Also lymphoma, lymphoepitheliomas (Schmincke's tumor), anaplastic carcinoma.

■ **Treatment**

Surgery, radiation.

2. Tumors of the Larynx (Malignant)

■ **Description**

Risk from **smoking** and **alcohol** synergistic.

■ **Symptoms**

Hoarseness, pain, dysphagia, odynophagia, cough, hemoptysis, halitosis.

■ **Diagnosis**

Direct laryngoscopy, pharyngoscopy, biopsy.

■ **Pathology**

Squamous cell carcinoma, neuroendocrine, salivary gland.

■ **Treatment**

Radiation, laryngectomy.

3. Tumors of the Larynx (Benign)

■ Symptoms

Hoarseness, later dyspnea, dysphagia, pain.

■ Diagnosis

Fiberoptic endoscopy.

■ Pathology

Papilloma (caused by papillomavirus), hemangioma, angiofibroma.

■ Treatment

Carbon dioxide laser (for papillomas).

4. Carcinoma of the Lung

■ Description

Produces 135,000 new cases per year in United States; 110,000 deaths. 80 to 90% associated with **smoking and passive smoke inhalation.** Occupational risks include **uranium, haloethers, arsenical fumes, asbestos. Asbestos and radon** (heavily insulated homes) may be cocarcinogens with cigarette smoke.

■ Symptoms

Cough, hemoptysis, weight loss, weakness, wheezing, fever, chest pain, superior vena cava (SVC) syndrome, Pancoast syndrome (superior sulcus tumor, with brachial plexus symptoms), and Horner's syndrome (sympathetic nerve involvement, with ptosis, meiosis).

■ Diagnosis

Chest x-ray (mass in lung; more in right lung and upper lobe). Need **tissue** via sputum cytology, bronchoscopic biopsy or brushings, trans-

bronchial biopsy or needle aspiration, thoracotomy. Screening chest x-rays are not of value in decreasing mortality.

■ Pathology

Four types make up 95%:

1. **Squamous cell**
2. **Adenocarcinoma**
3. **Large cell (large cell anaplastic)** and
4. **Small cell**

■ Treatment

Depends on stage and histology.

Non-small cell: TNM stage I and II: **surgery.**

Stage III: **surgery** and **irradiation.** Surgery results: 10 to 35% 5-year survival (squamous 37%, adeno 27%). Since very radiosensitive, give radiation therapy (XRT) in I, II, and III who do not have surgery. Unresectable (disseminated) non-small cell can be treated with XRT and **chemotherapy;** XRT also to palliate SVC syndrome, hemoptysis, cough, pain.

Chemotherapy: 30 to 40% response rate with **cisplatin** regimen.

Small cell lung cancer: very low survival. Treat with **chemotherapy** (very sensitive) and **irradiation.** Not a surgical disease. Useful programs include cyclophosphamide, methotrexate, lomustine (CCNU), doxorubicin, vincristine, and etoposide (VP-16). Radiation for palliation.

5. Metastases to the Lung

■ Description

Hematogenous and lymphatic spread.

■ Symptoms

Can be asymptomatic, dyspnea, chest pain, cough, cor pulmonale.

■ **Diagnosis**

Sputum cytology, bronchoscopy, thoracotomy.

■ **Treatment**

Treat the primary. Consider resection if solitary metastasis.

6. Mesothelioma

■ **Description**

Main primary pleural tumor. Benign or malignant. Malignant related to **asbestos** in 80 to 90%.

■ **Symptoms**

Cough, chest pain, dyspnea occur late.

■ **Diagnosis**

Malignant cells in pleural fluid or pleural biopsy.

■ **Pathology**

Benign associated with hypertrophic pulmonary osteoarthropathy and clubbing (responds to surgical removal).

■ **Treatment**

No known effective treatment. Prognosis very poor.

E. Digestive System

1. Salivary Gland Neoplasms

Most common is pleomorphic **adenoma** (benign). Malignancies include mucoepidermoid **carcinoma,** adenoid cystic carcinoma, adenocarcinoma.

■ **Symptoms**

Slow-growing mass leading to ulceration, invasion of nerves, numbness or facial paralysis.

2. Carcinoma of the Mouth

■ **Description**

Smoking and **alcohol** are risk factors. Tongue most common.

■ **Symptoms**

Painful indurated ulceration.

■ **Diagnosis**

Biopsy.

■ **Pathology**

Mostly **squamous,** with 20% chance of a **second head and neck cancer.**

■ **Treatment**

Radiation and surgery in combination can be curative. **Chemotherapy** in more advanced cases (methotrexate, bleomycin, cisplatin). Rehabilitation and prostheses important; 50% survival rate.

3. Carcinoma of the Esophagus

■ **Description**

Smoking and alcohol are risk factors.

■ **Symptoms**

Progressive **dysphagia,** steady, boring pain, halitosis, weight loss, cough after drinking fluid.

■ **Diagnosis**

Esophagogram, endoscopy with biopsy and brushings, CT of chest, chest x-ray.

■ **Pathology**

Squamous (more common; associated with head and neck cancer, lye strictures, inadequately treated achalasia).

Adenocarcinoma arises in columnar (Barrett's) epithelium (reflux esophagitis).

■ Treatment

Generally poor prognosis. Surgery: much morbidity. 5 to 6% 5-year survival with surgery or irradiation. Slightly better with combined modality.

4. *Carcinoma of the Stomach*

■ Description

Majority are malignant; 5% are lymphomas.

Decreasing in the United States. Common in Japan. Low incidence where colorectal cancer is high. Dietary factors may be important (nitrosamines). Vitamin C and refrigeration may cause decrease in gastric CA in United States. Other risk factors: blood group A, atrophic gastritis, pernicious anemia, adenomatous polyps, subtotal gastric resection for benign disease, immunologic deficiencies.

■ Symptoms

Early are asymptomatic. **Anorexia, weight loss, early satiety,** bloating, dysphagia, epigastric pain, vomiting.

■ Diagnosis

Epigastric mass, Virchow's node (left supraclavicular), Blumer's shelf. Recurrent thrombophlebitis (Trousseau syndrome), acanthosis nigricans. Air-contrast UGI x-rays. Endoscopy with biopsy and brush cytology.

■ Pathology

Usually **adenocarcinoma.** Spread to esophagus, liver, pancreas, transverse colon, lung, brain, bone.

■ Treatment

Surgery for cure or palliation. **Chemotherapy** for unresectable disease: 5-FU, doxorubicin (Adriamycin), mitomycin-C in combination (FAM). **Radiotherapy.**

5. *Carcinoma of the Pancreas*

■ Description

Slowly progressive, **highly malignant. Second most common GI tumor after colon.** Risk factors include smoking, high-fat, high-meat diet, exposure to manufacturing of paper, oil refining, gasoline.

■ Symptoms

Epigastric pain, weight loss, vomiting, hematemesis, melena, jaundice, palpable mass, palpable gallbladder (Courvoisier's sign), thrombophlebitis, psychiatric disturbances, diabetes, anemia, blood in stool, silver stools.

■ Diagnosis

Ultrasound and/or CT, followed by **needle aspiration.** If negative, ERCP (very sensitive and tissue for cytology helpful). The UGI is poor in early detection. Occasional amylase elevation.

■ Pathology

Usually adenocarcinoma. Occasionally endocrine tumors (apudomas and carcinoids).

■ Treatment

Usually non-resectable. Options: **surgery, chemotherapy,** and **radiation,** but **results are generally poor. Whipple's resection** (pancreaticoduodenectomy) for small focal mass lesions. High operative mortality; 5% 5-year survival. Chemotherapy of little value.

Some improved survival with radiation.

6. Carcinoma of the Biliary System

■ Description
Results of 70 to 80% in patients with cholelithiasis.

■ Symptoms
Obstructive jaundice, acute cholecystitis, palpable mass, right upper quadrant (RUQ) pain, or disseminated carcinoma.

■ Diagnosis
Ultrasound. Must distinguish from cholesterol polyp or stone.

■ Pathology
Adenocarcinoma.

■ Treatment
Surgery; 5% 5-year survival, even with optimal surgery.

7. Carcinoma of the Liver

■ Description
Uncommon, but **increasing in United States.** In parts of Asia, Africa, and Greece it is among the most common of malignant tumors. Usually in a **cirrhotic liver** (associated with **hemochromatosis** or **hepatitis** C and occasionally B). Also associated with **aflatoxins** from *Aspergillus flavus* (peanuts and grains).

■ Symptoms
Abdominal pain, mass, weight loss, deterioration of patient with cirrhosis.

■ Diagnosis
Ultrasound. Technetium 99m-sulfur colloid **scan.** Tumor "staining" on angiography. Elevated alkaline phosphatase and transaminase. **Needle biopsy, wedge biopsy** at laparotomy.

■ Pathology
Usually **hepatocellular carcinoma.**

■ Treatment
Median survival 6 months. **Hepatic resection** effective if early. **Chemotherapy** with doxorubicin (Adriamycin), 5-FU, cisplatin regimens yield 50% response rate, but minimal survival advantage.

8. Metastases to the Liver

Most hepatic tumors are **metastatic** in adults. Mostly stomach, colon, pancreas.

9. Carcinoma of the Colon

■ Description
A **disease of developed countries. Risk factors** include increased fat, animal protein, decreased fiber, increasing age, inflammatory bowel disease, family history of female genital or breast CA, history of colonic cancer or adenoma (especially villous adenomas), history of familial colon cancer syndromes (familial polyposis, Gardner syndrome, Peutz–Jeghers syndrome, generalized juvenile polyposis).

■ Symptoms
Silent; **bleeding,** obstruction, **change in bowel habits,** pain, symptoms of localized perforation. Right-side le-

sions rarely obstruct. Left-side poly-poid lesions cause diarrhea and sign of obstruction.

■ Diagnosis

In suspected case, **digital rectal exam** followed by **sigmoidoscopy,** and then **barium enema** or **colonoscopy.** Brushings and/or biopsy. Must distinguish from angiodysplasia, diverticulosis, benign tumors.

■ Pathology

About **60% occur from splenic flexure down.**

■ Treatment

Surgery with curative intent. **Radiation** preoperatively or for recurrent disease. **Chemotherapy** for metastatic disease (especially liver) with 5-FU. Evidence for effectiveness of adjuvant chemo in Duke's C colon carcinoma with 5-FU and levamisole. Follow with colonoscopy, carcinoembryonic antigen (CEA) (not good for screening).

■ Screening

See *American Cancer Society Recommendations for the Early Detection of Cancer in Asymptomatic People,* p. 97. High-risk patients require annual sigmoidoscopy beginning at puberty.

10. Carcinoma of the Rectum

If below the peritoneal reflection, it commonly recurs and postop radiation + 5-FU is recommended. Anal: chemotherapy + radiation is better than surgery.

11. Carcinoid Tumors

■ Description

Tumors that arise from **enterochromaffin cells** (Kulchitsky) and **produce biologically active amines and peptides** (serotonin, bradykinin, histamine, prostaglandins).

■ Symptoms

Cutaneous **flushing** (precipitated by alcohol, food, stress), facial telangiectasias, tachycardia and decreased blood pressure, headache after the flush, **diarrhea,** symptoms from peritoneal fibrosis, right-sided endocardial fibrosis (with congestive heart failure [CHF]). Bronchoconstriction and wheezing less common.

■ Diagnosis

Clinical suspicion; markedly **increased urinary 5-hydroxyindoleacetic acid (5-HIAA)** hepatomegaly. Of less help are CT, ultrasound, scans.

■ Pathology

Arise in ileum and metastasize to the liver. Excrete **serotonin** and 5-HIAA. Other carcinoids arise in appendix, rectum, stomach, bile duct, and so on.

■ Treatment

No treatment for mild symptoms. Symptomatic treatment (antidiarrheal agents, bronchodilators, nutritional support, for syndrome symptoms. Chemotherapy for the tumor. Surgery for obstruction and intussusception. Less than 5-year survival.

12. Polyps

■ **Description**

Importance: **bleeding** or **malignant potential.**

■ **Symptoms**

Asymptomatic, bleeding, pain, diarrhea.

■ **Diagnosis**

Endoscopy, biopsy.

■ **Pathology**

Four main types:

1. **Hyperplastic**—(majority of rectal polyps; not considered neoplastic).
2. **Tubular adenomas.**
3. **Villous adenomas**—(neoplastic; villous have high malignant transformation rate than tubular).
4. **Mixed type**—cancer rate much higher in larger polyps.

■ **Treatment**

Removal. Follow with colonoscopies.

13. Polyposis Syndromes

a. Familial polyposis. Autosomal dominant; will nearly all develop carcinoma.

■ **Treatment**

Subtotal colectomy.

b. *Gardner syndrome.* Dominantly transmitted; associated with bone tumors (osteomas), and soft tissue tumors (lipomas, sebaceous cysts, fibromas, fibrosarcomas); high malignant potential.

■ **Treatment**

Subtotal colectomy.

c. *Munro syndrome.* Colon adenomas plus central nervous system tumors; high malignant potential.
d. *Peutz–Jeghers syndrome.* Autosomal dominant; polyps plus mucocutaneous hyperpigmentation; low malignant potential.
e. *Generalized juvenile polyposis.* Autosomal dominant; hamartomas; possible increased carcinoma incidence.

F. Endocrine and Reproductive Systems

1. Pituitary Adenoma

■ **Description**

Form 90% of all pituitary tumors; **most are functioning; benign,** but may have aggressive growth pattern.

■ **Symptoms**

Variable **headaches, visual disturbances** (blindness, optic atrophy), temperature instability, hyperphagia, emotional disturbance, disturbed sleep patterns, hypopituitarism, hypogonadism.

■ **Diagnosis**

Enlarged sella by x-ray, **mass** on CT or MRI, visual fields, visual evoked response.

■ **Pathology**

Solid, with well-defined capsule.

■ **Treatment**

Transsphenoidal pituitary **surgery.** Optionally, can **irradiate.**

2. Thyroid Nodules and Cancer

2–1. Benign Nodules

■ Description

About 96% are benign.

■ Symptoms

Asymptomatic. Large functioning adenomas produce hyperthyroidism.

■ Diagnosis

Needle aspiration.

■ Pathology

Adenomas. Functioning nodules are very rarely carcinomas. Many cannot concentrate iodine and are "cold" nodules; 90% do not produce significant hormone.

■ Treatment

Follow *warm* (non-clinically thyrotoxic) nodules with **annual thyroid function tests (TFTs).** *Hot* (clinically toxic) nodules are treated with **surgery** or **radioactive iodine.**

2–2. Thyroid Cancer

■ Description

Risk factors include **childhood exposure to radiation,** and **heredity;** 11,000 cases per year; 1000 deaths; 3 to 4% of solitary thyroid nodules are cancer.

■ Symptoms

Thyroid nodule; symptoms of local invasion.

■ Diagnosis

Needle aspiration may reduce the need for surgery by 60%. Optionally, thyroid scanning and ultrasound, or thyroxine to suppress thyroid stimulating hormone (TSH).

■ Pathology

May occur as part of familial thyroid carcinoma (multiple endocrine neoplasia [MEN] Type II and III). *Four histologic types:*

1. **Papillary**—(the most benign and the most common; pathognomonic is the **psammoma body).**
2. **Follicular.**
3. **Medullary**—(produces calcitonin).
4. **Poorly differentiated**—(the most highly malignant).

■ Treatment

Needle aspiration; surgical resection (if hypo- or euthyroid) or **radiation therapy** with ^{131}I (if hyperfunctional); **thyroxine suppression;** irradiation and chemotherapy for thyroid lymphoma.

3. Adrenal Neoplasms

3–1. Cushing Syndrome

■ Description

A rare syndrome, due to primary adrenal tumor secreting cortisol (accounts for 15% of Cushing's).

■ Symptoms

Abdominal mass. **Obesity, plethora, hirsutism,** menstrual disorders, **hypertension, weakness** (hypokalemia), back pain (from osteopenia), **striae, acne,** depression, bruising.

■ Diagnosis

Use **24-hour urine free cortisol;** overnight 1 mg **dexamethasone-suppression test;** basal plasma ACTH levels. Tumor localization with CT and ultrasonography.

■ Pathology

Adenoma and carcinoma equally. Spread to liver and lung.

■ Treatment

Adrenalectomy, followed by **mitotane** for residual or non-resectable carcinoma. Alternately, metyrapone and aminoglutethimide. **Steroid replacement** therapy.

3–2. Pheochromocytoma

■ Description

Catecholamine-producing tumors that cause **hypertension.** Importance:

1. **The hypertension can be lethal.**

2. **The tumor may be carcinoma.**

3. The tumor could be part of a MEN (multiple endocrine neoplasia syndrome 1 or 2).

■ Symptoms

Headache, palpitations, diaphoresis that are **paroxysmal and associated with hypertension.**

■ Diagnosis

Clinical suspicion and **biochemical tests (plasma catecholamines** [norepinephrine and epinephrine]); unconjugated catecholamines, total metanephrines, or vanillylmandelic acid (VMA) in urine; study when drug-free and stress-free. CT scanning to localize. Radioisotope scanning of some help.

■ Pathology

Arise from chromaffin cells, usually adrenal medulla. Most release norepinephrine.

■ Treatment

Surgical removal preceded by 10 days of alpha-adrenergic antagonist (eg, prazosin).

4. Uterine Tumors

4–1. Fibroids (Leiomyoma)

About 25% of women have these. Most are asymptomatic.

■ Treatment

If excessive menstrual bleeding, significant pain, excessive size, or rapid growth, preferred treatment is **hysterectomy. Myomectomy** an option in young women.

4–2. Endometrial Carcinoma

■ Description

Only 40% is detected with Pap test. **High-risk women need annual endometrial sampling.** Postmenopausal bleeding requires endometrial sampling. *Risk factors:* estrogens, obesity, nulliparous state increase the risk. Combination oral contraceptives and sequential contraceptives reduce the risk.

■ **Pathology**

Adenoacanthoma; adenocarcinoma, secretory. Tumor markers: LASA (lipid-associated sialic acid); CA-125; NB/70K.

■ **Treatment**

Stage I: **wide total abdominal hysterectomy (TAH), bilateral salpingo-oophorectomy (BSO), pelvic node sampling,** possibly followed by ^{32}P intraperitoneally or **irradiation.**

5. Carcinoma of the Cervix and Cervical Dysplasia

■ **Description**

Risk factors are **multiparity, multiple sexual partners, human papillomavirus.**

■ **Symptoms**

Asymptomatic, bleeding, discharge.

■ **Diagnosis**

Pap smears. Should **do Pap every 3 years after two negative Paps done at yearly intervals** (annually if more than one sexual partner).

■ **Treatment**

Carcinoma-in-situ and superficial disease: endocervical **cone biopsy.** Microinvasive: **abdominal hysterectomy.** Advanced local: **radiation + surgery.** Metastatic: **cisplatin-based chemotherapy.**

6. Carcinoma of the Ovary

■ **Description**

Functioning tumors may cause reproductive abnormalities or altered sexual development. All ages, though usually postmenopausal.

■ **Symptoms**

Most are asymptomatic; bladder and rectal pressure symptoms; ascites, pain; periods of amenorrhea and excess vaginal bleeding; pseudopuberty; postmenopausal bleeding.

■ **Diagnosis**

Usually found on routine pelvic exam.

■ **Treatment**

Staging and treatment includes **abdominal hysterectomy, bilateral oophorectomy, lymph node sampling, omentectomy, peritoneal cytology and tumor removal.** Chemotherapy postop if tumor outside the ovary. Follow response with CA-125 marker; "second look" laparotomy to restage and debulk. Chemotherapy for residual tumor (cisplatin-based).

7. Carcinoma of the Vulva

Must biopsy early to help.

8. Neoplasms of the Vagina

Female offspring of women given **diethylstilbestrol** during pregnancy may get adenosis of vagina and have increased risk of vaginal cancer (adenocarcinoma, clear cell type).

9. Carcinoma of the Breast

■ **Description**

From 120,000 to 130,000 new cases per year; 11% of women will get it; 85% are older than 40 years old. *Risk factors:* prior breast cancer, family history, early menarche, late menopause, late or no pregnancy; moderate alcohol intake; radiation exposure; western society diet. Oral contraceptives do not increase the risk, nor does estrogen given for osteoporosis.

■ Symptoms

Painless lump. Hard, irregular mass, skin dimpling, or nipple retraction.

■ Diagnosis

Screening. See *American Cancer Society Recommendations for the Early Detection of Cancer in Asymptomatic People*, p. 97.

■ Diagnosis

Mammograms (90% accuracy), **fine-needle biopsy, excisional biopsy.**

■ Pathology

Assume distant metastases. Size of tumor, and presence of axillary nodes correlates with risk of recurrence. The presence of estrogen receptors (ER) and progesterone receptors (PR) indicates better prognosis. About 80% are infiltrating ductal; others are infiltrating lobular, medullary, comedocarcinoma, colloid carcinoma.

■ Treatment

Two steps: outpatient fine-needle biopsy or excisional biopsy under local; discuss options and do definitive treatment.

> *Stage I and II disease*—local resection (tylectomy [lumpectomy and axillary node dissection] or modified radical) followed by irradiation if local recurrence likely. Adjuvant chemotherapy if axillary metastases.
> *Lobular*—might do "mirror-image biopsy" rather than prophylactic mastectomy of opposite breast.
> *Resectable stage III*—do mastectomy.
> *Unresectable stage III* or **inflammatory** breast carcinoma—give chemotherapy followed by irradiation (and possible resection).

Stage IV (metastatic)—hormonal (bone, soft tissue, and mild pulmonary spread respond) or **chemotherapy** (liver, brain, and extensive lung).

9–1. Premenopausal

> If ER-positive, **hormonal** therapy with **tamoxifen** or oophorectomy; adrenalectomy or hypophysectomy. If ER-negative or refractory to endocrine therapy, **chemotherapy** (combinations produce 60 to 70% response, 10 to 15% complete remission) with such drugs as cyclophosphamide, 5-FU, methotrexate, vincristine, doxorubicin, and mitomycin-C.

9–2. Postmenopausal

> Tamoxifen if PR-positive; chemotherapy if resistant to hormone.
> *Adjuvant chemotherapy.* NIH Consensus says adjuvant chemotherapy (6 cycles) and hormonal therapy (tamoxifen) are effective in axillary node-positive patients (especially if ER+); optimal treatment has not been defined; should enroll patients in trials.
> *Follow response to therapy with CEA*

10. Gestational Trophoblastic Disease

■ Description

Proliferative trophoblastic growth that develops from pregnancy, usually from **molar pregnancy. Most choriocarcinomas are metastatic, most commonly to lungs.**

■ Symptoms

Abnormal **vaginal bleeding,** anemia, uterine enlargement, toxemia of pregnancy, hyperemesis gravidarum.

- **Diagnosis**

Workup should include human chorionic gonadotropin **(hCG) levels,** chest x-ray, ultrasound of abdomen, pelvis, and liver.

- **Pathology**

Includes the hydatidiform mole, invasive mole, choriocarcinoma. About 15% of mole pregnancies show localized uterine invasion.

- **Treatment**

Treat with **evacuation of pregnancy** and/or **chemotherapy** (methotrexate, actinomycin-D). Treat until hCG is normal; 100% cure rate in stages I to III, 85% in IV.

11. Neoplasms of Testes

11–1. Non-seminomatous

- **Description**

Germ cell tumors that include embryonal cell carcinomas, choriocarcinomas, and teratomas.

- **Symptoms**

Painless testicular **mass.** May have dyspnea, abdominal or back pain, gynecomastia, supraclavicular adenopathy, or ureteral obstruction.

- **Diagnosis**

Stage with CXR, CT chest and abdomen, AFP, β-hCG.

- **Treatment**

Inguinal orchiectomy and **retroperitoneal lymph node dissection** for staging and initial treatment, followed by **cisplatin-based aggressive chemotherapy**

combinations. Stage A and B: 99% cure rates. Stage C: 70% cure rate. **The** *preferred* **induction chemotherapy:** PVB-16B (PVB + etoposide) yields 83% CR. Radioresistant.

11–2. Seminoma

- **Description**

Rare; most are malignant, derived from germ cells, 20 to 35 years old. *Risk factor* is cryptorchidism.

- **Diagnosis**

Evaluate with alpha-fetoprotein (AFP), beta subunit of human chorionic gonadotropin (β-hCG), CT of abdomen and pelvis, possible lymphangiogram.

- **Treatment**

Radiosensitive. Inguinal orchiectomy and radiation produce 80 to 95% cure rates. If increased AFP, treat like non-seminomatous germ cell tumor (GCT).

G. Kidney and Urinary System

1. Hypernephroma (Renal Cell Carcinoma, Renal Adenocarcinoma, Grawitz's Tumor, Nephrocarcinoma)

- **Description**

Risk factors include pipe and cigar smoking, and maleness.

- **Symptoms**

Gross or microscopic **hematuria, flank pain, abdominal mass.** Symptoms of paraneoplastic syndrome (fever, hypertension, anemia, hepatic dysfunction [Stauffer syndrome]). Many unusual symptoms.

■ Diagnosis

Intravenous pyelogram (IVP), ultrasound, CT. Rule out renal vein thrombus complication.

■ Pathology

Three histologic types.

■ Treatment

Stage I, II, and IIIA require **radical nephrectomy** and yield 50 to 70% 5-year survival. No significant benefit from radiation, chemotherapy (including adjuvant) or immunotherapy, though progestational agents (medroxyprogesterone) produce regression (15 to 30% response rate) in metastatic disease. *Newer therapies:* **interferon** and **LAK cells** (created with interleukin-2) may yield 30 to 80% response rate.

2. Wilms' Tumor (Nephroblastoma)

■ Description

Most are under 4 years old.

■ Symptoms

Palpable mass, pain, hematuria, hypertension.

■ Diagnosis

Intravenous pyelogram (IVP), ultrasound or CT. Must distinguish from neuroblastoma (with urinary VMA).

■ Pathology

About 80% are localized and resectable.

■ Treatment

Limited disease: **surgery + chemotherapy** (doxorubicin, actinomycin D, vincristine) yields 85% disease-free

survival. Advanced disease: **irradiation + chemotherapy.**

3. Carcinoma of the Bladder

■ Description

About 49,000 new cases per year; men predominate. Chemical carcinogens are implicated (including those in cigarette smoke).

■ Symptoms

Hematuria, bladder irritability (frequency, dysuria).

■ Diagnosis

Cystoscopy and transurethral bladder **biopsy.**

■ Pathology

Transitional cell. Rarely squamous if *Schistosoma haematobium* infestation.

■ Treatment

Stage A: transurethral resection of bladder tumor (TURBT). **Cystoscopic surveillance** for multiple recurrences. **Intravesical chemotherapy:** thiotepa, doxorubicin, mitomycin-C, or BCG. *Stage B and C:* **pelvic lymphadenectomy and radical cystectomy.** *Metastatic disease:* **chemotherapy** (vinblastine, methotrexate, and cisplatin, with or without doxorubicin).

4. Benign Prostatic Hyperplasia

■ Description

The most common male neoplasm. Symptomatic in 50 to 75% of men older than 50.

■ Symptoms

Decreased caliber and force of stream, hesitancy, trouble stopping, postvoid dribbling, sense of incomplete empty-ing, urinary retention. Nocturia.

■ Diagnosis

Symptoms, rectal exam, urinalysis, culture, serum creatinine, prostate specific antigen or acid phosphatase. Intravenous pyelogram and cystoscopy.

■ Treatment

Initially usually just **observe. Surgery transurethral prostatic resection (TURP) for significant obstructive complications.** *New agent:* Finasteride shrinks gland, but clinical improvement in < 50% of patients.

5. Carcinoma of the Prostate

■ Description

Second leading cancer cause in males. No relationship to benign prostatic hypertrophy (BPH); little relationship to smoking or alcohol. Of 30,000 deaths per year, 30 to 50% of men older than 50 have at least a focus of adenocarcinoma of prostate.

■ Symptoms

Asymptomatic early, urinary retention symptoms, bone pain.

■ Diagnosis

Digital rectal exam, transrectal prostatitic ultrasound (TRUS), confirmation with transurethral ultrasound (TRUS)-guided **needle biopsy.** If positive, do **prostate specific antigen (PSA),** IVP, bone scan.

■ Pathology

About 50% of prostate nodules are malignant; **95% are adenocarcinomas.** Bone metastases common (pelvis,

lumbar spine, femurs, thoracic spine, ribs); lung and liver metastases the most common visceral spread.

■ Treatment

A1. Observation and rebiopsy.

A2 and B1. **Radical prostatectomy** if older than 70.

B2 and C. **TURP followed by radiation** (40% post-XRT impotence; 2% incontinence).

D (metastatic). **Hormonal therapy** (orchiectomy or LHRH analog or DES), which should be delayed until symptoms appear. **Chemotherapy** if hormone independent (investigational now).

Treating complications. **Radiation** for pain; **transfusion** for anemia.

After treatment. Follow with periodic digital rectal exam (DRE) and PSA.

H. Skin and Musculoskeletal Systems

1. Actinic Keratosis

■ Description

Precancerous lesions of atypical keratinocytes due to **sun injury. May evolve into squamous cell CA.**

■ Symptoms

Red, poorly marginated macules and papules with yellow-brown scales in sun-damaged skin.

■ Diagnosis

Biopsy.

■ Treatment

Liquid nitrogen or **topical 5-FU.**

2. Basal Cell Carcinoma

■ **Description**

Carcinoma of skin arising from the basal cell layer. Related to amount of ultraviolet and x-irradiation exposed to over one's life.

■ **Symptoms**

Opalescent waxy nodule, often ulcerated on exposed areas. Extensive local destruction, but rarely metastasize.

■ **Diagnosis**

Biopsy.

■ **Treatment**

Removal or destruction (curettage, electrodessication, scalpel excision, radiotherapy, cryotherapy). **Mohs' surgery,** a new technique used when recurrence likely.

3. Squamous Cell Carcinoma

■ **Description**

Malignant neoplasm of the keratinocytes. Ultraviolet light and x-irradiation are risk factors. More aggressive than basal cell CA (BCC) and may metastasize.

■ **Symptoms**

Hard, smooth, or verrucous nodules that often show hyperkeratinization.

■ **Diagnosis**

Biopsy.

■ **Treatment**

Removal.

4. Melanoma

■ **Description**

Cutaneous neoplasm of melanocytes and nevus cells. Sunlight and heredity (dysplastic nevus syndrome) may be risk factors.

■ **Symptoms**

Flat to nodular pigmented lesions.

■ **Diagnosis**

ABCDs = A (asymmetry), B (borders are irregular), C (color variegated), D (diameter > 6 mm). **Biopsy.**

■ **Pathology**

Several clinical presentations. One third arise from existing nevi ("the changing nevus"). Metastases more common with greater depth.

■ **Treatment**

Early disease—**surgery alone** (no added value from radiation or chemotherapy).

Metastatic disease—**chemotherapy,** yield 10 to 30% response rate.

5. Pigmented Nevi

■ **Description**

Benign accumulations of pigment-forming nevus cells. Appear early in life.

■ **Symptoms**

Uniformly pigmented, flat to nodular, symmetrical lesions.

■ **Diagnosis**

Appearance. Do not fit the ABCDs of melanoma, but **changing nevi are suspect.**

■ **Pathology**

Three forms: junctional nevi, compound nevi, intradermal nevi.

■ **Treatment**

None.

6. Hemangioma

■ **Description**

Benign proliferations of dermal vessels.

■ **Symptoms**

Flat to nodular, soft, red, blue, purple lesions.

■ **Pathology**

Small superficial vessels produce nevus flammeus and strawberry hemangiomas. Larger vessels produce cavernous hemangiomas.

■ **Treatment**

Many involute on their own and require no therapy. Rarely, cavernous hemangiomas consume platelets and cause the **Kasabach–Merritt syndrome.**

7. Osteosarcoma

■ **Description**

Arise from mesenchymal tissue. Uncommon; mostly in the young.

■ **Symptoms**

Pain, limitation of movement, swelling.

■ **Diagnosis**

Bone destruction and soft tissue mass. High alkaline phosphatase.

■ **Pathology**

Metastatic to lungs early. Aggressive.

■ **Treatment**

Wide excision (amputation) followed by **adjuvant chemotherapy** for 1 year, and resect isolated pulmonary metastases. *Metastatic disease:* good responses to chemotherapy (doxorubicin, high-dose methotrexate with citrovorum rescue, cisplatin, ifosfamide, decarbazine [DTIC]).

8. Metastases to Bone

High rate from **breast, lung, prostate, kidney, thyroid.** Metastatic more common than primary bone. **Bone scans** very sensitive in detection. Prostate 90% blastic; breast 50% blastic; lung 25% blastic. *Treatment:* **radiation;** open reduction and internal fixation of threatened or fractured bone.

I. Head and Neck Tumors

■ **Description**

Risk factors: tobacco and alcohol. Premalignant lesions include leukoplakia, erythroplakia.

■ **Pathology**

Usually squamous (epidermoid). Oral 44%; laryngeal 32%.

■ **Treatment**

Surgery and/or **irradiation.** Chemotherapy for palliation. *Advanced disease:* high response rates seen with chemotherapy (to include cisplatin and 5-FU).

BIBLIOGRAPHY

Brain MC, Carbone PP. *Current Therapy in Hematology–Oncology.* 4th ed. Philadelphia, Pa: BC Decker; 1992.

DeVita VT Jr, Hellman S, Rosenberg S. *Cancer: Principles and Practices of Oncology.* Philadelphia, Pa: Lippincott; 1989.

Larsen PR. The thyroid. In: Wyngaarden JB, Smith LH, Bennett JC, eds. *Cecil Textbook of Medicine.* 19th ed. Philadelphia, Pa: WB Saunders Co; 1992. Algorithm for Diagnostic Evaluation of Solitary Thyroid Nodule: Figure 216–10, p 1268.

Levin B, Murphy GP. Revision in American Cancer Society recommendations for the early detection of colorectal cancer. *CA-A Cancer Journal for Clinicians.* 1992;42(5):296–299.

Schein PS. *Decision Making in Oncology.* Toronto, Canada: BC Decker; 1989.

Williams WJ, Beutler E, Erster A (eds). *Hematology.* 4th ed. New York: McGraw-Hill; 1990.

Wilson JD, Braunwald E, Isselbacher KJ, et al. *Harrison's Principles of Internal Medicine.* 12th ed. New York: McGraw-Hill, Inc; 1991.

Woodley M, Whelan A. *Manual of Medical Therapeutics.* 27th ed. Boston, Mass: Little, Brown and Co; 1992.

Wyngaarden JB, Smith LH, Bennett JC. *Cecil Textbook of Medicine.* 19th ed. Philadelphia, Pa: WB Saunders Co; 1992.

CHAPTER 7

Immunology and Allergy

JOEL S. GOLDBERG, DO

I. HEALTH AND HEALTH MAINTENANCE

A. Epidemiology and Prevention of Food and Drug Reactions

■ **Description**

General information:

> Type 1 hypersensitivity reaction: anaphylaxis. *IgE mediated*
>
> Type 2 hypersensitivity reaction: cytotoxic-antibody (drug and transfusion reactions).
>
> Type 3 hypersensitivity reaction: immune complex (serum sickness, glomerulonephritis).
>
> Type 4 hypersensitivity reaction: cell mediated (delayed hypersensitivity, contact dermatitis).

1. Epidemiology

Includes a wide range of reactions (minimal to anaphylactic) to any food, medication, or foreign substance. No increased incidence by gender or geographic location. Shellfish, nuts, and milk products are common offenders (drugs include antibiotics, vaccines, hormones, dyes, and allergic extracts; foreign substances include venom from *Hymenoptera* insects).

> Allergic (eosinophilic) gastroenteropathy—rate disorder of immunoglobulin E (IgE) production and rapid-onset food allergy (nausea/vomiting, etc).
>
> Anaphylactic reactions—IgE antibody mediated (type 1), widespread organ disorder.
>
> Contact dermatitis—mediated via T-cell hypersensitivity.
>
> Drug reaction—mediated via IgE (penicillin anaphylaxis), T cell (contact dermatitis), immune complex (serum sickness), or cytotoxic-antibody systems (nephritis and Coombs'-positive hemolytic anemia).

2. Prevention

Includes allergy testing and allergen avoidance or desensitization. Accurate history taking and skin testing prior to medication use are important. Testing includes wheal-and-flare skin testing and radioallergosorbent test (RAST) serum testing. Patients with known allergies are advised to wear Medic Alert bracelets. Medical facility protocols to avoid drug allergy reactions, transfusion reactions, and so on. Use of preventive medication when risk of allergic reaction is significant (prednisone/benadryl prior to contrast dye injection).

B. HIV Infections and AIDS

1. Epidemiology

RNA retrovirus human immunodeficiency virus (HIV)-induced pandemic (possible 15 to 20% population infected in Africa, and cases throughout the world), with increased frequency in blacks/Hispanics (compared to population figures), and pockets of increased frequency among drug users noted (New York). Adult risk of infection by transfusions (including blood, blood products, factor VIII, needle sharing), broken skin/mucosal exposure, and vaginal/anal intercourse. Newborns and children by birth most often (infected mother), child abuse, *?* and blood products.

2. Impact

A significant public health concern with increasing frequency of reported acquired immunodeficiency syndrome (AIDS) cases (about 200 in 1982, about 82,000 in 1989), with resulting impact (medical, financial, social/psychological, legal) on the patients, the patient's families, the health care system (including social service, home health, and foster care systems), and the insurance industry.

AIDS remains 100% fatal (no vaccine/cure).

3. Screening

Screening includes detection of HIV infection by a ELISA (enzyme-linked immunosorbent assay), and confirmation by Western blot.

Screening of high-risk patients and blood products/blood donors is critical. Screening via voluntary screening sites, and by most insurance companies for life insurance policies, is in effect. Universal premarital or populace screening may prove costly, with low yield and increased false-positive reports.

United States blood donation centers began screening in March, 1985. Minimal transfusion-related HIV/AIDS risk remains, due to seronegative period between exposure to HIV and blood positivity detection (screening/refusing high-risk donors will help).

4. Prevention

Cornerstone is **education** (including safe sex, and effective use of condoms, types of high-risk behavior). Special effort to address high-risk groups (homosexuals, intravenous (IV) drug users/parenteral exposure, prostitutes, promiscuous individuals, hemophiliacs, partners of high-risk individuals) are needed. Education and regulation to protect health care workers and their patients (decontamination, gloves, reduction of needlesticks). Screening will provide both patient education/treatment and partner tracing/treatment. Distribution of condoms and bleach has been attempted. Distribution of sterile needles has been proposed. Medication zidovudine (AZT) to delay/improve HIV-related disease and AIDS. Vaccine under development.

C. Prevention of Newborn Hemolytic Disease

■ Description

Also termed **erythroblastosis fetalis**. Fetal **red blood cell antigens attacked by maternal immunoglobulin G (IgG)** (isoimmune disease) or **anti-A** or **anti-B** (ABO disease) **antibodies,** after transplacental passage.

Prevention includes maternal testing for **type, Rh, and antibody screen;** $Rh_o(D)$ immune globulin (RhoGAM) injection; more accurate screening for maternal sensitization/fetal disease (amniocentesis), with intervention (labor induction) as necessary.

Give Rh immune globulin injection for Rh-negative mothers (give at 28 weeks, within 3 days of delivery, and after bleeding or amniocentesis). *[handwritten: also in ectopic pregnancy]* If baby has positive Rh, give the mother another dose of Rh immune globulin after birth. Standard dose: 1 mL (300 mcg), will counteract 10 mL antigenic fetal cells.

Kleihauer test: determines amount of fetal cells in maternal serum. Perform after traumatic delivery to determine amount of Rh immune globulin to give.

D. Prevention of Transfusion Reactions

■ Description

Usually ABO incompatibility. Prevention includes proper blood-bank specimen handling and technique, along with accurate patient and specimen identification. Other factors include close patient observation during transfusion (major hemolytic reactions occur early during transfusion), and observation of the blood itself (abnormal color may indicate bacterial contamination).

Patient history of atopy or asthma may predispose to allergic transfusion reactions, so additional caution/observation is indicated. Pretransfusion treatment with antihistamines may be of value, along with the use of washed erythrocytes.

Patient history of multiple transfusions or pregnancies may predispose to febrile transfusion reactions. May try infusing leukocyte-depleted infusions (donor leukocyte antigens may result in the reaction).

Patient history and examination will assist in dictating rate and amount of volume to be infused (thus avoiding congestive heart failure).

E. Immunization

Passive (antibodies given for short-acting protection) or **active** (antigen given).

1. Infants and Children

[handwritten left margin:]
Birth — Hep B
2mo — Hep B, DPT OPV, HiB
4mo — DPT, OPV, HiB
6mo — DPT, Hep B OPV
12mo — varicella
15mo — MMR, HiB
18mo — DPT, OPV
4-6y — DPT, OPV
7-8 — MMR

Birth, 1 month and 6 months—hepatitis B vaccine.

2 months—diphtheria–pertussis–tetanus (DPT), poliovirus vaccine, live oral trivalent (TOPV), *Haemophilus* b conjugate vaccine (HIB).

4 months—DPT, TOPV, HIB.

6 months—DPT (polio for endemic areas only).

12 months—chickenpox (varicella) vaccine now available.

15 months—measles–mumps–rubella (MMR), HIB.

18 months—DPT, TOPV.

4 to 6 years—DPT, TOPV.

Middle school age—MMR 2.

2. Adults

Tetanus, diphtheria (Td) every 10 years.

Influenza (yearly in elderly, or chronic cardiopulmonary disease patients).

Pneumococcus vaccine (high-risk chronic cardiopulmonary disease, asplenia, diabetes, and elderly).

Hepatitis vaccine if in higher risk group.

Other specific vaccines for travel and/or work: rabies, cholera, typhoid.

3. Postexposure Hyperimmune Immunoglobulin

Hepatitis: hepatitis B immune globulin (HBIG).

Rabies: rabies immune globulin (RIG).

Tetanus: tetanus immune globulin (TIG).

4. Compromised Immune System Patients

Give ZIG (zoster immune globulin) to prevent chickenpox, if exposed.

Avoid live, attenuated vaccines (increased risk of paralysis with TOPV). **Avoid BCG vaccine.**

OK to give influenza, inactivated polio vaccine, and pneumococcal vaccines. *[handwritten:]* Also give MMR b/c measles is worse than vaccine

5. Severe EGG Allergy

AVOID INFLUENZA, MEASLES, and MUMPS VACCINES.

Additional Information. **Difference between DT and Td—Children with pertussis vaccine reaction are given DT. Children older than 7 and adults are given** Td vaccine (less diphtheria toxoid dose).

F. Prevention of Allergic-Related Morbidity

■ Description

Key is **education,** along with early detection (both of the disease and of hypoxia/respiratory distress), and treatment of asthma/allergic rhinitis.

Education includes avoiding specific triggers (sulfites, aspirin, home/environmental/occupational triggers, allergens and irritants, reflux).

Preventive treatment includes desensitization and medication.

Inhaled bronchodilators prior to exertion in exercise-induced asthma may prevent attacks. Cromolyn sodium and/or inhaled corticosteroids are effective as preventive therapy for asthmatics. Other considerations include evaluation and treatment of emotional components.

Early intervention may prevent ventilatory failure.

Allergic rhinitis prevention: avoidance, desensitization, antihistamines, nasal cromolyn sodium/corticosteroids.

II. MECHANISMS OF DISEASE, DIAGNOSIS, AND TREATMENT

A. Allergic Dermatopathies

1. Hereditary Angioneurotic Edema

■ **Description**

Rare, swelling disorder.

■ **Symptoms**

Slow-onset, swelling attacks without hives (lasting 1 to 4 days). *(deeper dermal swelling)*

no pruritis

■ **Diagnosis**

History and physical examination, lab studies (low C4 and C1 isonicotine hydrazine [INH]), **no hives present.**

■ **Pathology**

Autosomal dominant; C1 esterase inhibitor deficiency.

■ **Treatment**

Supportive; danazol.

Additional Information. Attacks may affect laryngeal area resulting in airway obstruction. Epinephrine/corticosteroids of little value.

2. Angioneurotic Edema

■ **Description**

Also termed **angioedema; more common.**

■ **Symptoms**

Swelling; may be associated with hives and pruritus.

■ **Diagnosis**

History and physical examination.

■ **Pathology**

Cutaneous anaphylaxis resulting from **IgE-mediated reaction** (though may also result from unknown causes).

■ **Treatment**

Antihistamines, epinephrine, corticosteroids.

3. Urticaria

■ **Description**

Hives; acute or chronic (more than 6 weeks' duration).

■ **Symptoms**

Hives (wheal and flare), pruritus. *central raised clearing c̄ erythema*

Flare *wheal*

■ **Diagnosis**

History and physical examination.

■ **Pathology**

Increased vascular permeability. *2° histamine release*

■ **Treatment** *→ diphenhydramine*

Antihistamines (hydroxyzine), epinephrine, corticosteroids, H$_2$ inhibitor (Tagamet).

Additional Information. Other urticarial triggers: **Cold, heat, sun, vibration/pressure.**

Most common physical urticaric disorder: dermographism.

pressure on skin results in urticaria!

B. Allergic Rhinitis, Hay Fever, and Asthma

1. *Allergic Rhinitis*

■ **Description**

Seasonal or continuous eye, nose, and throat symptoms.

■ **Symptoms**

Itchy nose/eyes, rhinitis, dry cough, and sneezing.

■ **Diagnosis**

History and physical examination, allergy testing (skin and/or RAST, including IgE level), nasal smear for eosinophils.

■ **Pathology**

Release of **histamine** (and other mediators) after allergen exposure in sensitized individuals.

■ **Treatment**

Avoidance, desensitization, antihistamines, nasal corticosteroids and/or cromolyn sodium.

Additional Information. **Child with purulent rhinitis: rule out foreign body.**

Head injury with rhinitis: rule out cerebrospinal fluid (CSF) leak.

Continuous rhinitis with normal nasal smear: rule out vasomotor rhinitis.

2. *Asthma*

■ **Description**

Reversible airway obstructive disorder.

■ **Symptoms**

Wheezing, cough and **dyspnea.**

■ **Diagnosis**

History and physical examination, chest x-ray, pulmonary function testing (pre- and postbronchodilator), provocation testing, allergy testing.

■ **Pathology**

Airway inflammation and hyperreactivity (triggered by allergen exposure or emotional/environmental factors).

■ **Treatment**

Education, chest physical therapy (PT), hydration, avoid inciting agents, cromolyn sodium, inhaled corticosteroids, bronchodilators (including theophylline, epinephrine, albuterol, and other beta$_2$-adrenergics), and anticholinergic medications.

[handwritten: also leukotriene inhibitors!]

Additional Information. **Child with large foul stools and wheezing: rule out cystic fibrosis.**

Wheezing with diarrhea and flushing: rule out carcinoid.

Child with unilateral sudden wheezing: rule out foreign body.

C. Immunologic Pulmonary Disease

1. *Hypersensitivity Pneumonitis*

■ **Description**

Allergic pulmonary disorder, from organic dust inhalation.

■ **Symptoms**

Cough, fever, chills (4 to 6 hours after exposure to offending allergen).

■ **Diagnosis**

History and physical examination, chest x-ray, pulmonary function testing, inhalation challenge testing, lung biopsy.

- **Pathology**

Immunologic reaction to dust inhalation. Includes wide variety of antigens (wood, hair, mold, trees).

- **Treatment**

Avoid inciting agent, bronchodilators, and corticosteroids.

2. **Allergic Bronchopulmonary Aspergillosis**

- **Description**

Hypersensitivity disorder.

- **Symptoms**

Fever, wheezing, cough, and dyspnea.

- **Diagnosis**

History and physical examination, chest x-ray, sputum examination and skin testing for *Aspergillus*, proximal bronchiectasis, and elevated IgE level.

- **Pathology**

Aspergillus fumigatus, may present in 15 to 20% of asthma patients.

can form a fungus ball in any cavitary lesion

- **Treatment**

Bronchodilators and corticosteroids.

3. **Goodpasture Syndrome**

- **Description**

Pulmonary hemorrhage and renal dysfunction.

- **Symptoms**

Hemoptysis, hematuria, cough, anemia, lethargy, proteinuria.

- **Diagnosis**

History and physical examination, **renal biopsy**, chest x-ray, **positive serum antiglomerular basement membrane antibody,** and antialveolar basement membrane antibody.

- **Pathology**

Antigen-antibody reaction. **Linear immunoglobin deposits noted on glomerular basement membrane.**

lung & kidney disease

- **Treatment**

Plasmapheresis, corticosteroids, and **cyclophosphamide.**

4. **Pulmonary Eosinophilia**

- **Description**

Loffler syndrome.

- **Symptoms**

Eosinophilia, cough, pulmonary infiltrates, or asymptomatic.

- **Diagnosis**

History and physical examination, serum for eosinophils.

- **Pathology**

Allergic reaction to various agents.

- **Treatment**

Symptomatic.

D. **Transfusion Reactions**

1. **ABO Incompatibility**

- **Description**

Major transfusion reaction **shortly after onset of transfusion.**

■ **Symptoms**

Shock, renal failure, fever/chills, hemorrhage.

■ **Diagnosis**

History and physical examination.

■ **Pathology**

Hemolysis. *resulting in hemoglobinuria & hypoxia (renal failure), hypotension*

■ **Treatment**

Stop transfusion, treat shock, corticosteroids, monitor urine output, supportive.

Additional Information. Delayed hemolytic transfusions may take place up to 3 weeks later.

2. **Allergic Transfusion Reactions**

■ **Description**

Allergy-mediated reaction, usually after 50% of unit infused.

■ **Symptoms**

Urticaria, pruritus.

■ **Diagnosis**

History and physical examination.

■ **Pathology**

Allergic response to plasma proteins.

May premedicate ē ASA Tylenol; & benadryl to prevent this

■ **Treatment**

Antihistamines, stop transfusion if reaction severe.

3. **Febrile Transfusion Reactions**

■ **Description**

Transfusion-related fever.

■ **Symptoms**

Fever/chills, headache.

■ **Diagnosis**

History and physical examination (history of prior transfusions commonly).

■ **Pathology**

Patient's antibodies react against donor antigens.

■ **Treatment**

Symptomatic treatment; discontinue transfusion if severe.

4. **Transfusion-related Infections**

Includes cytomegalovirus (CMV); non-A, non-B hepatitis; HIV; Epstein–Barr virus (EBV); bacterial; parasitic disease, and hepatitis B. *Hepatitis C*

Most common is non-A, non-B hepatitis *(Hepatitis C)*

5. **Other Transfusion Reactions**

Hypothermia: blood too cold. Hyperkalemia, volume overload, citrate intoxication.

E. **Immunologically Mediated Drug Reactions**

1. **Anaphylactic Shock**

■ **Description**

Acute, life-threatening allergic reaction.

■ **Symptoms**

Shock, hypotension, airway obstruction/bronchoconstriction, urticaria, angioedema.

■ Diagnosis

History and physical examination.

■ Pathology

Immediate hypersensitivity reaction, in individual with prior sensitization.

IgE mediated!

■ Treatment

Control airway, cardiopulmonary resuscitation **(CPR), epinephrine 1:1000 (0.3 to 0.5 mL subcutaneously),** repeat epinephrine **twice every 15 to 20 minutes, volume replacement,** corticosteroids, antihistamines, beta-agonists.

Additional Information. **Anaphylactoid reactions:** etiology is direct mediator *(histamine)* release (contrast dye for example), **presentation/treatment similar to anaphylaxis.**

2. Hemolytic Drug Reactions

■ Description

Hemolysis secondary to medication ingestion.

■ Symptoms

Dyspnea, hypotension, lethargy (symptoms of anemia).

■ Diagnosis

History and physical examination, serologic studies (direct Coombs').

■ Pathology

Etiology includes immune complex formation, medication antibodies, and autoimmune hemolytic anemia, methyldopa (Aldomet).

■ Treatment

Stop offending medication, corticosteroids have limited benefit in autoimmune-type hemolysis.

F. Autoimmune Disorders

1. Chronic Thyroiditis—Hashimoto's

■ Description

Thyroid inflammatory disorder, with female preponderance.

■ Symptoms

Pain, normal gland size or swelling, **hyperthyroidism or euthyroidism early, hypothyroidism** later in disease.

■ Diagnosis

History and physical examination, lab (elevated thyroid-stimulating hormone [TSH], **positive antimicrosomal antibody,** may have **positive antithyroglobulin antibody**), thyroid scan.

■ Pathology

Autoimmune disorder, with **lymphocytic infiltration** of the thyroid gland.

■ Treatment

Thyroid hormone replacement.

Additional Information. Thyroiditis types:

Acute: bacterial **(fever/pain).**
Subacute (de Quervain's) **viral? (fever/pain/large gland/high sed rate).**
Chronic (Hashimoto's): **autoimmune.** Chronic type also includes Reidel's thyroiditis (unknown cause). **Increased incidence of systemic lu-**

→ fibrosing/sclerosing thyroiditis

pus erythematosus (SLE), scleroderma and **pernicious anemia with Hashimoto's disease.**

Schmidt syndrome: **Hashimoto's disease plus Addison's disease.**

2. Graves' Disease

■ **Description**

Thyrotoxicosis disorder. **Most frequent etiology of hyperthyroidism.**

■ **Symptoms**

Thyrotoxicosis (tremor, weight loss, tachycardia, etc), and **goiter.** Ophthalmopathy and dermopathy may be present.

exophthalmos →   *↳ pretibial myxedema*

■ **Diagnosis**

low TSH   History and physical examination, **antithyroid antibodies,** elevated T_3, T_4, **thyroid scan: homogeneous uptake.**

■ **Pathology**

Autoimmune.

Ophthalmopathy c̄ dermopathy do not go away c̄
■ **Treatment** *Rx: 2° deposition of glycoproteins*

Beta-adrenergic blockers, followed by antithyroid medications (PTU, propylthiouracil methimazole [Tapazole]), surgery, or radioactive iodine.

3. Addison's Disease

■ **Description**

Adrenocortical insufficiency.

■ **Symptoms**

Weight loss, lethargy, hyperpigmentation, confusion, hypotension, nausea, dehydration, metabolic acidosis.

■ **Diagnosis**

History and physical examination, adrenocorticotropic hormone (ACTH) stimulation test (rapid and prolonged).

■ **Pathology**

Etiology most often idiopathic **(autoimmune),** or tuberculosis (TB).

■ **Treatment**

Acute: use IV glucocorticoids, fluids.

Chronic: prednisone and mineralocorticoid.   *(hydrocortisone)*

4. Pernicious Anemia

■ **Description**

Autoimmune B_{12}-deficiency disorder.

■ **Symptoms**

Symptoms of anemia, and neurologic disease (organic brain syndrome).

■ **Diagnosis**

History and physical examination (anemia/neurologic symptoms), positive **antiparietal cell and anti-intrinsic factor antibodies.**

■ **Pathology**

Vitamin B_{12} deficiency secondary to reduced intrinsic factor levels (resulting from gastric fundic gland injury).

■ **Treatment**

Parenteral B_{12}.

Additional Information. **Increased gastric carcinoma incidence.**

5. Idiopathic Thrombocytopenic Purpura (ITP)

■ Description

Acute or chronic thrombocytopenic disorder.

■ Symptoms

Acute: **purpura, petechiae, cutaneous bleeding** but gastrointestinal (GI) **bleed possible, splenomegaly.**

[handwritten: children; post-viral; self-limiting]

Chronic: **petechiae, bruising,** slow onset.

■ Diagnosis

[handwritten in left margin: No ALL in acute!]

By exclusion via history and physical examination, antiplatelet antibodies (usually research lab study), complete blood count (CBC) (otherwise normal), bone marrow examination (rules out other pathology).

■ Pathology

Immune disorder.

■ Treatment

Acute: supportive (avoid injury) or prednisone.

Chronic: prednisone, splenectomy, and immunosuppressives when other treatments fail.

Additional Information

Acute ITP: **usually children, often postviral,** self-limited disease usually.

Chronic ITP: **usually adults.**

6. Immune Hemolysis

6–1. Warm Autoimmune—Hemolytic Anemia

■ Description

Most frequent autoimmune anemia.

■ Symptoms

Anemia (asymptomatic slow onset, or rapid onset with chills/fever/back pain).

■ Diagnosis

History and physical exam (splenomegaly); **best test: positive direct Coombs,** serologic immunoglobulin and antiglobulin studies.

[handwritten: IgG antibody]

■ Pathology

Idiopathic or more often coexisting with other disease (infection, leukemia, etc).

■ Treatment

Corticosteroids, and/or splenectomy, immunosuppressives as final option. Control coexisting disorder.

6–2. Paroxysmal—Cold Hemoglobinuria

■ Description

Cold-induced hemolysis.

[handwritten: (happens more at night b/c likely to get cold then or in extremities!)]

■ Symptoms

Chills/muscle pains/hemoglobinuria after cold exposure.

■ Diagnosis

History and physical examination, **Donath–Landsteiner antibody present (IgG cold antibody).** *[handwritten: active <28°C]*

■ Pathology

Idiopathic or coexisting with disease (**syphilis, mononucleosis, measles**). *[handwritten: also mycoplasma infection]*

■ **Treatment**

Supportive, transfusion, **avoid cold.**

6–3. Cold-Agglutinin Disease

■ **Description**

Cold-induced hemolysis.

■ **Symptoms**

Hemolytic symptoms, acrocyanosis, splenomegaly.

■ **Diagnosis**

History and physical examination, serologic immunologic testing, **elevated cold agglutinin IgM antibodies.**

■ **Pathology**

Idiopathic (most cases) or coexisting with other disease (*Mycoplasma pneumoniae*, etc).

■ **Treatment**

Warm patient, treat coexisting disease.

6–4. Newborn—Hemolytic Disease

■ **Description**

Newborn immune hemolytic disorder (**erythroblastosis fetalis**).

■ **Symptoms**

Early-onset **jaundice**, anemia, kernicterus. (1st 24 hrs or born jaundiced)

■ **Diagnosis**

History and physical examination, prenatal lab studies, amniocentesis, **positive direct Coombs'.**

■ **Pathology**

Mother's antibodies (most often **D antigen Rh**), attack fetal blood cells.

■ **Treatment**

Predelivery: **fetoscopic transfusion.**

After delivery: **exchange transfusion**, phototherapy.

Additional Information

Direct Coombs': detects red (bound) blood cell surface antibody.

Indirect Coombs': serum antibody.

7. Chronic Active Hepatitis

■ **Description**

Chronic portal tract inflammation; also termed **autoimmune hepatitis.**

■ **Symptoms**

Lethargy, jaundice, ascites or extrahepatic symptoms (vasculitis, thyroiditis).

■ **Diagnosis**

History and physical examination, **liver biopsy**, elevated liver function tests (LFTs), **may have positive antinuclear antibody (ANA), and smooth-muscle antibody.**

■ **Pathology**

May be postviral (hepatitis B), medication (INH, methyldopa [Aldomet]), or of unknown/immune? etiology.

■ **Treatment**

Corticosteroids (better in autoimmune disease), interferon alpha (may be better in chronic active hepatitis B).

Additional Information. **Young person with chronic hepatitis: rule out Wilson's disease. Increased risk of cirrhosis and liver cancer with chronic HBV infection.**

8. Glomerulonephritis

■ Description

Glomerular disease, most often immune mediated.

■ Symptoms

Hematuria, edema, hypertension, lethargy, headache, proteinuria, oliguria. *(nephrotic syndrome has no HTN or hematuria!)*

■ Diagnosis

History and physical examination, **renal biopsy, urine analysis** (RBCs, casts, protein, WBCs), lab (poststreptococcal-reduced C3, C4).

■ Pathology

Proliferative glomerulonephritis noted poststreptococcal infection, with other bacteria, viruses, SLE, and vasculitis.

■ Treatment

Poststreptococcal: supportive, antibiotics, corticosteroids.

Other: steroids

9. Multiple Sclerosis

■ Description

Demyelinating central nervous system (CNS) disease.

■ Symptoms

Vertigo, lethargy, incoordination, incontinence, nystagmus, vision loss (optic neuritis), diplopia, internuclear ophthalmoplegia.

Suspect MS in young ♀ c̄ b/l optic neuritis!

■ Diagnosis

History and physical examination, magnetic resonance imaging (MRI), lumbar puncture (elevated CSF IgG), slowed **visual-evoked response** test.

oligoclonal bands

■ Pathology

Autoimmune?

■ Treatment

ACTH, prednisone, and immunosuppressive agents.

β interferon, copolymer, IVIG

10. Myasthenia Gravis

■ Description

Neuromuscular disorder.

■ Symptoms

Ptosis, diplopia, muscle use/repetition leading to fatigue (ocular/facial often).

■ Diagnosis

History and physical examination, electromyogram (EMG), **tensilon test** (improves strength).

■ Pathology

Immune **(positive acetylcholine-receptor antibodies).**

■ Treatment

Thymectomy, corticosteroids, anticholinesterase medications, also obtain computed tomography (CT) of chest to rule out thymoma.

Additional Information. **Rule out botulism, and Eaton–Lambert syndrome.**

11. *Pemphigus* vulgaris

■ **Description**

Unusual, possibly fatal skin disorder.

■ **Symptoms**

[handwritten: easily rupture involves mucous membranes elderly pt]

Multiple flaccid bullae, Nikolsky's sign (epidermal separation with pressure).

■ **Diagnosis**

History and physical examination, immunofluorescence testing, skin/lesion biopsy shows acantholysis.

[handwritten: bx shows intradermal antibody deposition]

■ **Pathology**

Unknown, but autoantibodies to epidermal antigen are present.

■ **Treatment**

Prednisone, fluids, antibiotics, immunosuppressives, gold.

G. Immunization Against Infectious Agents

See Sections I, E.

H. Connective Tissue Disorders

1. *Systemic Lupus Erythematosus*

■ **Description**

Multisymptom inflammatory immune disorder.

■ **Symptoms**

Malar/discoid rash, proteinuria, fever, arthritis, neurologic/psychiatric disease, vasculitis, alopecia, Raynaud's phenomenon, anemia, weight loss.

[handwritten: Bullous Pemphigoid]

■ **Diagnosis**

History and physical examination, skin biopsy, serologic tests (native anti-DNA antibody, ANA, antiphospholipid antibodies).

[handwritten: tense, deeper bullae; ⊖ Nikolsky's; no mucous involvent]

[handwritten: → Show disease even where no lesions!]

■ **Pathology**

Immune mediated with increased incidence in females, and those with positive family histories of SLE.

■ **Treatment**

Corticosteroids, immunosuppressives, antimalarials.

Additional Information. **Disorders that may coexist with SLE: psoriasis, porphyria cutanea tarda, Sjögren's syndrome.**

[handwritten: hydralazine gives SLE like syndrome]

2. *Juvenile Rheumatoid Arthritis (JRA)*

■ **Description**

Most frequent **childhood rheumatic disorder** (peak age 1 to 2 years). Also called **juvenile chronic arthritis.**

■ **Symptoms**

Asymmetric joint pain, tenderness and swelling, for more than 6 weeks' duration, fever, morning stiffness *[handwritten: (>1 hour)]*.

■ **Diagnosis**

History and physical examination, lab studies (sed rate, rheumatoid factor [RF], ANA, etc), x-ray.

■ **Pathology**

Autoimmune-induced synovitis—three types: systemic, polyarticular, and pauciarticular.

■ **Treatment**

Salicylates, non-steroidal anti-inflammatory drugs (NSAIDs), gold, anti-malarials, corticosteroids.

Additional Information. Systemic JRA: Still's disease; adenopathy, fever.

Polyarticular: 5 or more joints affected.

Pauciarticular: 4 or fewer joints, most frequent type, iridocyclitis is most significant complication.

3. Adult Rheumatoid Arthritis

■ **Description**

Chronic adult immune-mediated synovitis.

■ **Symptoms**

Symmetric joint swelling, morning stiffness, subcutaneous nodules, extraarticular symptoms (episcleritis, neuropathy, pulmonary fibrosis/pleuritis, vasculitis, lethargy).

■ **Diagnosis**

History and physical examination (with attention to American Rheumatism Association criteria), lab (RF, sed rate), x-ray (marginal erosions/osteoporosis), synovial fluid analysis.

■ **Pathology**

Chronic synovitis resulting from immune complex formation with joint/tissue injury.

■ **Treatment**

NSAIDs, corticosteroids, disease-modifying medications (gold, methotrexate, hydroxychloroquine, etc), therapy, physical therapy/occupational therapy (PT/OT), surgery.

Additional Information. Felty syndrome: RA, granulocytopenia, and splenomegaly.

4. Rheumatic Fever

■ **Description**

Poststreptococcal multisystem inflammatory disorder.

■ **Symptoms**

Major: polyarthritis, chorea, carditis, erythema marginatum and subcutaneous nodules.

Minor: fever, abnormal lab studies antistreptolysin-O [ASO] titer, C-reactive protein (CRP), sed rate, leukocytosis).

Must have hx strep infection ⊕ 2 Major or 1 major & 2 minor

■ **Diagnosis**

History and physical examination, streptococcal infection plus Jones criteria (two major symptoms or one major plus two minor).

■ **Pathology**

Multisystem tissue inflammation; a possible result of host versus streptococcal antigen reaction. *(M antigen?)*

■ **Treatment**

Penicillin (eliminates strep, but will not alter RF disease course), NSAIDs, prednisone (for carditis).

Additional Information *Must watch for dev. of MR, AS!*

Carditis—most dangerous symptom.

Joint complaints—most frequent symptom.

5. Scleroderma *(Progressive Systemic Sclerosis)*

■ **Description**

Multisystem connective tissue disorder (progressive systemic sclerosis).

■ Symptoms

Affects **skin/vascular** system (Raynaud's phenomenon), GI **tract, renal, pulmonary** and **cardiac systems.** Also anemia, dyspnea, and arthritis.

■ Diagnosis

History and physical examination, lab studies (single-strand RNA, ANA), biopsy.

■ Pathology

Increased skin and organ collagen deposition, along with vascular narrowing. May be localized (morphea), or generalized.

■ Treatment

Supportive, corticosteroids?

Additional Information

Most frequent cause for scleroderma death: renal disease.

Most frequent internal organ affected: esophagus.

6. *Polymyalgia Rheumatica*

■ Description

Rheumatologic disorder of the elderly.

■ Symptoms

Severe shoulder muscle and **pelvic girdle pain/stiffness,** fever, lethargy.

■ Diagnosis

History and physical examination **(no reduced joint motion),** lab studies **(high sed rate).**

■ Pathology

Human leukocyte antigen (HLA) associated.

■ Treatment

Corticosteroids: small dose, rapid relief.

Additional Information. **Temporal arteritis may coexist (diagnosis by temporal artery biopsy).**

  Be sure to **rule out multiple myeloma** (also high sed rate/back pain in elderly.

I. HIV Infection and AIDS

■ Description

Cell-mediated and humoral deficiency disorder.

■ Symptoms

Adenopathy, lethargy, fever, weight loss, opportunistic infections (in AIDS), rash, chronic diarrhea, hepatosplenomegaly.

■ Diagnosis

History and physical examination, serologic testing (ELISA test for antibodies to HIV, with Western blot confirmation).

■ Pathology

Viral-induced cell-mediated immunity disorder, reduced CD4 lymphocytes, with reduced host defense against infections/cancer.

■ Treatment

Preventive care, AZT, consult current literature. See Cell-Mediated Immunity Deficiency.

AIDS

■ Description

T-cell deficiency.

C
Raynaud's
E
S
T

■ **Symptoms**

Infections (chronic and recurring), persisting diarrhea.

■ **Diagnosis**

History and physical examination, lab (immunoglobins, CBC, T-cell evaluation), skin antigen testing (delayed response).

■ **Pathology**

T-cell deficiency.

■ **Treatment**

Preventive care (avoid infections). Avoid corticosteroid use, live virus vaccines, and transfusions (may cause graft-versus-host disease).

Additional Information. **DiGeorge syndrome: thymic aplasia, decreased T cells, most frequent sign is hypocalcemia,** congenital cardiac disease, **treat by thymus grafting.**

J. **Humoral Immunity Deficiency**

■ **Description**

Antibody-mediated immunity.

■ **Symptoms**

Infections, diarrhea.

■ **Diagnosis**

See Cell-Mediated Deficiency; reduced immunoglobins.

■ **Pathology**

B-cell deficiency.

■ **Treatment**

See Cell-Mediated Deficiency; also gamma globulin. Combined immunodeficiency disease.

■ **Description**

B-cell and T-cell disorder.

■ **Symptoms**

Severe infection, sepsis.

■ **Diagnosis**

History and physical examination, lab (reduced T cells and immunoglobins).

■ **Pathology**

X-linked disorder, of early (infant) onset.

■ **Treatment**

Symptomatic; treat infections.

K. **Transplantation Rejection**

■ **Description**

Immunological transplant rejection.

■ **Symptoms**

Fever, pain, lethargy. Dysfunction of transplanted organ.

■ **Diagnosis**

History and physical examination, additional studies (kidney: blood urea nitrogen [BUN], creatinine, renal biopsy).

■ **Pathology**

Lymphocyte- and antibody-induced reaction, with T-cell graft tissue injury (acute reaction). Renal transplant may also present as hyperacute or chronic reaction.

■ **Treatment**

Immunosuppressive medication (corticosteroids, cytotoxic medications, antimetabolites).

L. Neoplasms

1. Multiple Myeloma

■ **Description**

Plasma cell cancer.

■ **Symptoms**

Back pain, lethargy, pathologic fractures, renal disease.

■ **Diagnosis**

History and physical examination, lab studies (**serum protein electrophoresis, bone marrow,** serum/urine paraprotein, hypercalcemia), x-ray (lytic lesions, fractures).

■ **Pathology**

Paraprotein production.

■ **Treatment**

Chemotherapy.

2. Non-Hodgkin's Lymphoma

■ **Description**

Lymphocyte cancer.

■ **Symptoms**

Sweats, fever, adenopathy, weight loss, lethargy.

■ **Diagnosis**

History and physical examination, **lymph node biopsy.**

■ **Pathology**

A result of T-cell receptor and immunoglobin genetic translocation. May occur in both transplant and AIDS patients.

■ **Treatment**

Chemotherapy, with/without local irradiation.

BIBLIOGRAPHY

Ball GV. *Clinical Rheumatology*. Philadelphia, Pa: WB Saunders Company; 1986.

Behrman RE. *Nelson Textbook of Pediatrics*. 13th ed. Philadelphia, Pa: WB Saunders Company; 1987.

Bierman CW. *Allergic Diseases from Infancy to Adulthood*. 2nd ed. Philadelphia, Pa: WB Saunders Company; 1988.

Callen JP. *The Medical Clinics of North America, Collagen Vascular Diseases*. Vol. 73. Philadelphia, Pa: WB Saunders Company; 1989.

Cohen PT. *The AIDS Knowledge Base*. Waltham, Mass: The Medical Publishing Group; 1990.

Corless IB. *AIDS, Principles, Practices and Politics*. New York: Hemisphere Publishing Corporation; 1989.

Dieppe PA. *Atlas of Clinical Rheumatology*. Philadelphia, Pa: Lea and Febiger; 1986.

Lawlor GJ. *Manual of Allergy and Immunology, Diagnosis and Therapy*. 2nd ed. Boston, Mass: Little, Brown and Company; 1988.

Mindel A. *AIDS, A Pocketbook of Diagnosis and Management*. Baltimore, Md: Urban and Schwarzenberg, Inc; 1990.

Moskowitz RW. *Clinical Rheumatology*. 2nd ed. Philadelphia, Pa: Lea and Febiger; 1982.

Roitt IM. *Essential Immunology*. 7th ed. London: Blackwell Scientific Publications; 1991.

Stites DP. *Basic and Clinical Immunology*. 7th ed. Norwalk, Conn: Appleton and Lange; 1991.

CHAPTER 8

Injury and Toxicology

JOEL S. GOLDBERG, DO

I. HEALTH AND HEALTH MAINTENANCE

A. Epidemiology, Impact, and Prevention of Specific Disorders

1. Home Accidents

■ **Description**

Epidemiology involves <u>all age groups</u> and consists of a wide variety of hazards (<u>electrical, thermal, poisoning, and trauma</u>).

Impact includes large numbers of accidents, of both minor and major severity.

Prevention includes education, <u>preventive planning</u> (<u>bicycle helmets, toy/playground equipment checks, removal of dangerous objects/obstacles,</u> etc).

2. Workplace Accidents

■ **Description**

Epidemiology includes increased risk groups (meat cutters/packers, steelworkers, etc), along with all employees.

Impact is considerable in terms of numbers of individuals affected, degree of injury, residual injury/loss of work time, and financial impact on the patient, employer, and insurance industry.

Prevention includes both education and exercise of precautions (eye shield, hearing protection, hard hats, steel tip shoes, etc), and elimination of dangerous materials/practices and procedures.

3. Athletic Accidents

■ **Description**

Epidemiology includes home, school, recreational, and professional accidents.

Impact and type of injuries are multiple, including falls, trauma, thermal injury, sprains/strains, fractures, concussions, contusions, and death.

Prevention includes education, correction of both training and performance errors (spearing in football), providing protective equipment of correct fit.

4. Automobile Accidents and Drunk Driving

■ **Description**

Epidemiology includes all ages of society, with increased risk for both teenagers (drunk and reckless driving) and the elderly (visual impairment, cognitive functioning, and reaction time). Increased risk is associated with motorcycle and three-wheel all-terrain vehicle use.

Impact is significant, as automobile accidents account for 30% or more of accidental deaths.

Prevention includes education (driving, seatbelts, drugs/alcohol), reduced speed limits, better roads, improved roadway markings/median barriers, and abutment protection. Multiple other factors play a role, such as a larger size vehicle, air bags, collapsible steering wheel, and padded dash regulations. Drunk-driving prevention includes both education and modification of drinking age, along with effective legal deterrents (fines/jail terms).

5. Head/Spinal Cord Injury and Whiplash

■ **Description**

Epidemiology includes motor vehicle accidents (the major cause for these injuries), falls, child abuse, occupational, and trauma-induced accidents.

Impact includes significant morbidity/mortality, with possible residual neurologic and/or psychologic effects, and cognitive deficits including reduced intellectual functioning.

Prevention includes education, safety devices (automotive: air bags, seat/shoulder belt, padded dash, head rest; work: hard hats, etc), and behavior modification (avoidance of high-risk activities and/or behavior). Appropriate emergency care may prevent permanent neurologic sequelae (sandbag/stabilize head).

6. Chest or Abdominal Injuries

■ Description

Epidemiology most often cites motor vehicle accidents as the etiology. Blunt injury, occupational injury, falls, and trauma play a role. Increased incidence of trauma-related abdominal/chest injury in low socioeconomic areas.

Impact includes significant morbidity/mortality (due to coexisting cardiac and/or visceral injury). Pneumothorax/hemothorax, viscera and/or vascular tears are common.

Prevention involves driver education and vehicle safety modifications for automobiles. Community programs, education, job opportunity, and effective law enforcement reduce the incidence of street crime/trauma.

7. Ocular or Auditory Injury

■ Description

Epidemiology includes blunt ocular trauma (occupational, recreational, environmental), and ophthalmic foreign bodies and lacerations. Auditory injury may affect children (fireworks), teens (high-decibel music), and adults (occupational).

Impact includes the possibility of permanent visual or auditory impairment.

Prevention involves eye and ear protection along with education.

8. Drowning

■ Description

Epidemiology involves children most often.

Impact is significant as a frequent cause of accidents with associated mortality and possibility of residual neurologic damage. **Prevention** centers on education (parents and children), swimming instruction, water/boating safety, dangers of hyperventilation, dangers of drug/alcohol use, and cardiopulmonary resuscitation (CPR) training. Recognition of high-risk patients (epilepsy, syncope, divers, children, etc).

9. Aspiration

■ Description

Epidemiology suggests that both children and high-risk patients are at risk.

Impact includes high mortality.

Prevention includes identification and management of high-risk patients (postop, sedated/overdose, nasogastric [NG] tube patients, neuromuscular disorder patients), reduce gastric acidity (Zantac, etc). In children avoid grapes, hot dogs; check toys/objects for small parts, and maintain alertness. Instruction in the Heimlich maneuver.

10. Ingestion of Poisonous and Toxic Agents

■ Description

Epidemiology includes accidental overdose in both children and adults, and work/environmental toxicology and suicide in adolescents and adults.

Prevention includes education, awareness, and labeling of dangerous substances, prevention of child access (keep medication/toxins locked and in unaccessible location, "child-proof" containers), and easy access to emergency advice and/or treatment. Need to keep ipecac at home.

11. Gunshot Wounds and Stab Wounds

■ Description

Epidemiology demonstrates an increasing rate of violent crime, and increasing use of handguns/automatic weapons. Elevated level of crime in poor socioeconomic areas.

Impact includes an ever-increasing utilization of medical/emergency facilities, increasing financial burden on the medical/insurance system, and increasing morbidity/mortality, including innocent bystanders.

Prevention includes education, gun control(?), control of alcohol/drug use and abuse, law enforcement, and society efforts to reduce inner city neglect and populace anger.

B. Prevention of Burns

■ Description

Prevent burns through education, caution, and skin protection when working in hazardous environment.

C. Prevention of Thermal Injury

■ Description

Key points include education (increased heat disorders with alcohol, cystic fibrosis patients, dehydration, dark/non-breathing clothing, antipsychotics and diuretic use, high-humidity days), and need for increased fluid intake, and gradual heat acclimatization. Skin protection and early recognition of symptoms in frostbite and hypothermia patients is critical. Increased awareness for high-risk patients (elderly and children, alcohol/drug abuse, central nervous system [CNS] disease and sepsis) is important.

D. Child, Spouse, and Elder Abuse

■ Description

Epidemiology suggests that susceptible victims include children, spouses, and elders.

Impact is significant as a frequent society malady with great morbidity, mortality, and possible permanent psychological impact. Difficult to obtain accurate numbers of cases involved due to sensitivity of the subject, and reluctance of many abused individuals to tell their stories.

Prevention via physician and family education to obtain early diagnosis, and screen for potentially abusive parents (observe/evaluate mother for postpartum depression). High index of suspicion may be required. Medical history (abusers may have been abused themselves as children).

E. Sexual Abuse and Rape

■ Description

Epidemiology suggests that adolescents and young children are at risk for sexual abuse (usually by family member).

Impact is significant, and includes psychological impact for both sexual abuse and rape.

Prevention includes early recognition by health care workers, and education. Rape prevention includes patient education (how to avoid being a target), and self-defense.

F. Fire Prevention

■ Description

Prevention includes education (smoking in bed, proper flammables storage, etc), home precautions (smoke detector/fire extinguisher, fireplace glass screen, fire safety plan/escape route, upkeep of electrical system, etc).

G. Falls

■ **Description**

Affects children, elderly, and adults (workplace injury, seizure disorder patients, alcoholics), and is a frequent cause of accidental death. Significant morbidity/mortality associated with hip fractures.

Prevention in children includes childproofing the house, covering sharp corners, window locks, stair gates, and control of obstacles. In the elderly, medical/family assessment for need of cane/walker/wheelchair, medical treatment/control of contributing illness (Parkinson's disease, visual impairment, anemia, stroke, etc).

H. Insect- and Snake-Bite Prevention

■ **Description**

Prevention measures include avoidance of areas of infestation, and protective clothing (netting, snake boots, etc). Shake clothing/shoes before wear.

II. MECHANISMS OF DISEASE, DIAGNOSIS, AND TREATMENT

A. Fractures

1. Facial

■ **Description**

Fractures of the frontal bone, mandible, maxilla, orbits, or nose.

■ **Symptoms**

Pain, cerebrospinal fluid (CSF) rhinorrhea, diplopia, deformity, and ecchymosis.

Orbital fracture—swelling, difficulty with eye movement, vertical diplopia, and facial emphysema.
Frontal/ethmoid—may have CSF rhi-norrhea.
Nasal bones—deformity, epistaxis.

Mandible/maxilla—swelling, pain, airway compromise, jaw pain/deformity when opening/closing the mouth (abnormal occlusion).

■ **Diagnosis**

History and physical examination, x-rays.

■ **Pathology**

Trauma.

■ **Treatment**

Control airway and hemorrhage, antibiotics, fracture reduction.

Nasal—closed reduction for simple fracture, open reduction in severe fracture cases.
Maxillary—reduction, interdental wiring (simple fractures), orbital/zygoma wiring and traction (complex fractures).
Mandibular—internal fixation.
Orbital—surgical to resupport orbit.

2. Skull

■ **Description**

Closed (simple), or **open** (compound) fractures, of linear or depressed type.

■ **Symptoms**

Asymptomatic, or pain/swelling, CNS signs, CSF leak (nose or ears).

■ **Diagnosis**

History and physical examination, x-ray examination.

■ **Pathology**

Trauma.

■ **Treatment**

Use CPRs ABCs, then:

Simple linear. Observation.

Compound linear. Antibiotics.

Simple depressed. Surgical treatment (fragment elevation).

Compound depressed. Urgent surgical treatment.

Additional Information

Basilar skull fracture sign—cerebrospinal fluid in nose or ears.

Battle's sign—ecchymosis behind ear (mastoid fracture).

Raccoon eyes—orbital roof fracture/basilar fracture.

Linear fracture across middle meningeal artery—watch for epidural hematoma.

3. Vertebral Column

■ **Description**

Vertebral body fracture (wedging, body fracture), articular process fracture, transverse process fracture.

■ **Symptoms**

Pain, neurologic abnormalities.

■ **Diagnosis**

History and physical examination, x-ray examination, CT exam.

■ **Pathology**

Trauma.

■ **Treatment**

Simple compression fracture.

Brace—(some advocate surgical intervention, especially in young individual).

Initial cervical spine treatment—ensure airway, control shock/hemorrhage.

Unstable fracture or *progressing neurologic deficit*—cranial traction followed by surgical internal fixation.

Most other simple spinal fractures are treated with bracing or casting, with surgical intervention reserved for progressive neurologic symptoms.

4. Rib Cage

■ **Description**

Rib fracture.

■ **Symptoms**

Pain, increased with inspiration/palpation, ecchymosis.

■ **Diagnosis**

History and physical examination, x-ray examination.

■ **Pathology**

Trauma.

■ **Treatment**

need adequate pain management to prevent atelectasis & pneumonia

Simple rib fracture—analgesics, ice initially, injection of local anesthetic (into intercostal nerve) as an option.

Additional Information. Rib x-rays may be negative shortly after injury, yet show a "healing fracture" several weeks later. Rule out pneumothorax if patient remains dyspneic.

5. Pelvis

■ **Description**

Fracture of innominate bone (ilium, ischium, or pubis), sacrum.

■ **Symptoms**

Pain; history of injury.

■ **Diagnosis**

History and physical examination, **x-ray studies,** computed tomography (CT) exam.

■ **Pathology**

Trauma; via falls, motor vehicle accidents, sports injuries.

■ **Treatment**

Depends on multiple factors, with open reduction and internal fixation, traction, and external fixation as choices. Need to evaluate for coexisting injuries/trauma and treat accordingly.

Fracture ilium—rest.
Fracture anterior superior spine—surgery.
Fracture sacrum—rest/support.

Additional Information. **Most important complication of pelvis fracture: hemorrhage. Angiography/embolization may be required for severe persisting hemorrhage.**

(usually art. hemorrhage 2° ripping of vessels)

6. **Extremities**

6–1. *Tibia*

■ **Description**

Tibia fracture.

■ **Symptoms**

Pain.

■ **Diagnosis**

History and physical examination, **x-ray.**

■ **Pathology**

Trauma.

■ **Treatment**

Tibia shaft.

Closed reduction and cast.
Medial tibial condyle—open reduction and internal fixation (ORIF).
Lateral tibial condyle—external reduction.

6–2. *Fibula*

■ **Description**

Fracture fibula.

■ **Symptoms**

Pain and **swelling,** with retained ability to walk.

■ **Diagnosis**

History and physical examination, **x-ray exam.**

■ **Pathology**

Common. Rule out coexisting ankle injury.

■ **Treatment**

Walking cast/boot, followed by therapy.

6–3. *Femur*

■ **Description**

Fracture femur.

■ **Symptoms**

Pain, swelling, deformity.

■ **Diagnosis**

History and physical examination, **x-ray examination.**

■ **Pathology**

Significant trauma. **In child, rule out child abuse.**

■ **Treatment**

Femoral neck—long-term traction (usually in immobile patients) versus ORIF.
Femoral shaft—skeletal traction and **cast.**

Additional Information. **Complications of femoral neck fractures: avascular necrosis and nonunion** of fracture.

6–4. Radius

■ **Description**

Radius fracture.

■ **Symptoms**

Pain, reduced elbow joint motion.

■ **Diagnosis**

History and physical examination, **x-ray exam.**

■ **Pathology**

Fall on hand common.

■ **Treatment**

Radial head—hemarthrosis aspiration and mobilization if simple, **surgical (ORIF) if complete/displaced fracture.**
Distal radius undisplaced—cast 4 to 6 weeks, therapy.

Additional Information

Colles' fracture—fall on extended wrist, **fracture of distal radius and ulnar styloid** (volar angulation/dorsal displacement).
Smith's fracture fall on flexed wrist—(dorsal angulation/volar displacement).

6–5. Ulna

■ **Description**

Fracture ulna.

■ **Symptoms**

Pain, swelling, deformity.

■ **Diagnosis**

History and physical examination, **x-ray.**

■ **Pathology**

Trauma.

■ **Treatment**

Undisplaced—closed or open reduction.
Displaced—ORIF.

Additional Information. **Greenstick radius/ulna fractures in children: complete the break, then cast.**

6–6. Humerus

■ **Description**

Humerus fracture.

■ **Symptoms**

Pain, swelling.

- **Diagnosis**

History and physical examination, **x-ray exam.**

- **Pathology**

Trauma.

- **Treatment**

Humeral shaft/distal humerus—reduction (traction), then splint/sling.
Surgical neck of humerus—avoid immobilization, instead gentle range of motion; **ORIF for displaced tuberosity fracture.**

watch for brachial nerve injury

Additional Information. **Childhood medial/lateral epicondyle fractures.**

No displacement—splint elbow 90°.
Any displacement—**ORIF.**

B. **Sprains and Dislocations**

1. *Hands*

   1–1. *Distal Interphalangeal (DIP) Sprain*

   - **Description**

   Injury/sprain of DIP joint.

   - **Symptoms**

   Pain, difficulty with joint flexion or extension.

   - **Diagnosis**

   History and physical exam, x-ray examination.

   - **Pathology**

   Possible flexor/extensor tendon disruption.

- **Treatment**

Symptomatic (if able to flex/extend joint).

Additional Information. **Mallet finger: tendon disruption, with loss of joint extension. Treat with splinting in hyperextension, or surgery. Remember sprains involve ligament injury; strains affect muscle.**

1–2. **Proximal Interphalangeal (PIP) Dislocation**

- **Description**

Dislocation of PIP joint.

- **Symptoms**

Pain.

- **Diagnosis**

History and physical (displaced digit, motion loss), x-ray to rule out fracture.

- **Pathology**

Hyperextension, trauma.

- **Treatment**

Flexion splint 2 weeks.

Additional Information. For **PIP sprain:** splint—hyperextension injury, or collateral ligament sprain (flexion splint); extensor slip tear (splint in hyperextension).

1–3. **Metacarpophalangeal (MCP) Sprain**

- **Description**

Sprained finger or thumb MCP joint.

■ **Symptoms**

<u>Pain,</u> motion loss.

■ **Diagnosis**

History and physical exam, x-ray examination.

■ **Pathology**

Trauma.

■ **Treatment**

Splint.

Additional Information. **Gamekeep-er's thumb: the MCP joint of thumb sprained, affecting the ulnar collateral ligament. May need cast or surgical treatment.**

2. Ankle Sprain

■ **Description**

Ankle ligament injury.

■ **Symptoms**

Pain, swelling, ecchymosis.

■ **Diagnosis**

History and physical examination, x-ray studies.

■ **Pathology**

<u>Lateral pain</u>—injury to <u>anterior talo-fibular ligament.</u> May also include injury to fibulocalcaneal and posterior talofibular ligaments. <u>Medial pain</u>—deltoid ligament injury.

eversion injury - harder to tolto

inversion injury - more common

■ **Treatment**

<u>Rest, ice, compression, elevation</u> (<u>RICE</u>), non-steroidal anti-inflamma-tory drugs (<u>NSAID</u>s), <u>a</u>nkle splint sec-

ond-degree sprain; cast third-degree sprain. *(rupture of ~~tendo~~ ligament)*

3. Elbow

■ **Description**

Elbow sprain.

■ **Symptoms**

Pain on elbow extension.

■ **Diagnosis**

History and physical exam, x-ray examination.

■ **Pathology**

Sprain by extension injury.

■ **Treatment**

<u>Ice, sling.</u>

Additional Information. **Elbow disloca-tion—check vascular/neurologic sta-tus; urgent reduction indicated, then splint.**

4. Shoulder

■ **Description**

Sprain or dislocation injury.

■ **Symptoms**

Shoulder pain, protruding acromion/shoulder deformity with anterior dis-location.

■ **Diagnosis**

History and physical examination, x-ray exam.

■ **Pathology**

Anterior-inferior dislocation most common (in young patients).

■ **Treatment**

Dislocation—urgent reduction (slow traction, Kocher maneuver, or reduction under anesthesia). Other dislocations include posterior and inferior.

Mild sprain—prevent external rotation for 6 weeks; sling.

5. Spine

■ **Description**

Spinal strain, sprain, and dislocation.

■ **Symptoms**

Pain. Increased pain with muscle stretch (strain). Head in extension or tilted, muscle spasm and more pain (sprain). Stiff neck/back.

■ **Diagnosis**

History and physical exam, x-ray examination.

■ **Pathology**

Trauma, flexion/extension injury (cervical spine); overuse common in thoracic/lumbar spine injury.

■ **Treatment**

Cervical spine—protect from further injury (sandbag/collar/etc) until evaluation complete.
Strain—use NSAIDs, heat, rest, muscle relaxants.
Sprain—similar to strain; rule out fracture; may add traction, cervical collar.
Dislocation—sandbag neck, call neurosurgeon!
Thoracic/lumbar spine—rest, moist heat, NSAIDs, muscle relaxants, rehabilitation.

C. Burns, Electrical Injuries, and Thermal Injuries

1. Burns

■ **Description**

Thermal skin injury.

■ **Symptoms**

Erythema (minor; first degree), blisters (split thickness; second degree). Pain (first-/second-degree burns). No pain (third-degree).

■ **Diagnosis**

History and physical examination.

■ **Pathology**

Thermal skin/tissue injury (total epidermis destruction, with partial dermis destruction in second degree). Total epidermis and dermis destruction in third-degree burn.

■ **Treatment**

Remove patient from source of burn, clean/debride burn, fluids (Ringer's initially), antibiotics, tetanus toxoid, grafting.

Additional Information. **Rule of nines to estimate burn extent: each leg is 18%, each arm is 9%, body front is 18%, back is 18%, head is 9%, groin, 1%.**

2. Electrical Injuries/Burns

■ **Description**

Burns and trauma secondary to electrical injury.

■ Symptoms

Entry/exit wound (high-voltage, lightning). Massive tissue and bone destruction.

■ Diagnosis

History and physical examination.

■ Pathology

Massive tissue necrosis.

■ Treatment

Remove patient from source safely, CPR, fluids, clean/debride burns, surgical evaluation (fasciotomy, amputation).

3. Thermal Injuries

3–1. Frostbite

■ Description

Most severe cold injury.

■ Symptoms

Tissue cold/hard without feeling.

■ Diagnosis

History and physical examination; affected area may be white (superficial injury) or firm and frozen (deep injury).

■ Pathology

Skin/tissue damage from ice crystal formation. May be superficial or deep. Line of demarcation may develop.

■ Treatment

Rapid rewarming; surgical evaluation/amputation.

→ c̄ lukewarm H_2O

3–2. Hypothermia

■ Description

Reduced core temperature (under 35°C). $<35°C$

■ Symptoms

Lethargy, coma, hypotension, confusion.

■ Diagnosis

History and physical examination, core temperature, ECG (Osborne wave, elevated J-point; bradycardia; arrhythmias), flat electroencephalogram (EEG).

■ Pathology

Reduced core temperature from cold exposure resulting in decreased cardiac output, hypotension.

■ Treatment

Use CPR, core rewarming (heated oxygen), warming blankets.

Additional Information

Hypothermia complications—disseminated intravascular coagulation (DIC), pneumonia. Hypothermic death—cannot declare dead unless patient rewarmed.

3–3. Heatstroke

■ Description

Most severe type of heat injury.

■ Symptoms

Confusion, elevated core temperature with or without diaphoresis, tachycardia, hot skin.

■ **Diagnosis**

History and physical, **core temperature high,** combined with CNS signs.

■ **Pathology**

Tissue injury from elevated temperature; with children and elderly at most risk.

■ **Treatment**

Urgent cooling (water spray/ fans/ice packs).

Additional Information

Heat cramps—cramps from salt depletion; skin cool; give fluids/salt, keep cool.
Heat exhaustion—salt/water loss; nausea/weakness/headache/ thirst; give fluids/salt, keep cool.
Complications of heat stroke —disseminated intravascular coagulation rhabdomyolysis, acidosis.

D. **Lacerations**

■ **Description**

Skin/soft tissue injury.

■ **Symptoms**

As in description.

■ **Diagnosis**

History and physical examination.

■ **Pathology**

Traumatic skin injury.

■ **Treatment**

Irrigation and debridement, antibiotics, tetanus toxoid, and primary closure (maintaining minimal wound tension, and evert wound edges). Use 1 to 2% lidocaine for anesthesia (with epinephrine, except for digits, and end organs). Remove facial sutures in 3 to 5 days. All other areas, 7 to 14 days.

Additional Information. **Human bites— increased infection with primary closure.**

E. **Chest, Abdominal, and Pelvic Injuries**

1. *Pneumothorax*

■ **Description**

Air in pleural space.

■ **Symptoms**

Dyspnea, chest pain. Tachycardia and hypotension may present in tension pneumothorax.

■ **Diagnosis**

History and physical examination (absent breath sounds, decreased tactile fremitus, hyperresonance), **chest x-ray.**

■ **Pathology**

A result of blunt or penetrating trauma (including iatrogenic trauma). May also be spontaneous, in patients with pulmonary disease, or menses associated (catamenial).

■ **Treatment**

Small (under 15%)/**stable pneumothorax—observe.**

Urgent tension pneumothorax—insert large-bore needle into second intercostal space, midclavicular line (MCL).

Tube thoracostomy—use fifth intercostal space, anterior axillary line.

2. Hemothorax

■ Description

Blood in pleural space.

■ Symptoms

Dyspnea, chest pain.

■ Diagnosis

History and physical examination (absent breath sounds), chest x-ray.

■ Pathology

Trauma, or spontaneous.

■ Treatment

Chest tube (32 to 40 French, with 20-cm water suction).

Open thoracotomy—for persisting hemorrhage, or massive initial blood loss.

Inadequate hemothorax drainage results in fibrothorax.

3. Flail Chest

■ Description

Respiratory paradox with inspiration, secondary to multiple rib fractures.

■ Symptoms

Paradoxical chest wall motion, respiratory distress.

■ Diagnosis

History and physical (chest palpation), x-ray examination.

■ Pathology

Etiology: several ribs fractured, each in multiple places, resulting in reduced vital capacity and respiratory distress.

■ Treatment

Intubation, and positive pressure ventilation with positive end-expiratory pressure (PEEP).

Additional Information. Pericardial tamponade symptoms—diminished heart tones, narrow pulse pressure, ECG with low voltage. Also Beck's triad (hypotension, reduced cardiac tones, high central venous pressure [CVP]).

4. Perforation of Viscus

■ Description

Traumatic abdominal injury.

■ Symptoms

Pain, abdominal rigidity, peritoneal irritation, reduced/absent bowel sounds.

■ Diagnosis

History and physical examination (peritoneal irritation, shoulder pain, reduced/absent bowel sounds). X-rays, CT scan, diagnostic peritoneal lavage, exploratory laparotomy.

■ Pathology

Trauma.

■ **Treatment**

Laparotomy and surgical repair.

> **Spleen**—repair or splenectomy. _(1st ; 2nd degree observe)_
> **Colon**—repair (resect if severe injury).
> **Stomach**—repair.

Additional Information

> **Blunt abdominal trauma—spleen most often injured.**
>
> **Penetrating abdominal trauma—small bowel most often injured.**
>
> **Positive peritoneal lavage criteria—red blood cells over 20,000 (in penetrating injury), or RBC over 100,000 (in blunt injury).**

F. Drowning

■ **Description**

Asphyxia from water aspiration or water-induced laryngospasm.

■ **Symptoms**

Wheezing, tachypnea, vomiting, pulmonary edema, or **unconsciousness, shock,** and **cardiac arrest.**

■ **Diagnosis**

History and physical examination.

■ **Pathology**

Dry (laryngospasm) or water-induced asphyxia results in hypoxia and brain damage.

■ **Treatment**

Urgent CPR and 100% oxygen. Remember to continue CPR in hypothermic/prolonged cold-water submersion victims.

G. Thermal Injury

■ **Description**

See Section C.

H. Insect and Snake Bites

■ **Description**

Insect/snake envenomation.

■ **Symptoms**

Insect bite—**mild erythema to anaphylaxis/hypotension.**

Snake bite—**pain, swelling,** hemorrhage, weakness, DIC, possible systemic signs (lethargy, vomiting, shock).

■ **Diagnosis**

History and physical examination.

■ **Pathology**

Insects. *Hymenoptera* **species** commonly. _bumblebee, hornet, yellowjacket, wasp_

Snakes—in United States, **pit vipers** are **responsible for poisonous bites** (copperhead, rattlesnake, water moccasin), and are toxic to cardiac, vascular, and/or hematologic systems.

■ **Treatment**

(do not pinch/squeeze)

Insect bite—remove stinger, ice, diphenhydramine hydrochloride (Benadryl). *Anaphylaxis.* **Epinephrine (1:1000 0.4 mL subcutaneously),** CPR, antihistamines, prednisone.

Snake bite—**tourniquet, antivenin.**

Additional Information

> **Black widow spider—red hourglass design on abdomen; diffuse muscle spasm/cramping typical;**

treat by cleaning wound, give tetanus toxoid, muscle relaxant, antivenin.

Brown recluse spider—violin design on back; possible skin necrosis; treat by cleaning wound, and give tetanus toxoid.

I. Motion Sickness

■ **Description**

Aberrant reaction to motion.

■ **Symptoms**

Diaphoresis, nausea, vomiting.

■ **Diagnosis**

History and physical examination.

■ **Pathology**

Etiology in **vestibular-visual mismatch.**

■ **Treatment**

Antihistamines, or scopolamine. Avoid inciting etiology; vestibular training.

J. Head, Eye, and Ear Injury

1. Concussion

■ **Description**

Head injury, including unconsciousness, without physical brain damage.

■ **Symptoms**

Brief loss of consciousness, headache, nausea, and vomiting.

■ **Diagnosis**

History and physical examination, x-ray, CT scan. *r/o brain injury*

■ **Pathology**

Head trauma.

■ **Treatment**

Observation (neurologic watch).
neuro exam q 2°

2. Subdural Hematoma

■ **Description**

Subdural space hemorrhage.

■ **Symptoms**

After prolonged time from injury: lethargy, headache, seizures.

■ **Diagnosis**

History and physical examination, x-ray (CT/MRI).

■ **Pathology**

Trauma resulting in vein or brain tear/hemorrhage.

■ **Treatment**

Surgical, observation in some cases (small bleed/high-risk patient).

3. Epidural Hematoma

■ **Description**

Hemorrhage outside of the dura.

■ **Symptoms**

Shortly after injury: lethargy, headache, seizures. May have brief loss of consciousness (lucid interval).

■ **Diagnosis**

History and physical examination, x-ray (CT/MRI).

- **Pathology**

Trauma-induced artery or vein tear (**middle meningeal** artery/vein **common**).

- **Treatment**

Urgent surgery.

4. Ocular Injury

- **Description**

Eye injury via chemicals, or trauma.

- **Symptoms**

May have **pain, vision loss,** subconjunctival hemorrhage. If light flashes noted, rule out retinal detachment.

- **Diagnosis**

History and physical examination, ophthalmoscopic and slit-lamp examination.

- **Pathology**

Chemicals—chemical conjunctivitis, blindness.
Trauma—hyphema, laceration, abrasion.

- **Treatment**

Hyphema—anterior chamber hemorrhage (ophthalmologist's evaluation needed as soon as possible).
Chemicals—irrigation with normal saline.
Corneal abrasion—antibiotic ointment, patch.
Corneal laceration—**patch, refer to ophthalmologist.**

5. Auditory Injury

- **Description**

Pinna, external ear canal, and tympanic membrane injury.

- **Symptoms**

Swelling, pain, hearing loss, vertigo, and hemorrhage.

- **Diagnosis**

History and physical examination, and audiometric exam, x-ray skull/temporal bone (rule out associated fracture).

- **Pathology**

Trauma.

- **Treatment**

Tympanic membrane perforation—if small, supportive treatment (cotton earplug, systemic antibiotic for infection); if large, surgical treatment.
Noise-induced hearing loss—no treatment (except hearing aid).

Additional Information. Trauma may cause subperichondral hematoma. Calcified hematoma results in **cauliflower ear.** Prevent with early drainage.

K. Industrial and Occupational Dermatitis

- **Description**

Pathology/dermatitis secondary to industrial/occupational chemical, physical, thermal, and toxin exposure.

- **Symptoms**

Pruritus, inflammation, erythema, blisters.

- **Diagnosis**

History and physical examination, skin biopsy, allergic patch test.

- **Pathology**

Skin contact with foreign agent resulting in dermatitis. **Contact dermatitis most frequent.**

- **Treatment**

Remove from source, antihistamines, topical/systemic corticosteroids.

L. Anaphylactic Shock

- **Description**

Systemic severe **IgE-induced** allergic reaction.

- **Symptoms**

Hypotension, urticaria, dyspnea, tachycardia, and pruritus.

- **Diagnosis**

History and physical exam.

- **Pathology**

Mast cell/basophils release histamine, platelet-activating factor and arachidonic acid.

- **Treatment**

Use **CPR/control airway, epinephrine** (1:1000 0.3 to 0.5 mL subcutaneously), diphenhydramine hydrochloride (Benadryl), **fluids, dopamine, beta-agonists, corticosteroids.**

M. Poisoning

1. *Acetaminophen*

   - **Symptoms**

   Hepatic failure, nausea/vomiting, hepatic necrosis.

   - **Diagnosis**

   Blood acetaminophen level.

   - **Treatment**

   Ipecac or gastric lavage, antidote is *N*-acetylcysteine (Mucomyst).
   must be given c̄/in 24 hours

2. *Tricyclic Antidepressants*

   - **Symptoms**

   Transient hypertension, then hypotension, tachycardia/arrhythmias, seizures, anticholinergic symptoms.
   ~~hallucination,~~

   - **Diagnosis**

   History and physical examination, blood level, ECG.

   - **Treatment**

   Ipecac or gastric lavage, charcoal, NG tube suction, sodium bicarbonate, physostigmine, phenytoin sodium (Dilantin).

3. *Sedatives*

   - **Symptoms**

   Lethargy, confusion, coma, hypotension.

   - **Diagnosis**

   History and physical examination, blood drug level.

■ **Treatment**

Control airway, activated charcoal (if patient awake), supportive care.

4. Stimulants

■ **Symptoms**

Euphoria, dilated pupils, hypertension, tachycardia, hyperactivity, psychosis.

■ **Diagnosis**

History and physical examination, blood drug level.

■ **Treatment**

Supportive, charcoal. **Emesis may cause seizures.**

5. Cocaine

■ **Symptoms**

Agitation, hyperthermia, hypertension, cardiac arrhythmia, tachycardia, seizures, pulmonary edema.

■ **Diagnosis**

History and physical examination, blood drug level.

■ **Treatment**

Supportive treatment, control airway.

6. Phencyclidine (PCP)

■ **Symptoms**

Nystagmus, lethargy, incoordination, violent behavior, self-destructive behavior.

■ **Diagnosis**

History and physical examination, blood drug level.

■ **Treatment**

Control airway, activated charcoal, supportive therapy.

7. Alcohol

■ **Symptoms**

Methanol. [drunk s̄ smell of EtOH]
Blurry vision, headache, vomiting.
Ethanol. Incoordination, diplopia, drunk!

■ **Diagnosis**

History and physical examination, blood alcohol level.

■ **Treatment**

Methanol—ipecac, antidote (ethanol), sodium bicarbonate.
Ethanol—ipecac, sodium bicarbonate.

8. Solvent Sniffing

■ **Symptoms**

GI irritation, CNS symptoms. Skin injury.

■ **Diagnosis**

History and physical examination.

■ **Treatment**

Supportive treatment, control airway, oxygen. Ipecac for massive ingestion only.

Additional Information [except meperidine]

Narcotics—pinpoint pupils, hypotension; give naloxone hydrochloride (Narcan).

Barbiturates—respiratory depression, hypotension; supportive care, charcoal and alkalinization of urine.

9. *Heavy Metals, Arsenic*

■ Symptoms

GI symptoms, arrhythmia, CNS symptoms, skin bronzing, Mee's lines, vomiting, garlic odor (bitter almond odor for cyanide).

■ Diagnosis

History and physical examination, x-ray abdomen (arsenic, lead, and iodides may be radiopaque).

■ Treatment

Charcoal/emesis, dimercaprol (BAL).

Additional Information

> **Lead**—vomiting, lethargy, blue gum line; lavage, then use ethylenediaminetetraacetic acid (EDTA).
> **Mercury**—give milk, gastric lavage, then dimercaprol (BAL).

10. *Carbon Monoxide*

■ Symptoms

Headache, confusion, nausea, dyspnea, **cherry-red skin.** Chronic exposure associated with parkinsonism.

■ Diagnosis

History and physical examination (cyanosis), elevated blood carboxyhemoglobin.

■ Treatment

Remove from source, oxygen.

11. *Diethyltoluamide (DEET)*

■ Symptoms

CNS symptoms/seizures, coma, hypotension, GI irritation.

■ Diagnosis

History and physical examination.

■ Treatment

Emesis/gastric lavage.

Additional Poisonings

> **Iron**—gastric lavage with Fleet's phospho-soda, parenteral deferoxamine.
> **Aspirin**—causes respiratory alkalosis, and metabolic acidosis.
> **Drugs visible on x-ray**—heavy metals, phenothiazines, iodides, and chloral hydrate.

III. PRINCIPLES OF MANAGEMENT

A. Traumatic Injury

■ Description

Use CPR, **control airway, treat urgent problems** (large pneumothorax, hemorrhage, etc), **oxygen, IV line, fluids/meds, history and physical examination, x-ray/ lab studies.**

B. Shock

■ Description

Use CPR, **control airway, history and physical exam, fluids** (caution with cardiogenic shock, check CVP and output), **vasopressors (dopamine), lab studies, corticosteroids,** diuretic (protects kidneys), buffers, antibiotics (septic shock).

C. Burns

■ Description

Use CPR, **cool burn, clean/debride burn, history and physical exam, determine area of burn, topical antibiotic, loose gauze wrap on non-adhering dressing. Severe burns: use CPR/airway control, fluid replacement (monitor CVP and output), NG tube, pain and sepsis con-**

trol (morphine), surgical treatment (grafting, etc).

D. Poisoning

■ Description

Use **CPR, maintain airway, history and physical exam, lab studies, gastric lavage/emesis, antidote** after lavage, **supportive care, laboratory work-up.** Avoid ipecac with caustic ingestions, and in somnolent patient. If antidote available, do not give charcoal in addition.

E. Child Abuse, Sexual Abuse, Rape

■ Description

History and physical examination, medical treatment, documentation of evidence and appropriate reporting, psychological evaluation/support, separation from danger (child abuse), and **long-term care plan.**

BIBLIOGRAPHY

Ballenger JJ. *Diseases of the Nose, Throat, Ear, Head, and Neck.* 14th ed. Philadelphia, Pa: Lea & Febiger; 1991.

Behrman RE. *Nelson Textbook of Pediatrics.* 13th ed. Philadelphia, Pa: WB Saunders Company; 1987.

Birnbaum JS. *The Musculoskeletal Manual.* Orlando, Fla: Academic Press Inc; 1982.

Bryson PD. *Comprehensive Review in Toxicology.* 2nd ed. Rockville, Md: Aspen Publishers Inc; 1989.

Cailliet R. *Neck and Arm Pain.* 3rd ed. Philadelphia, Pa: FA Davis Company; 1991.

D'Ambrosia RD. *Musculoskeletal Disorders, Regional Examination and Differential Diagnosis.* 2nd ed. Philadelphia, Pa: JB Lippincott Company; 1986.

Dreisbach RH. *Handbook of Poisoning: Prevention, Diagnosis and Treatment.* 12th ed. Norwalk, Conn: Appleton & Lange; 1987.

Goldfrank LR. *Toxicologic Emergencies.* 4th ed. Norwalk, Conn: Appleton & Lange; 1990.

Hardy JD. *Textbook of Surgery.* 2nd ed. Philadelphia, Pa: JB Lippincott Company; 1988.

Rockwood CA. *Fractures in Adults.* 3rd ed. Vols. 1 and 2. Philadelphia, Pa: JB Lippincott Company; 1991.

Schroeder SA. *Current Medical Diagnosis and Treatment.* 30th ed. Norwalk, Conn: Appleton & Lange; 1991.

Turek SL. *Orthopaedics Principles and Their Application.* 4th ed. Vols. 1 and 2. Philadelphia, Pa: JB Lippincott Company; 1984.

Upton AC. *The Medical Clinics of North America, Vol. 74, Environmental Medicine.* Philadelphia, Pa: WB Saunders Company; March 1990.

CHAPTER 9

Infectious and Parasitic Diseases
JOEL S. GOLDBERG, DO

Answers to Dr Baskin Questions:

   #6 D

   #7 C

   #8 A

   #9 C

   #10 C

   #11 B   prerenal
              BUN/Cr >20, Urine Osm > 300, FE$_{Na}$ <1, spot U$_{Na}$ <20   Ucre/Pcre high

   #12 B   Urinary anion gap: (Na+K) - Cl ; high chloride in feces ↑NH$_3$ so no problem c̄ kidney

   #13 B

   #14 B

   #15 C   5 stages of diabetic nephropathy : must do bx to find out b/c takes years

   #16

   #17

   #18

   #19

   #20

   #21

   #22

   #23

   #24

I. HEALTH AND HEALTH MAINTENANCE

A. Economic and Social Impact

- **Description**

Consider financial and social impact of infection and costs involved in infection control and treatment.

B. Disease Occurrence Patterns

- **Description**

Be aware of geographic, demographic, and temporal patterns of disease occurrence. Examples: increased temperature/humidity may allow mosquito vector to survive, also fungal infections. Geographic area may be a building, city, or school district. Demographic patterns play a role (poverty/sanitation, education/hygiene).

C. Surveillance

- **Description**

Reporting of disease and death-certificate information allows collection and analysis of epidemiologic information. Determination of leading causes of death and disability allows increased focus on areas in need of preventive/treatment planning.

D. Community Measures

- **Description**

Consider the need for sanitation, education, school health and immunization programs, investigation/control of outbreaks.

E. Individual Preventive Measures

- **Description**

Education, immunization, sanitation/hygiene, safe sex, home and occupational disease exposure.

F. Isolation and Reverse Isolation

- **Description**

Protection of medical personnel by eliminating contact with infectious patient and contaminated material (may be blood, urine, body secretions, feces, etc). Centers for Disease Control (CDC) guidelines list necessary precautions for specified disorder.

G. Surgical Infection Prevention

- **Description**

Sterility of procedure and physician (gowns, gloves, etc), prophylactic antibiotics, pulmonary toilet, irrigation, and adequate surgical technique.

H. Infants, Elderly, and Impaired Immunity

- **Description**

Importance of prevention, need for early intervention to prevent rapid disease spread in these patients, need to look for age-specific disorders, and disorders typical in impaired-immunity cases.

II. EPIDEMIOLOGY

A. Nervous System Infections

1. Meningitis

Etiology in **central nervous system (CNS) trauma, bacteria spread** from other infections.

Impact: significant fatality rate and possible **neurologic sequelae.**

Prevention by **immunization (*Haemophilus influenzae*)**, carrier elimination (meningococcal, **rifampin**), early detection and treatment of disease (Lyme, tuberculosis [TB]).

2. Poliomyelitis

Epidemiology: <u>fecal–oral</u> transmission of **poliomyelitis virus.**

Prevention by immunization (Sabin, oral live virus; **Salk,** inactivated vaccine), has resulted in dramatic reduction of cases.

3. Tetanus

Clostridium tetani in soil and feces. **More infection in poor nations.**

   Impact: greater mortality in elderly.

   Prevention: immunization. May give passive immunization with 250 U tetanus immune globulin.

4. Rabies

Epidemiology: wild animals most **common cause,** and incidence increasing. **Transmission via saliva, rarely respiratory** (cave exploration), and a few cases by corneal transplant.

   Impact: recovery unlikely.

   Prevention: immunization for at-risk individuals (rabies vaccine), avoiding exposure, and postbite treatment (**rabies immune globulin** and **rabies vaccine** given).

5. Neurosyphilis

Untreated syphilis may result in neurosyphilis (5 to 10%).

   Impact: may include **meningitis, paresis, posterior column degeneration (tabes dorsalis**), and **Argyll–Robertson pupil** (small, no light reaction).

   Prevention: treatment of **asymptomatic**-stage patient (**cerebrospinal fluid [CSF] pleocytosis,** elevated protein and positive serology). Also, treatment of primary- and secondary-stage disease.

6. Ophthalmia Neonatorum

Etiology in *Neisseria gonorrhoeae,* chlamydia, hemophilus, and staph.

   Impact: keratitis.

   Prevention: one percent **silver nitrate,** erythromycin.

B. Respiratory Infections

1. Influenza

Epidemiology: type A (pandemics), **most virulent, in animals** and humans. **Type B** (epidemics), and **Type C** (sporadic), mostly in humans.

   Increased winter incidence.

   Impact of **type B: pneumonitis, croup,** congestive heart failure (CHF), death, Reye syndrome.

   Prevention: vaccination or **amantadine.** Treat with amantadine.

2. Diphtheria

Epidemiology: respiratory epidemic **spread** in low socioeconomic areas typical. Carriers contribute to infection. Disease **mostly in children.**

   Impact: death (**myocarditis,** pulmonary obstruction).

   Prevention: immunization.

3. Pertussis

Epidemics every several years, reduced morbidity/mortality lately.

   Impact: may include **death** and complications (pneumonia, superinfection (**severe cough, hypoxia**).

   Prevention: immunization.

4. Tuberculosis

Increased incidence in low socioeconomic areas with **prevention by chemoprophylaxis** of **positive reactors** isonicotine hydrazine (INH), **vaccination** (BCG: Bacille Calmette-Guérin), **screening.**

5. Streptocococcal Pharyngitis

Respiratory transmission common, **carrier** may convey infection, **peak late winter.**

   Impact: rheumatic fever, glomerulonephritis, scarlet fever, and complication of peritonsillar abscess.

Prevention: penicillin if positive culture, or preventive treatment of rheumatic/scarlet fever contacts.

6. Pneumococcal Pneumonia

Epidemiology: respiratory transmission, increased incidence in chronic disease, immunosuppressed and splenectomized patients, and alcoholics. **Asymptomatic carriers** common, disease produced when defenses down. Complications include **empyema** and **shock.**

Prevention: immunization, especially for chronic cardiac/pulmonary disease, diabetics, elderly, S/P splenectomy.

C. Digestive Infections

1. Mumps

Epidemiology: Children typically, common in confined areas (military, hospitals), **respiratory spread.** Complications include **meningitis, deafness, orchitis,** nephritis, pancreatitis, encephalitis.

Prevention: live attenuated vaccine.

2. Botulism

Epidemiology: Higher incidence with **home canning/curing** of food. **Type A most severe. Types A, B (meat), type E (fish).**

Impact: may include fatal disease by muscular respiratory insufficiency.

Prevention: education about food preparation, canning, smoking, storage, and refrigeration, **heat food 60°C for 30 minutes. Botulism spores in honey—do not give to infants** (floppy baby disease).

3. Salmonella

Epidemiology: food/water transmission usually. Salmonella found in nearly all animals. *S. typhi* only in humans. Increase in poor socioeconomic areas, and with coexisting disease.

Impact: high morbidity/mortality **in underdeveloped countries, infants, elderly.** Complications include myocarditis, gastrointestinal (GI) bleed, pneumonia, meningitis.

Prevention: food/food handler testing/control. Water sanitation, turtle-shipping law, hygiene, treatment/follow-up/isolation of active cases. **Typhoid vaccine** in high-risk cases.

4. Shigella

Epidemiology: fecal/oral/insect transmission, increase in low socioeconomic areas, **mostly children. Rarely food/water vector.** Children/elderly/coexisting disease patients more likely to suffer dehydration.

Prevention: sanitation, fly control, hygiene, education.

5. Typhoid Fever

Epidemiology: water/food transmission from infected person.

Impact: greater in developing nations. Complications include **colon perforation/hemorrhage,** pneumonia, phlebitis.

Prevention: carrier treatment, typhoid vaccine partially effective.

6. Cholera

Epidemiology: water/food transmission to humans.

Impact: high mortality by shock, renal failure, acidosis, **if untreated.**

Prevention: immunization partially effective.

7. Viral Hepatitis

Epidemiology: type A (fecal/oral/food/water), no chronic infection state, and 1-month incubation. **Type B (parenteral/blood/body fluid exchange),**

carrier possible, 1- to 6-month incubation.

Impact: **hepatocellular carcinoma,** polyarteritis, with **type B. Fulminant hepatitis,** death, with **type A.**

Prevention in **type A: immune serum globulin** (pre-exposure in close contacts, postexposure if at high risk), **hygiene, sanitation.**

Prevention in **type B: immunization, postexposure hepatitis B immune globulin (HBIG),** education, hygiene. **Newborn immunization. Non-A, non-B: parenteral transmission** (transfusions), 1- to 2-month incubation.

8. Amebiasis

Epidemiology: greater incidence in poor socioeconomic/sanitation areas with **food/water transmission** and cyst ingestion.

Impact: **liver/lung abscess** as well as clonic mucosa.

Prevention: **water purification,** treat asymptomatic cyst carriers.

9. Giardiasis

Epidemiology: transmission by water/fecal/oral modes, **more in children, cyst survives water chlorination,** increased incidence in poor socioeconomic groups. On homosexual population seen transmitted by anal sex.

Impact: **malabsorption** and **travelers' diarrhea** agent often.

Prevention: hygiene, water (iodine tablets, boiling if traveling), safe sex, and carrier treatment.

10. Hookworm

Epidemiology: increase in tropics/inadequate sanitation. **Larvae enter exposed skin.**

Impact: large numbers of persons affected worldwide, **anemia.**

Prevention: wearing shoes, sanitation/waste disposal.

11. Pinworm

Epidemiology: children usually, hand/mouth transmission, increased family/school infections, **incidence not related to socioeconomic factors.**

Impact: **most frequent US worm infection.**

Prevention: hygiene.

12. Toxicogenic Escherichia coli Infection

Epidemiology: children commonly.

Impact: **number 1 cause of travelers' diarrhea.**

Prevention: doxycycline or trimethoprim sulfamethoxozole.

D. Cardiac Infections

1. Bacterial Endocarditis

Epidemiology: **acute infection** (vegetation) **after bacteremia, chronic** with pre-existing cardiac pathology (congenital disease/mitral valve prolapse). **More in elderly, children uncommon.**

Impact: chronic disease and death.

Prevention: **antibiotics** before/after bacteremic-inducing procedure.

2. Prosthetic Valve Infection

Epidemiology: **aortic valve more likely,** with *Staphylococcus epidermidis* most often.

Impact: **incidence 3%** with **50% mortality.**

Prevention: **prophylactic antibiotics.**

E. Sexually Transmitted Diseases (STDs)

1. HIV Infection/AIDS

Epidemiology: initially IV-drug users, homosexual men, and Haitians. Additionally, heterosexuals, recipients of transfusions, hemophiliacs, infants born to human immunodeficiency virus (HIV)-positive mothers.

Impact: worldwide fatal disease, social/sexual behavior changes, health system/financial burden. Prevent by education, blood precautions, safe sex.

2. Gonorrhea

Epidemiology: sexual transmission.

Impact: septic arthritis, prostatitis, pelvic inflammatory disease (PID), infertility.

Prevention: asymptomatic case treatment, education, condom.

3. Chlamydial Infection

Epidemiology: sexual transmission.

Impact: common STD agent, resulting in PID. Also, **newborn inclusion conjunctivitis.**

Prevention: screening, education, treatment of partners.

4. Chancroid

Epidemiology: poor socioeconomic area STD.

Impact: worldwide infection.

Prevention: carrier treatment/ screening, condom.

5. Syphilis

Epidemiology: sexual/congenital/parenteral transmission. Also kissing (if oral lesions present).

Impact: complications of **late syphilis** (CNS, cardiac, blindness, etc.).

Prevention: screening, education, public health programs.

6. Urinary Tract Infection

Epidemiology: more common with urinary stasis, structural lesions, reflux, intercourse, pregnancy. **Females more common, except in neonates.**

Impact: large numbers of people infected, risk of complications, and economic concerns.

Prevention: education, catheter care, antibiotics.

F.   Other Infectious Disorders

1. Rubella

Epidemiology: transmission by **respiratory droplets,** mild in children, periodic epidemics prior to vaccine (every 6 to 9 years).

Impact: includes fetal risk if pregnant in first trimester (congenital rubella syndrome, **cataracts, heart defects, deafness, microcephaly**).

Prevention: live attenuated rubella vaccine.

2. Rubeola

Epidemiology: respiratory transmission, children usually, extremely contagious.

Impact: complications include death, pneumonia, encephalitis, keratitis, and otitis media.

Prevention: live measles virus vaccine, two doses now advised.

3. Chickenpox

Epidemiology: mostly children, **most common children's exanthem,** respiratory and direct-contact transmission, incubation 2 to 3 weeks.

Impact: Reye syndrome, pneumonia, encephalitis, death, hospital/medical costs, and potential fetal anomalies.

Prevention: varicella-zoster immune globulin in high-risk patients.

4. Rocky Mountain Spotted Fever

Epidemiology: usually young males, **tick bite** transmission (wood/dog tick), but **bite may not be recalled.** Incubation 1 week.

Impact: death, shock, disseminated intravascular coagulation (DIC).
Prevention: avoiding tick bites and tick control.

5. Malaria

Epidemiology: transmission by mosquito/parenteral protozoa injection.
Impact: many deaths yearly.
Prevention: draining swamps, mosquito protection, **chloroquine** 500 mg weekly, 2 weeks before exposure, to 6 weeks after. If **chloroquine-resistant-strain area, give fansidar** (pyrimethamine/sulfadoxine).

III. MECHANISMS AND DISEASE DIAGNOSIS/TREATMENT

A. General Aspects

1. Bacteremia and Septicemia

■ **Description**

Spread of infection to the bloodstream (bacteremia), septicemia includes symptoms.

■ **Symptoms**

Fever, chills, hypotension, hypothermia, shock. Rash (**ecthyma gangrenosum,** with *Pseudomonas* and others).

■ **Diagnosis**

Blood culture.

■ **Pathology**

Complex. Usually **gram-negative bacteria. Endotoxin** may cause symptoms/shock.

■ **Treatment**

Antibiotics, supportive (fluids, pressors), corticosteroids?

2. Toxic Shock Syndrome

■ **Description**

Toxin-producing staph infection.

■ **Symptoms**

Fever, rash, hypotension, dermal peeling of palms and soles (skin desquamation).

■ **Diagnosis**

History and physical, tampon use, culture (vagina/blood).

■ **Pathology**

Toxin of *Staphylococcus aureus,* by tampon or wound infection. (Not exclusive of *Staph.* infection, also seen with certain *Strep.* infections, although not frequent).

Can also occur in children & other types of pt.!

■ **Treatment**

Antibiotics (β-lactamase-resistant, antistaphylococcal), remove tampon.

3. Antimicrobial Susceptibility and Resistance

■ **Description**

Germs may develop antimicrobial resistance via multiple methods, which may be genetic or non-genetic in nature. Antimicrobial agents may be bacteriostatic (inhibit germ replication), or bactericidal. Attack on germs may involve cell membrane breakdown, disruption of enzyme-substrate reactions, enzyme protein alterations, and others. Antibiotic susceptibility testing by **dilution** and **diffusion** tests.

Leptospirosis: petechiae, liver & kidney failure

B.   Infectious and Parasitic Disease

1. Eyes

1–1. Ophthalmia Neonatorum

- **Description**

Newborn conjunctivitis.

- **Symptoms**

Purulent conjunctivitis before 1 week old.

- **Diagnosis**

History and physical examination, culture.

- **Pathology**

Etiology in *Neisseria gonorrhoeae, Chlamydia, Hemophilus*.
↳ *rarer*

- **Treatment**

Antibiotics. Prevent by 1% silver nitrate. *@ birth!*

1–2. Bacterial Conjunctivitis

- **Description**

Conjunctival inflammation.

- **Symptoms**

Exudate, itching, eyelid edema.

- **Diagnosis**

History and physical exam, **conjunctival scraping** and **culture.**

- **Pathology**

Wide etiology possible.

- **Treatment**

Antibiotics. Topical and/or systemic.

1–3. Viral Keratoconjunctivitis

- **Description**

Corneal infection/inflammation.

- **Symptoms**

Red, painful eye especially in children, may be minimal symptoms also.

- **Diagnosis**

History and physical exam.

- **Pathology**

Herpes simplex most common in children, also other viruses including adenovirus (common with adult infections).

- **Treatment**

Trifluridine (Viroptic).

2. Ears

2–1. External Otitis

- **Description**

External auditory canal inflammation. "Swimmer's ear."

- **Symptoms**

Pain, drainage, itching.

- **Diagnosis**

History and physical examination. Culture.

- **Pathology**

Staphylococcus epidermidis, other bacteria, fungal. **If chronic, suspect** *Pseudomonas.*
   Malignant otitis, suspect *Pseudomonas* or *Proteus.* *(esp diabetics)*

■ **Treatment**

Topical and (if necessary) systemic antibiotics.

2–2. Otitis Media

■ **Description**

Middle ear inflammation.

■ **Symptoms**

Fever, hearing loss, pain.

■ **Diagnosis**

History and physical examination.

■ **Pathology**

Streptococcus pneumoniae common. Multiple other agents possible. Common in children with eustachian tube dysfunction as possible etiology.

■ **Treatment**

Antibiotics (amoxicillin).

2–3. Mastoiditis

■ **Description**

Mastoid air cell inflammation.

■ **Symptoms**

Fever, pain, hearing loss, postauricular swelling/erythema, pinna displaced.

■ **Diagnosis**

History and physical, x-ray studies.

■ **Pathology**

Spread from otitis media.

■ **Treatment**

Antibiotics, myringotomy, mastoidectomy.

3. Nervous System

3–1. Meningitis

■ **Description**

Brain/spinal cord membrane inflammation.

■ **Symptoms**

Fever/nuchal rigidity/headache/ vomiting. **Brudzinski's sign:** cervical motion elicits pain. **Kernig's sign:** painful hamstring stretch.

■ **Diagnosis**

History and physical. Examination of CSF (bacteria: low glucose, elevated protein; viral: normal glucose, slightly elevated protein).

■ **Pathology**

Spread of germs to the CNS via the blood. Common germs: up to 1 month of age, *E. coli,* and group B strep; 1 month to age 6, *H. influenza* type b, *Streptococcus pneumoniae* and *Neisseria meningitidis;* older than 6, *S. pneumoniae* and *N. meningitidis.*

■ **Treatment**

Antibiotics.

3–2. Brain Abscess

■ **Description**

Local intracranial infection.

■ **Symptoms**

Headache, mental changes, nausea/vomiting.

■ **Diagnosis**

History and physical examination, computed tomography (CT) scan, lumbar puncture.

■ **Pathology**

Anaerobic bacteria common. May extend from ear/sinuses, follow injury, or be blood-borne from other areas (lung).

■ **Treatment**

Antibiotics IV, surgical drainage.

3–3. **Spinal Epidural Abscess**

■ **Description**

United States Medical Licensing Examination (USMLE) infrequent disease with early intervention to prevent paraplegia.

■ **Symptoms**

Local severe back pain changing to radicular pain, then weakness. Fever and local tenderness also.

■ **Diagnosis**

History and physical examination, x-rays, CT, lumbar puncture.

■ **Pathology**

Blood-borne spread from skin and other sites (dental work), by *Staphylococcus aureus* usually.

■ **Treatment**

Surgical drainage, antibiotics.

3–4. **HIV Infection/AIDS**

■ **Description**

Acquired immunodeficiency syndrome (AIDS) is HIV positivity with opportunistic infections and weight loss.

■ **Symptoms**

HIV infection: may be asymptomatic, or multiple system complaints (oral candidiasis, hairy leukoplakia, herpes simplex, etc).
AIDS: weight loss, diarrhea, opportunistic infections, fever.

■ **Diagnosis**

History and physical, serologic testing (enzyme-linked immunosorbent assay [ELISA] HIV, Western blot to confirm).

■ **Pathology**

Sexual, parenteral, and vertical transmission of HIV virus, resulting in immunodeficiency. Target of HIV is CD4 lymphocyte.

■ **Treatment**

Zidovudine (AZT). Treat individual infections (herpes simplex, acyclovir; cryptococcal meningitis, amphotericin B; *Pneumocystis carinii*, trimethoprim/sulfamethoxazole; toxoplasmosis, pyrimethamine).

3–5. Poliomyelitis

■ Description

Spinal cord inflammatory disorder.

■ Symptoms

Fever, headache, weakness, sore throat. Muscle wasting, lower motor neuron lesion, vomiting.

■ Diagnosis

History and physical examination. Examination of CSF. Stool/throat/fecal culture. Serologic testing to confirm.

■ Pathology

Poliomyelitis virus transmitted by fecal/oral means, resulting in non-paralytic and paralytic (spinal and bulbar) polio. If only flu-like symptoms, termed abortive polio.

■ Treatment

Symptomatic.

3–6. Rabies

■ Description

Viral encephalitis.

■ Symptoms

Hydrophobia (laryngeal spasm with drinking or just sight of water), paresthesia/pain at bite site. Hyperactivity, ascending paralysis.

■ Diagnosis

History and physical, animal bite. Check animal's brain for rabies. Also via state lab: search for rabies virus/antigen by neck skin/cornea biopsy, and serologic screening (for antirabies antibody).

■ Pathology

Transmission by virus in saliva.

■ Treatment

Pray! (rabies is usually fatal), supportive care. Also, early post-exposure vaccination with rabies vaccine and rabies immune globulin are effective in prevention.

3–7. Herpes Zoster

■ Description

Varicella-zoster virus infection in sensory ganglia.

■ Symptoms

Vesicular eruption in dermatome distribution, pain.

■ Diagnosis

History and physical examination. Viral culture.

■ Pathology

Varicella-zoster virus.

■ Treatment

Acyclovir, systemic corticosteroids may reduce chance of postherpetic neuralgia.

3–8. Herpes Simplex

■ Description

Type 1 usually non-genital. Type 2, genital.

- **Symptoms**

Group of vesicles on erythematous patch. Fever, tender lymph nodes.

- **Diagnosis**

History and physical examination, Tzanck smear positive for multinucleated giant cells.

- **Pathology**

Incubation one week. Skin/mucosa/skin transmission.

- **Treatment**

Acyclovir.

3–9. Tetanus

- **Description**

Neurotoxin-induced muscle spasm disorder.

- **Symptoms**

Tonic muscle spasms (jaw, trismus/lockjaw), trismus sardonicus: trismus-induced facial sneer. Opisthotonos, tetanospasms.

- **Diagnosis**

History and physical examination.

- **Pathology**

Clostridium tetani produces neurotoxin. Several days to 3 weeks incubation, after germ entry via wound.

- **Treatment**

Supportive, tetanus immune globulin, and penicillin G.

3–10. Viral Encephalitis

- **Description**

Meningeal CNS inflammation/infection. *Brain parenchyma = encephalitis*

- **Symptoms**

Stiff neck, headache, seizures, CNS alterations, fever, vomiting. Symptoms may be subclinical or severe in nature.

Herpes gives personality ∆/o

- **Diagnosis**

History and physical, CSF culture/examination (increased protein/pressure), throat/fecal viral cultures.

bloody CSF in herpes

- **Pathology**

Vast etiology (arboviruses, enteroviruses).

temporal lobes in herpes

- **Treatment**

Supportive (herpes simplex, give acyclovir).

3–11. Toxoplasmosis

- **Description**

Protozoan infection.

- **Symptoms**

Usually asymptomatic; fever, headache, myalgia, adenopathy. Congenital infection (microcephaly, seizures, retinochoroiditis).

- **Diagnosis**

Serologic testing, blood exam for cysts/trophozoites. History and physical.

■ **Pathology**

Infection with *Toxoplasma gondii* usually by **cyst ingestion** (cat litter/soil/undercooked meat. **Pregnant women must avoid all three**). Also, transplacental.

■ **Treatment**

Pyrimethamine plus sulfadiazine.

4. Nose and Throat

4–1. Common Cold

■ **Description**

Self-limited, upper respiratory tract infection.

■ **Symptoms**

Coryza (runny nose), cough, sneezing, sore throat.

■ **Diagnosis**

History and physical examination.

■ **Pathology**

Rhinoviruses, coronaviruses, and others.

■ **Treatment**

Symptomatic.

4–2. Sinusitis

■ **Description**

Paranasal sinus infection.

Maxillary, facial, ethmoid

■ **Symptoms**

Facial headache/pressure, teeth/eye pain, nasal congestion/blockage.

■ **Diagnosis**

History and physical examination (purulent nasal discharge, swollen nasal mucosa, tenderness to percussion, etc). X-ray studies.

■ **Pathology**

Bacterial (*Streptococcus pneumoniae*), viral, by germ spread or sinusal ostia blockage.

■ **Treatment**

Antibiotics.

4–3. Pharyngitis

■ **Description**

Pharynx inflammation.

■ **Symptoms**

Fever, sore throat, pharyngeal/tonsil exudate may be present.

■ **Diagnosis**

History and physical, throat culture.

Strep pharyngitis = palatal petechiae

■ **Pathology**

Bacterial, viral, and other.

■ **Treatment**

Bacterial, antibiotics. Non-bacterial, supportive.

4–4. Peritonsillar Abscess

■ **Description**

Peritonsillar space abscess.

■ **Symptoms**

Pain, dysphagia, drooling.

■ **Diagnosis**

History and physical exam, throat/aspirate culture. Laboratory studies (complete blood count [CBC], mono screen, etc).

■ **Pathology**

Usually **group A beta-hemolytic strep,** from tonsillopharyngitis spread. **Most common pharyngitis complication.**

■ **Treatment**

Aspiration/incision and drainage (I and D), antibiotics.

4–5. Acute Laryngotracheitis

■ **Description**

Spasmodic croup (laryngotracheitis).

■ **Symptoms**

Barking cough, coryza, fever, air hunger, inspiratory stridor.

improves ō cold air

■ **Diagnosis**

History and physical, cultures.

■ **Pathology**

Viral (parainfluenza virus) usually.

■ **Treatment**

Humidification, airway control, antibiotics if bacterial.

4–6. Pertussis

■ **Description**

Acute respiratory tract disease.

■ **Symptoms**

Coughing, whoop, fever, after 5- to 10-day incubation.

may vomit after coughing or have seizure (2° hypoxia)

■ **Diagnosis**

Clinical. Catarrhal then paroxysmal stages, culture.

■ **Pathology**

Bordetella pertussis.

■ **Treatment**

Supportive, erythromycin, ampicillin.

4–7. Diphtheria

■ **Description**

Upper respiratory tract infection.

■ **Symptoms**

Purulent nasal discharge, tonsillar membrane, fever, cervical adenopathy, nausea/vomiting.

■ **Diagnosis**

Clinical, sore throat with green/gray pharyngeal membrane.

■ **Pathology**

Corynebacterium diphtheriae.

■ **Treatment**

Diphtheria antitoxin (DAT), and penicillin or erythromycin. Penicillin or erythromycin for carrier state.

4–8. Epiglottitis

■ Description

Bacterial supraglottic inflammation. "Cherry-red epiglottis."

■ Symptoms

Fever, sore throat, respiratory distress, drooling, dysphagia.

Stridor

■ Diagnosis

Clinical. Improper examination may result in laryngeal spasm/cardiorespiratory arrest. Also controlled exam, blood culture, lateral neck x-ray.

DO NOT upset this kid!

■ Pathology

Haemophilus influenzae type B.

■ Treatment

Airway control, antibiotics.

take the kid to OR c̄ mom & do exam under anaesthesia!

5. Lungs

5–1. Bronchitis

■ Description

Bronchial inflammation.

Inflammation of larger airways

■ Symptoms

Productive cough, fever, headache, sore throat, hemoptysis.

■ Diagnosis

History and physical. Chest x-ray to rule out other pathology.

■ Pathology

Etiology in bacteria or viruses.

■ Treatment

Supportive. Antibiotics if condition not improving.

5–2. Bronchiolitis

■ Description

Childhood respiratory disease, usually younger than age 2.

Inflammation of small airways

■ Symptoms

Respiratory distress, wheezing, runny nose. Tachypneic and irritable infant.

possibly flaring & retractions

■ Diagnosis

History and physical exam. Chest x-ray (hyperinflation).

■ Pathology

Respiratory syncytial virus most often.

■ Treatment

Antibiotics for secondary infection/pneumonia, ribavirin (Virazole), oxygen, theophylline.

if bad infection

5–3. Pneumonia

■ Description

Lung parenchyma inflammation/infection.

■ Symptoms

Bacterial fever/chills, cough with purulent/bloody sputum.

Mycoplasma—gradual onset, headache, myalgia, cough, fever.

Chlamydia—infants, conjunctivitis, cough.

■ Diagnosis

History and physical, sputum culture/Gram stain, chest x-ray, blood culture. Mycoplasma, cold agglutinins/antibody titer.

■ Pathology

Viral (influenza A **common in adults**), **bacterial,** fungal, **mycoplasma,** and *Chlamydial* infection via blood spread, inhalation or aspiration.

■ Treatment

Chlamydia treated with **tetracycline.** Mycoplasma treated with erythromycin.

Additional Information. Pneumococcal pneumonia occurs with reduced host defense (alcoholic, coma, CHF, smoking, etc). Chest x-ray (CXR) shows lobar pneumonia, and air bronchogram.

> **Klebsiella: Friedlander's pneumonia, necrotizing (alcoholics, diabetics).**
>
> **Legionella:** pneumonia with **high fever, mental changes, diarrhea.** Treat with **erythromycin.**

pneumococcus classically has rusty sputum

5–4. Pulmonary Abscess and Empyema

■ Description

Local area of pus in lung (abscess), or pleural space (empyema).

■ Symptoms

Putrid sputum, cough, fever, weight loss.

■ Diagnosis

History and physical, chest x-ray, thoracentesis/culture.

■ Pathology

Mostly anaerobic bacteria cause empyema and abscess, **due to aspiration** of oral flora most often.

■ Treatment

Antibiotics and drainage.

5–5. Tuberculosis

■ Description

Pulmonary and extrapulmonary disease.

■ Symptoms

Pneumonitis and **hilar node infection (Ghon complex), fever, weight loss,** coughing. *night sweats*

■ Diagnosis

Positive tuberculin reaction or chest x-ray, may have no symptoms, sputum acid-fast stain.

■ Pathology

Mycobacterium tuberculosis by **respiratory transmission.**

■ Treatment

Use four-drug therapy for at least six weeks (until culture sensitivities are back), then narrow coverage to 3 to 2 drugs depending on the clinical scenario and drugs sensitivities, **for 6 months: isoniazid, ethambutol, rifampin, or pyrazinamide; (streptomycin 1 to 2 months).** Monitor for drug hypersensitivity reactions! *Attention:* on HIV positive patients need to use sensitivities strictly.

5–6. Histoplasmosis

■ Description

Systemic mycosis.

■ Symptoms

After 1- to 2-week incubation, **flulike illness, or asymptomatic,** erythema nodosum, hepatosplenomegaly.

■ Diagnosis

History and physical, blood culture, skin biopsy, serologic testing, elevated sed rate. Skin test may be positive for years, so cannot use it to confirm active infection. **Disseminated disease: think HIV.**

■ Pathology

Pulmonary infection (also skin, liver, spleen), by *Histoplasma capsulatum* via **spore inhalation,** from **bird/bat droppings.**

■ Treatment

Amphotericin B or ketoconazole. If mild disease, no treatment.

5–7. Coccidioidomycosis

■ Description

Fungal (mycotic) infection (San Joaquin Valley fever).

■ Symptoms

Flulike illness, arthralgias, or asymptomatic erythema nodosum.

■ Diagnosis

Serologic testing, sputum culture, elevated sed rate, skin biopsy, skin test may be positive for years.

■ Pathology

Inhalation of *Coccidioides immitis* **spores,** usually blacks/Filipinos.

■ Treatment

Mild, no treatment. More severe, **amphotericin B or ketoconazole.**

May cause serious disease in HIV⊕ pt

5–8. Pneumocystosis

■ Description

Pneumocystis carinii pneumonia.

■ Symptoms

Fever, cough, dyspnea.

hypoxia which just won't improve

■ Diagnosis

History and physical, culture/open lung biopsy (**use Gomori's** methenamine silver nitrate stain), hypoxemia.

■ Pathology

Prevalence in **debilitated/altered immune** patients of protozoan infection.

HIV ⊕

■ Treatment

Trimethoprim-sulfamethoxazole (can add steroids) if hypoxia present) also **pentamidine isethionate.**

6. Cardiovascular System

6–1. Endocarditis

■ **Description**

Endocardial infection of acute (under several weeks), or chronic duration.

■ **Symptoms**

Fever, murmur, anemia. Multiple other symptoms possible including **splinter hemorrhages,** *(2° septic emboli)* **Osler nodes** (red finger-tip bumps), **Janeway lesions** (red macules on palms/soles), **Roth spots**, weight loss, **petechiae.**

■ **Diagnosis**

History and physical, blood culture, echocardiogram.

■ **Pathology**

Acute often *Staphylococcus aureus* (drug use typical). **Chronic** often *Streptococcus viridans* (oral surgery). **Mitral valve most common site,** pulmonic least common; (in **drug users, tricuspid valve more common**). Platelets/fibrin form on abnormal area, then bacteria attach.

■ **Treatment**

Consult current literature. *Streptococcus,* **procaine penicillin G and streptomycin.** *Staphylococcus,* **nafcillin and gentamicin** (watch for MRSA). Also, note association of *Streptococcus bovis and colon cancer.*

7. Gastrointestinal System

7–1. Mumps

■ **Description**

Mumps virus infection.

■ **Symptoms**

After 2-week incubation, **fever, headache, enlarging parotid** (bilateral in 75%).

■ **Diagnosis**

History and physical, serologic testing/viral isolation.

■ **Pathology**

Contagious mumps virus (a paramyxovirus) infection, only in humans.

■ **Treatment**

None. Isolation.

7–2. Herpetic Gingivostomatitis

■ **Description**

Common oral herpes infection.

■ **Symptoms**

May be **asymptomatic,** or **fever, vesicles, and ulcers, adenopathy.**

■ **Diagnosis**

History and physical examination, cytologic smear, serologic testing.

■ **Pathology**

Herpes simplex virus, children often.

■ **Treatment**

Symptomatic, or acyclovir.

7–3. Candidiasis

■ Description

Mycotic infection (also termed moniliasis).

■ Symptoms

Vaginal itch/white thick discharge, diaper erythema and satellite lesions, balanitis, mucosal disease with esophageal symptoms common.

■ Diagnosis

History and physical, KOH preparation, endoscopy.

■ Pathology

Superficial fungal infection or fungemia/disseminated disease (rule out HIV).

■ Treatment

Amphotericin B Antifungal. Topical and/or oral medication.

7–4. Thrush

■ Description

Oral fungal infection.

■ Symptoms

Removable white mouth patches, plaque, halitosis.

■ Diagnosis

History and physical exam, KOH preparation.

■ Pathology

Candida albicans overgrowth. Culture not helpful; candida normally present.

■ Treatment

Nystatin mouth rinse and/or oral antifungal.

7–5. Retropharyngeal Abscess

■ Description

Retropharyngeal infection.

■ Symptoms

Fever, neck extension.

■ Diagnosis

History and physical exam, palpation, culture.

■ Pathology

Spread of infection from local area (sinus, nose, etc).

■ Treatment

Incision and drainage, antibiotics.

7–6. Food Poisoning

■ Description

Illness from ingestion of germ-contaminated food.

■ Symptoms

Nausea, vomiting, diarrhea, after food ingestion.

■ Diagnosis

Food/stool culture and toxicologic studies. History and physical exam.

■ Pathology

Numerous organisms (viral, bacterial) and toxins.

■ **Treatment**

Symptomatic, may treat specific bacterial isolate (*Clostridium difficile*, vancomycin by mouth).

7–7. Botulism

■ **Description**

Ingestion of food containing toxin-producing bacillus.

■ **Symptoms**

Nausea, vomiting, **dysphagia, diplopia, progressive paralysis** hours to days after ingesting bad fish/meat or canned product.

■ **Diagnosis**

History and physical, toxin in serum/stool/food. **Differs from myasthenia gravis by negative Tensilon test.**

■ **Pathology**

Clostridium botulinum, under anaerobic conditions produces neurotoxin. May be food- or soil-contaminated wound also (gas producing infection).

■ **Treatment**

Trivalent antitoxin (A, B, E), supportive treatment.

7–8. Viral Gastroenteritis

■ **Description**

"Stomach virus."

■ **Symptoms**

Vomiting, diarrhea, fever.

■ **Diagnosis**

History and physical, viral culture, serologic studies.

■ **Pathology** → winter

Rotavirus most common. Also, Norwalklike agents and others.

summer

■ **Treatment**

Supportive.

7–9. Typhoid

■ **Description**

Enteric fever.

■ **Symptoms**

Fever, cough, headache, constipation or **diarrhea, lethargy, bacteremia, delirium.**

■ **Diagnosis**

History and physical exam, **positive diagnosis by blood culture,** presumptive by stool/urine culture, agglutinin titer, abdominal "rose spots."

■ **Pathology**

Salmonella typhi, Gram-negative bacteria.

■ **Treatment**

Chloramphenicol (watch out for aplastic anemia).

7–10. Salmonella

■ **Description**

Enterobacteria infection.

- **Symptoms**

Fever, diarrhea, slow pulse, hepatosplenomegaly (enteric fever, *S. typhi*). Nausea, fever, cramps, bloody diarrhea (gastroenteritis, *S. enteritidis*), bacteremia or asymptomatic carrier.

- **Diagnosis**

History and physical, stool culture, negative blood culture with enteritis, may be positive with enteric fever.

- **Pathology**

Gram-negative rods, colon mucosa damage, endotoxin(?).

- **Treatment**

If mild, none. Otherwise ampicillin or chloramphenicol. Trimethoprim-sulfamethoxazole also used.

7–11. Shigella

- **Description**

Bacillary dysentery.

- **Symptoms**

Abdominal pain, tenesmus, bloody stool, cramping, fever.

- **Diagnosis**

History and physical, proctoscopy, stool culture. *Thayer-Martin Media*

- **Pathology**

Colon epithelial cell lining damage, usually superficial mucosa only. May transfer antibiotic resistance by conjugation.

- **Treatment**

Trimethoprim-sulfamethoxazole.

7–12. Toxicogenic Escherichia coli Infection

- **Description**

Diarrheal illness.

- **Symptoms**

Watery diarrhea, abdominal pain. **Enteroinvasive strains present like *Shigella*.**

- **Diagnosis**

Culture, serologic testing.

- **Pathology**

Escherichia coli producing exotoxin resulting in colon mucosa fluid secretion.

- **Treatment**

Hydration, try tetracycline.

7–13. Clostridial Infection

- **Description**

Toxin-producing germs.

- **Symptoms**

Gas gangrene: pain at wound infection, bullae, tissue gas, hypotension. *tissue crepitus*

- **Diagnosis**

History and physical exam, gram stain, culture.

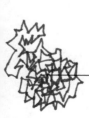

■ **Pathology**

Clostridium tetani, see Tetanus section; *C. perfringens*, see Gas gangrene; *C. botulinum*, see Botulism section; *C. difficile*, see Pseudomembranous colitis.

■ **Treatment**

Gas gangrene: debridement, penicillin G.

7–14. Cholera

■ **Description**

Self-limited infectious diarrhea.

■ **Symptoms**

Dehydration, **shock, severe watery diarrhea** ("rice-water stools").

■ **Diagnosis**

History and physical exam, culture.

■ **Pathology**

Vibrio cholerae (producing enterotoxin), **but not invasion of gut epithelium.** Gram-negative rod.

■ **Treatment**

Fluid replacement (lactated Ringer's).

7–15. Pseudomembranous Enterocolitis

■ **Description**

Antibiotic-induced colitis.

■ **Symptoms**

Watery diarrhea, tenesmus, cramps.

■ **Diagnosis**

History and physical, recent antibiotic use, stool for *C. difficile* toxin.

■ **Pathology**

Clostridium difficile.

■ **Treatment**

Stop antibiotic; *give* metronidazole, or vancomycin *(oral not IV)*.

7–16. Amebiasis

■ **Description**

Intestinal parasite infection.

■ **Symptoms**

Bloody diarrhea, pain, tenesmus, may have no fever.

■ **Diagnosis**

Stool exam for trophozoites/cysts, serologic testing.

■ **Pathology**

Trophozoite invades gut mucosa. *Entamoeba histolytica,* **colon;** *Giardia lamblia,* **small bowel.**

■ **Treatment**

Flagyl.
    Also: *Cryotosporidium,* rule out HIV. *Shigella* similar to amebiasis, but fever usually present.

7–17. Giardiasis

■ **Description**

Small-bowel protozoan infection.

■ **Symptoms**

Watery stools, foul odor, no blood/mucus. If chronic, malabsorption/weight loss.

■ **Diagnosis**

Stool exam, **string test, duodenal aspiration.**

■ **Pathology**

Giardia lamblia in small intestine produce epithelial/mucosa damage.

■ **Treatment**

Quinacrine hydrochloride (Atabrine), or **metronidazole hydrochloride (Flagyl).**

7–18. Hookworm and Pinworm

■ **Description**

Intestinal nematode infection.

■ **Symptoms**

Hookworm: cough, anemia, pruritis, weight loss.
Pinworm: pruritis ani at night.

■ **Diagnosis**

Hookworm: eosinophilia, anemia (microcytic/hypochromic), low albumin, stool exam.
Pinworm: scotch tape test, no eosinophilia.

■ **Pathology**

Hookworm: *Ancylostoma duodenale* or ***Necator americanus.***

> **Cycle:** eggs in feces reach soil; larvae form; larvae enter skin/blood/then lungs; larvae swallowed reach intestine.

Pinworm: *Enterobius vermicularis.*

■ **Treatment**

Hookworm: **mild infection,** none; severe, **mebendazole (Vermox),** or **pyrantel pamoate.**
Pinworm: **same meds.**

7–19. Appendicitis

■ **Description**

Vermiform appendix inflammation.

■ **Symptoms**

Abdominal pain shifting from periumbilical to right lower quarter (RLQ), anorexia, nausea.

■ **Diagnosis**

History and physical exam, moderate leukocytosis.

■ **Pathology**

Appendix lumen obstruction, (usually fecalith), superimposed infection (*E. coli* common) often.

■ **Treatment**

Surgery.

7–20. Diverticulitis

■ Description

Diverticula inflammation and perforation.

■ Symptoms

Left lower quadrant (LLQ) pain, rectal bleeding, constipation, chills/fever.

■ Pathology

Diverticula lumen obstruction.

Risk of perforation so watch carefully

■ Treatment

If mild, medical (nothing by mouth [NPO], antibiotics), otherwise surgical resection.

7–21. Intra-abdominal Abscess, Hepatic/Subphrenic

■ Description

Hepatic abscess: local collection of pus in liver. Intra-abdominal abscess includes subphrenic abscess.

■ Symptoms

Hepatic abscess: fever, right upper quadrant (RUQ) pain, jaundice. Intra-abdominal abscess fever, elevated diaphragm, leukocytosis, pain.

■ Diagnosis

History and physical, ultrasound, CT, gallium scan, **positive Hoover's sign (x-ray sternochondral widening).**

■ Pathology

Escherichia coli common.

■ Treatment

Antibiotics and surgery.

7–22. Viral Hepatitis

■ Description

Type A: infectious.

Type B: "serum." Viral infection with liver inflammation.

■ Symptoms

Fever, malaise, nausea, pruritus, dark urine, anorexia, jaundice. Type A has more rapid onset, younger patients. Type B more severe.

■ Diagnosis

A: hepatitis A virus (HAV) in stool, anti-HAV immunoglobulin M (IgM) in serum.

B: hepatitis B surface antigen (HBsAg) is first marker.

■ Pathology

Viral.

■ Treatment

A: none, treat complications.

Acute B: none.

Chronic B: corticosteroids, azathioprine.

Additional Information. **Hepatitis B.**

Acute	+HBsAg	+HBeAg	+Anti-HBc
Convalescent	–HBsAg	–HBeAg	+Anti-HBc
Carrier	+HBsAg	–HBeAg	+Anti-HBc

<u>HBeAg is a marker for infec</u>tivity. **Delta** agent is found only in hepatitis B patients, and is associated with increased chronic hepatitis risk. *Also more fulminant course*

7–23. Cholecystitis

- **Description**

Gallbladder inflammation.

- **Symptoms**

Right upper quadrant (RUQ) pain, nausea/vomiting, fever.

- **Diagnosis**

History and physical, plain films, ultrasound of gallbladder, DISIDA scan.

- **Pathology**

Cystic duct obstruction.

- **Treatment**

Initially medical, then surgery.

7–24. Choledocholithiasis

- **Description**

Common duct stones.

- **Symptoms**

Right upper quadrant **(RUQ) pain, fever, jaundice (Charcot's triad),** nausea/vomiting, shock.

- **Diagnosis**

History and physical, endoscopic retrograde cholangiography (ERCP).

- **Pathology**

Bile obstruction. **Obstructive jaundice: common duct stone most often etiology.**

- **Treatment**

Cholecystectomy and choledochostomy.

8. Urinary Tract and Reproductive System

See OB-GYN (Chapter 13) for discussion of gonorrhea, chlamydia, syphilis, chancroid, urethritis, vulvovaginitis, Bartholin's gland abscess, salpingitis/pelvic inflammatory disease (PID), endometritis.

8–1. Prostatitis

- **Description**

Prostate inflammation.

- **Symptoms**

Chills/fever, low back/pelvic pain, dysuria, urgency, discharge.

- **Diagnosis**

History and physical exam, culture of urethra/urine/prostatic fluid. Prostate **boggy and large.**

- **Pathology**

Escherichia coli, may also be non-bacterial.

- **Treatment**

Antibiotics (sulfamethoxazole-trimethoprim [Bactrim] and others).

8–2. Epididymitis

■ **Description**

Epididymis inflammation.

■ **Symptoms**

Scrotal enlargement and pain.

■ **Diagnosis**

History and physical, less pain with scrotal elevation (unlike torsion), pyuria, urine culture.

■ **Pathology**

Bacterial ascending infection, often E. coli.

■ **Treatment**

Scrotal support, antibiotics.

8–3. Orchitis

■ **Description**

Testicular inflammation.

■ **Symptoms**

Enlarging and **tender testicle**, mostly unilateral.

■ **Diagnosis**

History and physical examination.

■ **Pathology**

May result from mumps virus. Also trauma, metastatic disease.

■ **Treatment**

Symptomatic. Ice, elevation

8–4. Pyelonephritis

■ **Description**

Kidney infection/inflammation.

■ **Symptoms**

Flank pain, fever/chills, dysuria, costovertebral angle (CVA) tenderness, vomiting, malaise.

■ **Diagnosis**

History and physical examination, urinalysis (UA), urine culture.

■ **Pathology**

Escherichia coli most often, by ascending infection.

■ **Treatment**

Antibiotics, increase fluids.

8–5. Abscess: Renal, Pelvic, Perinephric

■ **Description**

Local collection of pus.

■ **Symptoms**

Tenderness at CVA, **fever/chills** if **renal**. Same, but slow onset if perinephric.

■ **Diagnosis**

History and physical, x-ray (including intravenous pyelogram [IVP]), gallium scan, ultrasound.

■ **Pathology**

Escherichia coli usually when urinary tract spread. Staphylococcus aureus, hematogenous spread.

Common complication of peritonitis, **pelvic abscess.** (esp appendicitis!)

■ **Treatment**

Intrarenal: antibiotics (antistaphylococcal).
Pelvic/perinephric: drainage and antibiotics.

9. Skin; Musculoskeletal System

Chickenpox, rubella, measles, Rocky Mountain Spotted Fever, cellulitis, carbuncle, dermatophytosis, viral warts, see *Dermatology,* **Chapter 2.**

9–1. Lymphangitis

■ **Description**

Bacterial infection spread.

■ **Symptoms**

Red streak extending from wound; fever, adenopathy.

■ **Diagnosis**

History and physical exam, blood culture.

■ **Pathology**

Mostly hemolytic strep; rule out cat-scratch fever. (Pasturella multicoda)

■ **Treatment**

Antibiotics.

9–2. Necrotizing Fasciitis and Gangrene

■ **Description**

Fascia inflammation/infection, with fascial plane germ dissection.

■ **Symptoms and Diagnosis**

See *Clostridia* section.

■ **Pathology**

Anaerobic strep and *Staphylococcus aureus* often.

■ **Treatment**

Antibiotics and surgical incisions.

9–3. Osteomyelitis

■ **Description**

Bone inflammation/infection.

■ **Symptoms**

Fever, bone/soft tissue signs (joint pain, warmth, erythema).

■ **Diagnosis**

① in all 3 phases →

History and physical exam, **bone scan, bone aspiration**, blood culture, x-ray (may be negative).

■ **Pathology**

Mostly **children,** with **hematogenous spread.** *Staphylococcus aureus* **most common.** Tibia/fibula and lumbar area common. **Sickle cell** *Salmonella* **association.**

■ **Treatment**

Parenteral antibiotics 4 to 6 weeks, surgery (debridement).

9–4. Septic Arthritis

■ **Description**

Joint inflammation/infection.

- **Symptoms**

Fever/chills, hot/tender joint, monoarthritis.

- **Diagnosis**

History and physical, **arthrocentesis**, complete blood count (CBC), sed rate, synovial fluid culture/gram stain, x-ray.

- **Pathology**

Staphylococcus aureus **most common.** Infants age 1 to 2, *H. influenzae*. Gonorrhea in young sexually active patients.

- **Treatment**

Antibiotics as per culture.

C. **Other Infectious and Parasitic Disorders**

1. *Lyme Disease*

    - **Description**

    Spirochetal disease.

    - **Symptoms**

    Rash (erythema migrans), chills, fever, myalgia in stage 1. Carditis/meningitis in stage 2. Arthritis in stage 3.

    - **Diagnosis**

    History and physical. May have no history of bite or rash. Lyme titer (ELISA), and Western blot confirmation.

    - **Pathology**

    Borrelia burgdorferi via deer tick *(Ixodes dammini).*

- **Treatment**

Doxycycline.

2. *Malaria*

    - **Description**

    Protozoal infection.

    - **Symptoms** (in cycles)

    High fever and chills. Headache, nausea, multiple other symptoms possible.

    - **Diagnosis**

    History and physical exam, **peripheral smear exam.**

    - **Pathology**

    Plasmodium species infection (falciparum, malariae, vivax, ovale).

    - **Treatment**

    Chloroquine phosphate. If resistant, give quinine sulphate and pyrimethamine.

IV. PRINCIPLES OF MANAGEMENT

A. **Acute Problems**

- **Description**

Perform complete history and physical, obtain necessary cultures, x-ray studies, and/or serologic testing. Institute presumptive therapy when unable to wait for test reports, based on exam, patient's age, likely organism, and so on. Consider special needs and need for early diagnosis/intervention with infants, elderly, and impaired-immunity patients. Consider typical germs responsible for disease in these particular groups.

B. Chronic Problems

■ Description

With fever of unknown origin, document fever, obtain routine lab/x-ray studies, look for common etiology first. Consider psychosocial impact on the patient of chronic infectious/parasitic disease.

See general principles of care in Chapter 12, Section VI.

C. Ethical and Legal Issues

■ Description

Diagnosis of HIV; remember to obtain patient's written request for testing, be aware of current laws pertaining to chart/information release, consider family/social/financial impact.

See General Principles of Medical Care in Chapter 12, Section VI.

BIBLIOGRAPHY

Bass JB, et al. Treatment and Tuberculosis Infection in Adults and Children. *Am Rev Resp Dis:* May 1994; 1359–74.

Beaver PC. *Clinical Parasitology.* 9th ed. Philadelphia, Pa: Lea & Febiger; 1984.

Bennett JE. *Principles and Practice of Infectious Disease.* 3rd ed. New York: Churchill Livingstone; 1990.

Braude AI. *Infectious Disease and Medical Microbiology.* 2nd ed. Philadelphia, Pa: WB Saunders Co; 1986.

Civetta JM. *Critical Care.* 2nd ed. Philadelphia, Pa: JB Lippincott Co; 1992.

Fields BV. *Virology.* New York: Raven Press; 1985.

Finegold SM. *Anaerobic Infections.* Chicago, Ill: Year Book Medical Publishers; 1986.

Hoeprich PD. *Infectious Disease.* 4th ed. Philadelphia, Pa: JB Lippincott Co; 1989.

Lambert HP. *Infectious Diseases Illustrated. An Integrated Text and Color Atlas.* Philadelphia, Pa: WB Saunders Co; 1982.

Mandell GL. *Principles and Practice of Infectious Disease.* 3rd ed, New York: John Wiley and Sons; 1991.

Schillinger D. *Infections in Emergency Medicine.* Vol. 2. New York: Churchill Livingstone; 1990.

Schroeder SA. *Current Medical Diagnosis and Treatment.* 31st ed. Norwalk, Conn: Appleton & Lange; 1992.

Thoene JG. *Physicians Guide to Rare Diseases.* Montvale, NJ: Dowden Publishing Company, Inc; 1992.

Youmans GP. *The Biologic and Clinical Basis of Infectious Disease.* 3rd ed. Philadelphia, Pa: WB Saunders Co; 1989

CHAPTER 10

Musculoskeletal and Connective Tissue Disease

JOEL S. GOLDBERG, DO

I. HEALTH AND HEALTH MAINTENANCE

A. Exercise, Fitness, and Conditioning

■ **Description**

Benefits of exercise include stress reduction, prevention of osteoporosis, maintaining and/or increasing strength, improving cardiovascular fitness, joint mobility and flexibility. High-repetition exercise with low weight resistance builds endurance and tones. Low repetition with heavy weights improves strength/muscle size.

B. Prevention of Disability Due to Osteoporosis

■ **Description**

Risk factors include **early menopause, alcohol use, chronic disease/malnutrition, small size/weight, lack of exercise.**

Impact as a significant health concern with vast numbers of affected individuals at increased fracture risk; resulting morbidity/mortality (15% of hip fractures result in death); and tremendous financial/medical resource costs.

Prevention involves dietary and lifestyle modifications (increase calcium intake to 1.5 g daily, weight-bearing exercise, quit smoking, etc), and estrogen use (0.6 mg conjugated estrogen daily).

C. Degenerative Joint and Disc Disease

■ **Description**

Epidemiology may relate to **aging, genetics, and/or injury.** Degenerative joint disease (DJD) is **common.**

Impact in chronic pain and disability is significant. May be asymptomatic in many individuals.

Prevention includes maintenance of flexibility, weight reduction, education regarding proper body mechanics for exercise/weight lifting and work. Avoiding occupational overuse/trauma and early treatment of associated metabolic/systemic disorders (hyperparathyroidism) are other considerations.

D. Prevention of Disability Due to Musculoskeletal Disorders

1. Frozen-Shoulder Syndrome

■ **Description**

Avoid shoulder immobilization, though fibrosis of the shoulder capsule may have no clear etiology in immobilization or injury.

2. Shoulder–Hand Syndrome (Reflex Sympathetic Dystrophy)

■ **Description**

Avoid disability via **early mobilization/therapy**, local anesthetic injection, or sympathetic block.

3. Immobilization

■ **Description**

Avoidance of immobilization is critical in prevention of musculoskeletal disease progression and complications.

4. Low Back Pain

■ **Description**

Prevention of low back pain includes control of weight, education in body mechanics and posture for exercise and work, stretching and conditioning exercise, and strengthening of abdominal muscles.

E. Prosthetic and Orthotic Devices

■ **Description**

Orthotic devices reduce joint stress, provide patient mobility where previous joint weakness/injury prevented ambulation, and may prevent/correct joint deformity (juvenile rheumatoid arthritis). Prosthetic devices for use by amputees provide physical and emotional benefits.

In early prosthetic infections, *Staphylococcus aureus* is the most common pathogen.

II. MECHANISMS OF DISEASE, DIAGNOSIS, AND TREATMENT

A. Infections

1. Osteomyelitis

■ **Description**

Bone inflammation, with usual etiology in infection.

■ **Symptoms**

Persisting backache (lumbar vertebral disease), spinous process/bony tenderness, fever/chills.

■ **Diagnosis**

History and physical exam, blood culture, bone aspiration, x-ray, bone scan, computed tomography (CT) scan, elevated sed rate.

Bone scan - ⊕ in all 3 phases

■ **Pathology**

Etiology by **hematogenous spread** (*Staphylococcus aureus* **most common**), and direct joint infection (open fracture, trauma). Direct infection extension is possible, as in postoperative infection.

Salmonella in Sickle cell

■ **Treatment**

Antibiotics.

Additional Information. **Acute osteomyelitis—more common in children, usual site is long bone metaphysis.**

2. Septic Arthritis

■ **Description**

Joint infection, usually in patient with coexisting illness or debilitated state.

■ **Symptoms**

Joint pain/swelling/motion limitation, fever/chills, redness.

■ **Diagnosis**

History and physical exam, **blood/joint fluid culture, lab (complete blood count** [CBC], sed rate), x-ray.

■ **Pathology**

May be bacterial (*Staphylococcus aureus* **most frequent older adult** (and childhood) **germ,** with gonococcus (GC) more common in ages 20 to 50), viral, fungal; **most frequently by hematogenous spread; risk factors include** drug abuse (pseudomonas), chronic disease/cancer, and prior joint pathology.

■ **Treatment**

Antibiotics, and perhaps surgical drainage.

Additional Information. **Septic hip arthritis—children most often, hip pain** and **lack of motion, surgical drainage is necessary.** Gonococcal arthritis—usually presents with tenosynovitis, multiple migratory arthralgias, and **skin pustules. Treat with ceftriaxone.**

emerge b/c can cause perm. damage

3. Lyme Disease

■ **Description**

Tick-borne multisystem disorder.

■ **Symptoms**

Initial presentation includes **fatigue, fever, erythema chronicum migrans (may present without rash also),** and **headache.** Neuritis, neuropathy, en**cephalopathy,** and **arrhythmias** after the initial symptoms (stage 2). **Stage 3 symptoms** include **arthritis,** and **central nervous system (CNS) disease.**

■ **Diagnosis**

History and physical examination, serologic testing.

■ **Pathology**

Spirochetal infection by *Borrelia burgdorferi* **via** *Ixodes dammini* **tick.**

■ **Treatment**

Tetracycline or doxycycline. More difficult to treat in later stages. If child or patient unable to take tetracycline, use amoxicillin.

4. *Gonococcal Tenosynovitis*

■ **Description**

Tendon sheath inflammation. A common manifestation of disseminated GC infection.

■ **Symptoms**

Tenosynovitis, pain, inflamed/red joint, fever, migratory polyarthritis, and wrist/knee/ankle arthritis.

■ **Diagnosis**

History and physical exam, blood/ joint culture.

■ **Pathology**

Gonococcal infection/inflammation.

■ **Treatment**

Penicillin G, or ceftriaxone.

B. Degenerative Disorders

1. *Degenerative Joint Disease and Arthralgia*

■ **Description**

Chronic inflammatory joint disorder.

■ **Symptoms**

Pain, brief morning stiffness.

■ **Diagnosis**

History and physical examination (Heberden's, distal and Bouchard's, proximal nodes on the hands), x-ray (narrowed joint cartilage, osteophytes, and ossicles).

■ **Pathology**

Cartilage damage/erosion, with bone cyst/osteophyte lesions, and bone hypertrophy.

■ **Treatment**

Tylenol may be just as effective

Aspirin, non-steroidal anti-inflammatory medications, rest, weight reduction, physical therapy modalities, joint replacement.

2. *Degenerative Disc Disease and Low Back Pain*

■ **Description**

Disc-space narrowing, with resulting signs and symptoms.

■ **Symptoms**

Back pain, loss of full motion, stiffness, referred pain, muscle spasm.

■ **Diagnosis**

History and physical exam, x-ray (including CT/magnetic resonance imaging [MRI] for disc and cord-compression evaluation).

■ **Pathology**

Etiology unknown, but **aging** (osteoarthritis), **trauma,** and **heredity** play a role.

■ **Treatment**

Aspirin, non-steroidal anti-inflammatory drugs (NSAIDs), physical therapy, back support, corticosteroid injection, weight reduction, rest, surgery.

Additional Information. **Herniated disc: most at L-4 to L-5 (weak big toe) and L-5 to S-1 (reduced Achilles reflex).**

C. **Neurologic Disorders**

1. *Carpal Tunnel Syndrome*

   ■ **Description**

   Nerve entrapment syndrome.

   ■ **Symptoms**

   Fingertip and/or **hand numbness/ weakness,** and **pain.**

   ■ **Diagnosis**

   History and physical (Tinel's [wrist percussion] and Phaelan's [wrist flexion] signs), electromyogram (EMG) and nerve conduction velocity (NCV) study.

   ■ **Pathology**

   Median nerve compression. Noted with overuse, and in myxedema, rheumatoid arthritis, pregnancy, injuries, amyloid disease, and others.

   ■ **Treatment**

   Rest, wrist splint, corticosteroid injection, surgery (nerve release).

2. *Charcot Joint*

   ■ **Description**

   Neuropathic joint.

■ **Symptoms**

Joint swelling with little or no pain.

■ **Diagnosis**

History and physical, x-ray.

■ **Pathology**

Lack of proprioception, resulting in joint injury. **Most frequent etiologies include diabetes and syphilis.**

■ **Treatment**

Joint immobilization.

3. *Poliomyelitis*

   ■ **Description**

   Infantile paralysis.

   ■ **Symptoms**

   Fever, gastrointestinal (GI) and central nervous system (CNS) symptoms (meningeal irritation, muscle weakness/spasm, encephalitis), respiratory paralysis.

   ■ **Diagnosis**

   History and physical exam, spinal fluid examination.

   ■ **Pathology**

   Polio virus resulting in CNS injury.

   ■ **Treatment**

   Supportive treatment, bed rest, physical therapy.

4. *Cerebral Palsy*

   ■ **Description**

   Motor function abnormality.

■ **Symptoms**

Mental retardation, ataxia, incoordination, spasticity/flaccidity.

■ **Diagnosis**

History and physical examination.

■ **Pathology**

Cerebral injury (**birth injury most frequent cause**) resulting in uncontrolled nerve signal production. May be **athetoid** or **spastic** in type.

■ **Treatment**

Physical therapy, spasm reduction (treatment via medication, bracing, and/or surgery).

D. **Congenital and Inherited Disorders**

1. *Congenital Hip Dislocation*

Description

Hip subluxation or dislocation.

■ **Symptoms**

Hip click (see the following), hip joint stiffness on exam.

■ **Diagnosis**

History and physical exam (**Ortolani's maneuver: hip click with flexion/abduction**), x-ray, lack of 90° hip abduction.

Barlow's also

■ **Pathology**

Risk factors include family history of congenital hip dislocation, breech babies, and infants with other orthopedic disorders.

1st ♀ in breech!

■ **Treatment**

Pavlik harness (will flex and abduct hips).

2. *Phocomelia*

■ **Description**

Hand or foot directly connected to the trunk.

■ **Symptoms**

Orthopedic structural abnormality.

■ **Diagnosis**

History and physical exam, x-ray.

■ **Pathology**

Noted with drugs (thalidomide).

■ **Treatment**

None.

Additional Information

Sprengel deformity—failure of scapula descent, treat with surgery.
Pectus excavatum—indented lower sternum, treat surgically if necessary.

3. *Osgood–Schlatter's Disease*

■ **Description**

Apophysitis.

■ **Symptoms**

Tibial tubercle tenderness and lump.

■ **Diagnosis**

History and physical exam, x-ray.

■ **Pathology**

Traction of patellar tendon results in inflammation. Common in active, fast-growing child.

■ **Treatment**

Rest, aspirin.

4. Osteochondritis Dissecans

■ **Description**

Disorder in which articular cartilage loses blood supply.

■ **Symptoms**

Knee pain, patellar tenderness, or elbow pain.

■ **Diagnosis**

History and physical exam, x-ray (joint mouse).

■ **Pathology**

Avascular necrosis, usually of medial femoral condyle, in teenage males.

■ **Treatment**

Non-weight-bearing, casting, and surgery.

5. Slipped Capital Femoral Epiphysis

■ **Description**

Adolescent hip disorder.   *Black & fat*

■ **Symptoms**

Groin/thigh pain, and limp in adolescent.

■ **Diagnosis**

History and physical exam, **x-ray evaluation.**

■ **Pathology**

Sliding epiphyseal plate, with hormonal etiology(?).

■ **Treatment**

Surgical (pinning).

6. Legg–Calvé–Perthes Disease

■ **Description**

Hip necrosis disorder. "Osteochondritis Deformans."

■ **Symptoms**

Hip or knee pain and limp.

■ **Diagnosis**

History and physical exam, x-ray exam.

■ **Pathology**

Femoral head avascular necrosis (probably due to hip effusion/pressure cutting off blood supply to femoral head), typically in children ages 5 to 10.

■ **Treatment**

Weight bearing only in abduction (casting), surgery.

7. Transient Synovitis

■ **Description**

Most frequent disorder causing childhood hip pain.

■ **Symptoms**

Hip pain, low-grade fever.

■ **Diagnosis**

History and physical, x-ray, joint aspiration (negative).

- **Pathology**

Etiology unknown, viral(?). Typically in children ages 3 to 6.

- **Treatment**

Bed rest, aspirin.

Additional Information. **If temperature high, or elevated white blood cells (WBC)/sed rate: consider patient to have a septic joint.**

8. In-Toeing

- **Description**

Gait abnormality.

- **Symptoms**

In-toeing gait (neutral position to 30° out-toeing is normal).

- **Diagnosis**

History and physical exam.

- **Pathology**

Metatarsus adductus deformity—forefoot adduction (front of foot turns in), passively correctable, treat with foot stretching (casting if not passively correctable).

Tibial torsion—inward tibia rotation with knee straight but whole foot pointing inward (thigh-foot angle normally neutral to 10° outward), no treatment or night splinting.

Femoral anteversion—internal hip rotation over 80°, no treatment.

- **Treatment**

As in pathology.

E. Metabolic and Nutritional Disorders

1. Osteoporosis

- **Description**

Osteopenia (decreased bone mass).

- **Symptoms**

Fractures (vertebral compression T-12, L-1, common), **pain** (may increase with activity).

- **Diagnosis**

History and physical exam, single/dual energy photon absorption, metacarpal/vertebrae x-ray (thick end plates/fractures), normal alkaline phosphatase.

- **Pathology**

May be primary (postmenopausal), or secondary (drugs/alcohol, nutritional, and endocrine).

- **Treatment**

Avoid inactivity; estrogens and calcium reduce bone turnover. Fluoride and calcium increase bone mass.

Additional Information. **Rule out multiple myeloma** (serum protein electrophoresis, bone marrow study, etc), **which may present like osteoporosis.** Osteomalacia: inadequate bone mineralization; a result of renal disease or malabsorption; **bones are soft, with elevated serum calcium and elevated alkaline phosphatase.**

2. Gout

- **Description**

Monoarticular arthritis.

- **Symptoms**

Pain, redness, swelling, and **warm joint.**

■ **Diagnosis**

History and physical exam, **positive aspiration for rodlike birefringent urate crystals,** serum uric acid.

■ **Pathology**

Hyperuricemia with crystal deposition in joints; **first metatarsalphalangeal (MTP) joint most often.** *big toe!*

■ **Treatment**

> **Acute**—colchicine.
> **Chronic**—allopurinol and colchicine.

3. Pseudogout

Description

Crystal deposition disorder.

■ **Symptoms**

Acute joint inflammation.

■ **Diagnosis**

History and physical exam, x-ray **(chondrocalcinosis-cartilage calcification), calcium pyrophosphate crystals in aspirate.**

■ **Pathology**

Monoarticular; knee joint common.

■ **Treatment**

With NSAIDs, treat coexisting disease, colchicine (?).

4. Rickets

■ **Description**

Inadequate bone mineralization, in growing bone.

■ **Symptoms**

Craniotabes (soft skull), frontal bossing, lethargy, rachitic rosary (large costochondral junction bumps), bowlegs, potbelly.

■ **Diagnosis**

History and physical examination, **x-ray (frayed/widened bone ends, pseudofractures),** elevated alkaline phosphatase.

■ **Pathology**

Due to vitamin D deficiency (poor intake, malabsorption) **and/or rapid growth; growing plates affected,** so a **disease of children.**

■ **Treatment**

Vitamin D, and light.

Additional Information. Phenytoin sodium (Dilantin) and phenobarbital affect vitamin D metabolism, and may predispose to rickets. Other causes: liver and renal disease. Harrison's groove sign: abdominal groove at diaphragm insertion site; typical of rickets.

F. Inflammatory and Immunologic Disorders

1. Polymyalgia Rheumatica (PMR)

■ **Description**

Inflammatory disorder of elderly.

■ **Symptoms**

Hip and shoulder muscle pain/stiffness in elderly patient.

■ **Diagnosis**

History and physical exam, **elevated sed rate.** Both **x-rays** and **muscle biopsy are normal.**

■ **Pathology**

Inflammatory disorder.

■ **Treatment**

Corticosteroids give rapid relief.

Additional Information. **Complications of PMR include temporal arteritis** (may result in blindness).

Fibromyalgia: normal sed rate (see the following).

2. Fibromyalgia

■ **Description**

Also termed **fibrositis.**

■ **Symptoms**

Multiple trigger points, irregular sleep pattern, anxiety/depression/ hysteria, widespread achiness.

■ **Diagnosis**

History and physical exam, classic trigger points (**superior** or **inferior medial scapula border are common** points).

■ **Pathology**

Unknown.

■ **Treatment**

Trigger-point injection, patient education, cyclobenzaprine.

3. Lupus Arthritis

■ **Description**

Polyarthritis, without destructive joint disease.

■ **Symptoms**

Arthralgias (hip joints and hands typically), **Raynaud's phenomenon,** morning stiffness, myalgias.

■ **Diagnosis**

History and physical exam, serologic testing **(antibody to native DNA, antinuclear antibodies [ANA]).**

■ **Pathology**

More common in young women.

■ **Treatment**

Rest, NSAIDs, corticosteroids.

Additional Information

Psoriatic arthritis: joint damage and **opera glass deformity on x-ray.**

Gouty arthritis: proximal great toe joint and hands.

4. Polymyositis, dermatomyositis

■ **Description**

Skeletal muscle inflammatory disorder.

■ **Symptoms**

Weak muscles proximally, arthralgias, **heliotrope (eyelid) rash,** dysphagia.

■ **Diagnosis**

History and physical examination, **elevated muscle enzymes, muscle/skin biopsy,** abnormal emg study.

■ **Pathology**

Abnormal muscle biopsy (degenerated/regenerated muscle fibers).

■ **Treatment**

Rest, corticosteroids, and methotrexate if they fail.

Additional Information. **Dermatomyositis is polymyositis plus a rash.**

Coexisting malignancy may be present with both **polymyositis** and **dermatomyosis.**

No ocular muscle problems with polymyositis or dermatomyositis (unlike myasthenia gravis).

5. Rheumatoid Arthritis

■ Description

Symmetrical inflammatory disorder.

■ Symptoms

Rheumatoid nodules, joint swelling/ heat/inflammation, worse after resting, pleural effusion, lethargy, fever.

■ Diagnosis

History and physical exam, x-ray, elevated sed rate and rheumatoid factor.

■ Pathology

Etiology unknown.

■ Treatment

Rest and therapy, NSAIDs, corticosteroids, and **disease-modifying drugs** (gold and hydroxychloroquine [Plaquenil]; methotrexate and penicillamine for more severe cases).

Additional Information. **Therapy side effects:**

Gold—rash, liver/renal abnormalities, hematologic disorders.
Methotrexate—marrow toxicity, teratogenic.
Penicillamine—rash, hematologic toxicity, teratogenic.
Hydroxychloroquine—rash, retinal damage.

6. Juvenile Rheumatoid Arthritis

■ Description

Still's disease.

■ Symptoms

High fever, joint deformity, iridocyclitis, rash.

■ Diagnosis

History and physical examination (arthritis of one or several joints for more than 3 months, splenomegaly, etc), x-ray, **may have negative rheumatoid factor and ANA.**

■ Pathology

Chronic synovitis of unknown etiology. **Pauciarticular type 1 is the most common type.**

■ Treatment

Aspirin, physical therapy, **corticosteroids** (intra-articular or systemic), gold salts.

7. Ankylosing Spondylitis

■ Description

Young adult arthritic disorder.

■ Symptoms

Back pain and stiffness, joint pains and swelling.

■ Diagnosis

History and physical exam (reduced chest expansion), **positive HLA-B27,** elevated sed rate, x-ray (sacroiliitis).

■ Pathology

More common in young males.

■ Treatment

Use **NSAIDs, aspirin,** physical therapy.

8. Bursitis

■ Description

Bursa inflammation.

■ Symptoms

Non-tender swelling (prepatellar) or pain (hip). Other common sites include elbow and shoulder.

■ Diagnosis

History and physical exam.

■ Pathology

Bursa inflammation from overuse, abnormal joint motion, trauma.

■ Treatment

Rest, NSAIDs, physical therapy, aspiration (with/without corticosteroid injection).

9. Tendonitis General Information

■ Description

Tendon inflammation.

■ Symptoms

Pain at tendon insertion, or along tendon.

■ Diagnosis

History and physical exam.

■ Pathology

Inflammation of bone-to-muscle connection (tendon); secondary to overuse or abnormal mechanics.

■ Treatment

Rest, physical therapy, NSAIDs, corticosteroid injection.

10. Tendonitis Iliotibial Band Syndrome

■ Description

Knee area tendonitis.

■ Symptoms

Distal and lateral knee pain.

■ Diagnosis

History and physical exam, positive pain with stretching leg/hip on affected side (Ober's sign). Pain worse with stairs.

■ Pathology

Etiology in stretching and overuse of tendon, resulting in inflammation.

■ Treatment

Use NSAIDs, physical therapy, corticosteroid injection, adjust mechanical factors (shoes, terrain, activity level, etc), stretching.

11. Achilles Tendonitis

■ Description

Achilles tendon inflammation.

■ Symptoms

Pain along heel/Achilles tendon.

■ Diagnosis

History and physical exam, pain at or just above Achilles tendon insertion.

■ Pathology

Etiology related to short tendon mechanical/gait factors, and overuse.

■ **Treatment**

Use NSAIDs, correct mechanical dysfunction, heel lift, calf stretching, therapy.

12. Patellar Tendonitis

■ **Description**

Jumper's knee.

■ **Symptoms**

Pain around patella.

■ **Diagnosis**

History and physical exam, **patellar tendon tenderness.**

■ **Pathology**

Overuse and **jumping sports** resulting in quadriceps contraction and tendon inflammation.

■ **Treatment**

Use NSAIDs, rest, physical therapy, stretching.

G. Neoplasms

1. Osteosarcoma

■ **Description**

Most frequent primary bone cancer.

■ **Symptoms**

Pain, lethargy, limping, metastatic signs (usually lungs).

■ **Diagnosis**

History and physical exam, **x-ray (long bone metaphysis destruction)**, biopsy, elevated alkaline phosphatase. *Sunburst*

■ **Pathology**

Osteoid production by the tumor, which is **usually near knee joint; in 15- to 30-year-old age group.**

■ **Treatment**

Surgery (may include amputation), **plus chemotherapy.**

2. Osteoid Osteoma

■ **Description**

Benign bone tumor.

■ **Symptoms**

Pain (worse at night). *No relief c̄ tylenol ⊕ relief c̄ ASA*

■ **Diagnosis**

History and physical examination, **pain relieved by aspirin,** x-ray (**sclerotic area with central lysis), biopsy.**

■ **Pathology**

Affects young individuals.

■ **Treatment**

Surgical removal.

3. Osteochondroma

■ **Description**

Most frequent benign bone tumor.

■ **Symptoms**

Asymptomatic or pain.

■ **Diagnosis**

History and physical examination, x-ray (pedunculated tumor), biopsy.

■ **Pathology**

Most common site: femur.

■ **Treatment**

Surgical removal.

4. Ewing's Sarcoma

■ **Description**

Malignant round-cell **childhood bone tumor.**

■ **Symptoms**

Pain, fever, swelling, and tenderness.

■ **Diagnosis**

History and physical exam, **x-ray (dia-physeal tumor), bone biopsy.**

■ **Pathology**

Femur most often.

■ **Treatment**

Radiation plus chemotherapy.

5. Hypertrophic Osteoarthropathy

■ **Description**

Pulmonary and **arthritis syndrome.**

■ **Symptoms**

Arthritis, clubbing, diaphoresis.

■ **Diagnosis**

History and physical examination, **x-ray (periostitis).**

■ **Pathology**

Etiology unknown; lung cancer/ chronic obstructive pulmonary dis-ease (COPD) often present.

■ **Treatment**

Treat primary condition, NSAIDs, cor-ticosteroids, therapy.

H.   Other Disorders

1. Frozen-Shoulder Syndrome

■ **Description**

Adhesive capsulitis.

■ **Symptoms**

Pain, reduced glenohumeral motion.

■ **Diagnosis**

History and physical.

■ **Pathology**

Adhesions, and shoulder capsule fi-brosis.

■ **Treatment**

Range-of-motion exercise, shoulder capsule injections, NSAIDs.

2. Sudeck's Atrophy

■ **Description**

Reflex sympathetic dystrophy.

■ **Symptoms**

Burning pain, skin changes (temper-ature/color), **edema.**

■ **Diagnosis**

History and physical exam, **x-ray (patchy decalcification).**

■ **Pathology**

Posttraumatic sympathetic nerve dis-order; with reflex vasospasm-induced symptoms.

■ **Treatment**

Use NSAIDs, physical therapy, and corticosteroid injection.

3. Dupuytren's Contracture

■ **Description**

Finger flexion deformity.

■ **Symptoms**

Lump in the hand; contracture of fourth or fifth fingers, in flexion.

■ **Diagnosis**

History and physical examination.

■ **Pathology**

Thick palmar fascia, of unknown etiology.

■ **Treatment**

Surgical.

Additional Information. **Positive association with cirrhosis, diabetes, and epilepsy.**

4. Carpal Tunnel Syndrome

■ **Description**

Compression syndrome.

■ **Symptoms**

Hand paresthesia and pain.

■ **Diagnosis**

History and physical examination (Phalen's test [wrist flexion] and Tinel's test [percussion of nerve, thenar eminence atrophy]), EMG and NCV study.

■ **Pathology**

Median nerve compression (hypothyroidism, overuse, trauma, pregnancy, etc).

■ **Treatment**

Rest, splinting, physical therapy, corticosteroid injection, surgical release.

5. Chondromalacia Patellae

■ **Description**

Knee pain syndrome.

■ **Symptoms**

Anterior knee pain; worse with hills/steps, and distance running.

■ **Diagnosis**

History and physical exam (crepitus), x-ray, arthroscopic examination.

■ **Pathology**

Increased softening and roughness of cartilage under patella.

■ **Treatment**

Rest, NSAIDs, physical therapy including quadriceps strengthening.

6. Paget's Disease of Bone

■ **Description**

Bone disorder; more common in elderly; osteitis deformans.

■ **Symptoms**

Symptoms depend on area of bone affected. May be asymptomatic or bone deformity, pain arthritis, and fractures.

■ **Diagnosis**

History and physical exam, **elevated alkaline phosphatase, bone scan, x-ray.**

■ **Pathology**

Excessive/overactive osteoclasts.

■ Treatment

Use NSAIDs, and **antiresorptive agents (calcitonin, bisphosphates, and plicamycin).**

Additional Information. **Complications of Paget's—osteogenic sarcoma, spinal cord compression, and high-output congestive heart failure (CHF) (affected bone has higher blood flow).**

7. Eosinophilic Granuloma

■ Description

Reticuloendothelial proliferative disorder.

■ Symptoms

Vertebral collapse, **pain.**

■ Diagnosis

History and physical examination (tenderness, swelling), **x-ray,** biopsy.

■ Pathology

Single destructive eosinophilic/histiocytic infiltrate in bone; most often childhood disorder.

■ Treatment

Surgical removal of lesion; low-dose radiation and corticosteroids have been tried.

8. Shin Splints

■ Description

Painful lower leg disorder.

■ Symptoms

Lower leg pain, medial or lateral location.

■ Diagnosis

History and physical examination.

■ Pathology

Posterior tibialis periostitis (medial leg pain), and anterior tibialis strain (lateral leg).

■ Treatment

Rest, NSAIDs, physical therapy, stretching, control mechanical dysfunctions.

Additional Information. **Do x-ray and/or bone scan to rule out stress fracture.**

9. Cervical Sprain

■ Description

Whiplash.

■ Symptoms

Patient initially relates neck pain (then relates his attorney's name and telephone number).

■ Diagnosis

History and physical examination, x-ray, and CT/MRI to rule out disc disease (if indicated).

■ Pathology

Hyperextension and flexion injury.

■ Treatment

Rest, cervical collar, NSAIDs, and physical therapy.

10. Thoracic Outlet Syndrome

■ Description

Arm pain disorder from compression of nerve/vascular structures.

■ **Symptoms**

Hand/arm/back numbness and pain; may be positional.

■ **Diagnosis**

History and physical exam (positive Adson's test), Doppler study, x-ray.

■ **Pathology**

Anatomic neurovascular compression.

■ **Treatment**

Exercises, physical therapy, surgical rib/muscle resection.

11. Pulled Elbow

■ **Description**

Childhood painful elbow disorder.

■ **Symptoms**

Elbow pain, arm held flexed.

■ **Diagnosis**

History (child pulled by arm), and physical. No fracture on x-ray examination.

■ **Pathology**

Subluxed radius head.

■ **Treatment**

Push back head of radius with arm supinated.

12. Metatarsalgia

■ **Description**

Foot pain disorder.

■ **Symptoms**

Foot pain.

■ **Diagnosis**

Area under second metatarsal head is tender.

■ **Pathology**

Overuse, or faulty mechanics.

■ **Treatment**

Use NSAIDs, arch support, moist heat, and shoe padding.

13. Acromioclavicular (AC) Separation

■ **Description**

Shoulder pain disorder, after fall/injury.

■ **Symptoms**

Shoulder pain, history of fall/injury.

■ **Diagnosis**

History and physical (AC tenderness), weight-bearing x-ray (elevated end of clavicle).

■ **Pathology**

Injury to AC and coracoclavicular ligaments.

■ **Treatment**

Sling if mild (first-degree without separation on x-ray), sling 6 weeks for second-degree injury (second-degree, separation not greater than clavicle width), and conservative or internal fixation for third-degree (greater AC separation).

14. *Lateral Epicondylitis*

■ **Description**

Tennis elbow.

■ **Symptoms**

Elbow pain, increasing with activity.

■ **Diagnosis**

History and physical exam (lateral epicondyle tender, and pain on resisting patient's attempts on hand/middle finger dorsiflexion).

■ **Pathology**

Overuse of forearm muscles creates inflammation at tendon insertion.

■ **Treatment**

Rest, NSAIDs, physical therapy, tennis elbow support, corticosteroid injection, and surgery.

I. Neurologic Exams

1. *Lower Extremity*

■ **Description**

L-3—quadriceps muscle.

L-4—patella reflex.

L-5—great toe dorsiflexion, sensation at web of great and first toes.

S-1—Achilles reflex, gastrocnemius muscle and plantar flexors.

2. *Cervical Region*

■ **Description**

C-5—deltoid muscle, biceps tendon reflex.

C-6—biceps/thumb muscle, biceps tendon reflex.

C-7—affects triceps muscle, triceps reflex, grip strength, sensation index/middle fingers.

C-8—intrinsic hand muscles.

BIBLIOGRAPHY

Ball GV. *Clinical Rheumatology*. Philadelphia, Pa: WB Saunders Co; 1986.

Birnbaum JS. *The Musculoskeletal Manual*. Orlando, Fla: Academic Press; 1982.

Cailliet R. *Neck and Arm Pain*. 3rd ed. Philadelphia, Pa: FA Davis Co; 1991.

Callen JP. *The Medical Clinics of North America, Cutaneous Manifestations of Collagen Vascular Disease and Related Conditions*. Vol. 73. Philadelphia, Pa: WB Saunders Co; September, 1989.

Connolly JF. *The Management of Fractures and Dislocations: An Atlas*. 3rd ed. Philadelphia, Pa: WB Saunders Co; 1981.

D'Ambrosia RD. *Musculoskeletal Disorders*. 2nd ed. Philadelphia, Pa: JB Lippincott Co; 1986.

Dieppe PA. *Atlas of Clinical Rheumatology*. Philadelphia, Pa: Lea & Febiger; 1986.

Enneking WF. *Musculoskeletal Tumor Surgery*. New York: Churchill Livingstone; 1983.

Morrissy RT. *Pediatric Orthopedics*, Vols. 1 and 2. 3rd ed. Philadelphia, Pa: JB Lippincott; 1990.

Niwayama G, Resnick D. *Diagnosis of Bone and Joint Disorders*. 2nd ed. Philadelphia, Pa: WB Saunders Co; 1988.

O'Donoghue DH. *Treatment of Injuries to Athletes*. 4th ed. Philadelphia, Pa: WB Saunders Co; 1984.

Turek SL. *Orthopedics: Principles and Their Application*. Vols. 1 and 2. 4th ed. Philadelphia, Pa: JB Lippincott; 1984.

CHAPTER 11

Neurology

JOEL S. GOLDBERG, DO

I. HEADACHE

ominous signs:
- *HA + focal neurologic deficit*
- *progressive HA*
- *HA c̄ papilledema*
- *wakes pt from sleep*
- *HA c̄ N|V*

A. Migraine – 10% population

■ **Description**

Migraine c̄ aura
Classic migraine—**unilateral throbbing headache with aura.**

Migraine s̄ aura
Common migraine—subtle onset, no aura, represents 80% of cases.

■ **Symptoms** *onset! ⇒ may not stay unilateral*

hours (2-5)
Unilateral, throbbing, visual and autonomic disturbances, nausea. **Vertebral basilar** migraine may present with ataxia, vertigo, dysarthria.

■ **Diagnosis**

onset childhood, adolescence or early adulthood
Typical symptoms in young adult, **positive family history** often, 75% cases are women. Increased incidence of motion sickness and infantile colic.

■ **Pathology**

Vasomotor changes.

■ **Treatment**

Acute (abortive)
- *ergot*
- *imitrex (Suma-triptan)*
- *DOC: seratonin agonist*

Prophylactic (≥ 2|mo)
- *β blockers*
- *Ca++ chan. blockers*

Ergot alkaloids, preventive treatment with **beta-blockers, methysergide** (potential for **r**etroperitoneal fibrosis with long-term use), calcium channel blockers, antidepressants, non-steroidal anti-inflammatory drugs (NSAIDs), cyproheptadine, avoid alcohol, tyramine (cheese), chocolate, citrus, onions, and nitrite.

B. Cluster

■ **Description**

Vascular headache, **histamine cephalgia, Horton's headache.**

■ **Symptoms**

not throbbing
20-30 min
Severe pain in short episodes without aura, for weeks to months, then remits, ipsilateral lacrimation, nasal congestion.

typically described as behind or around the eye (unilateral)
(+) Horner's syndrome (ptosis, miosis)
(+) rhinorrhea, lacrimation

■ **Diagnosis**

Typical symptoms, **men more often** (95%), **worse with alcohol** and sleep.

■ **Pathology**

Autonomic dysfunction.

■ **Treatment**

#1!
Similar to migraine, also **prednisone**, oxygen, lithium. *↳ during attack*

C. Temporal Arteritis (Giant Cell)

■ **Description**

Inflammatory systemic illness in elderly.

■ **Symptoms**

Temporal headache, vision loss, malaise.
Jaw claudication

■ **Diagnosis**

Biopsy, elevated sed rate.
(May miss lesion)

■ **Pathology**

Lymphocyte and **giant-cell infiltrates** in cranial arteries.

■ **Treatment**

Corticosteroids.

D. Benign Intracranial Hypertension, *Idiopathic Intracranial HTN*

■ **Description**

Called **pseudotumor cerebri.**

■ **Symptoms** *→ no focal neurologic deficits*

Those of increased intracranial pressure without tumor **headache, papilledema.**
big worry – visual loss 2° b/l papilledema

■ **Diagnosis**

Headache and papilledema without tumor, more common in **obese females.** Ob-
multiparous

tension-type headache
excessive contraction of scalp muscles
b/c nonthrobbing, long lasting (weeks, months)
rx: analgesics
muscle relaxants
biofeedback

tain computed tomography (CT) scan, MRI *no mass!* and electroencephalogram (EEG); if both OK, lumbar puncture. → ↑opening pressure

■ **Pathology**

Unknown, but may be seen in tetracycline and corticosteroid use.
also in Vitamin A excess

■ **Treatment**

Lumbar punctures, prednisone. • optic nerve sheath fenestration
Remove cause if possible
• lumboperitoneal shunt

E. Trigeminal Neuralgia

■ **Description**

Also called **tic douloureux.**

■ **Symptoms**

Brief episodes of **pain in fifth cranial nerve distribution,** third and second divisions.

■ **Diagnosis**

Onset after 40, more often in women, may coexist with multiple sclerosis (MS); history is diagnostic, may have facial trigger points.

■ **Pathology**

Compression of trigeminal nerve in the posterior fossa.

■ **Treatment**

Phenytoin, carbamazepine, baclofen, surgery.

II. DIZZINESS

A. Syncope and Presyncope

Impending loss of consciousness secondary to inadequate cerebral perfusion. Etiology vascular or cardiac, not neurologic. May be due to hyperventilation, orthostatic hypotension, vasovagal, micturition.

B. Dysequilibrium

Disorder of balance system, dizziness when standing and walking, multiple possible central nervous system (CNS) causes. Chronic and common in elderly.

C. Vertigo

Sensation of movement, due to abnormality of the peripheral or central vestibular system pathways. Nystagmus may be present. Peripheral nystagmus is unidirectional and suppressed by fixation. Central nystagmus may be multidirectional and is never suppressed by fixation. Ménière's disease: hearing loss, tinnitus, and vertigo. Perilymph fistula: oval window tear resulting in vertigo aggravated by change in head position, sneezing, noises. Other disorders resulting in vertigo include vestibular neuronitis, labyrinthitis, posttraumatic, brainstem transient ischemic (TIA), MS, posterior fossa tumor, and basilar artery migraine.

III. EPILEPSY – *2 or more seizures s̄ explainable caus*

A. Generalized Epilepsy → *both hemispheres from beginning*

1. Grand mal—tonic and/or clonic, loss of consciousness, postictal confusion, no true aura, major motor activity present.
   Synchronous contractions 2-3 min

2. Petit mal—brief loss of consciousness or twitching or repetitive swallowing/facial movements, minor motor activity, EEG positive for three per second spike and slow wave pattern. Drug of choice: ethosuximide.
   10-15 sec

3. Myoclonic—single or multiple body jerks or spasms without loss of consciousness.

4. Atonic seizures—drop attacks secondary to diffuse brain disease.
   poor prognosis

>30 min = status epilepticus → neurologic emergency when tonic/clonic
→ start c̄ diazepam (valium) or lorazepam (Ativan), then give phenytoin (Cerebrix)
then phenobarb
then general anaesthesia — Drug of choice for
→ grand mall

5. **Infantile spasms**—sudden flexion of **neck and trunk**, etiology in perinatal infection, trauma, and brain disease, possible salaam movements. *Rx: ACTH, Depakene*

also assoc. c̄ tuberous sclerosis so be sure to r/o T.S

assoc. c̄ diffuse brain injury & mental retardation

6. **Atypical absence**—absence spell followed by brief **tonic seizure**. *Rx: Depakene*

7. **Lennox–Gastaut syndrome**—atypical absence spells in a patient with **neurologic deficits, slow EEG spike** and **wave** patterns along with a generalized seizure disorder.

8. *Febrile seizures*
6mo – 6yo – brief (few min) generalized seizure, no post ictal, high fever, no focal neurologic signs, ⊕ fam hx; no sequelae EEG → diffuse slowing. ⅓ never recur; ↑ risk of recurrence if < 1yo

B. Focal Epilepsy (Partial)

1. **Jacksonian** seizures—**involuntary spreading movements without loss of consciousness.**

2. **Uncinate fits**—complex partial seizures with **olfactory aura.** *→ LOC*

May look like absence but absence should stop by adolescence

3. **Temporal lobe (psychomotor, limbic)**—aura and complex partial seizure of temporal lobe structures. *Rx: Tegretol*

partial simple → no Δ in MS
complex: Δ in mental status

4. **Sylvian** or **Rolandic**—childhood partial seizure where EEG shows **centrotemporal** spikes. ✱

Additional Information. **Todd's postictal paralysis** reflects a **partial seizure** having taken place. **Note** that **focal epilepsy** represents the **most common seizure type** with **complex partial** most often secondary to local cortical discharge; **aura present.**

C. Seizure Medication — *Rx cause first! then sx*

1. **Treatment of generalized tonic/clonic seizures**

a. **Diphenylhydantoin (Dilantin).** **Ataxia** and **sedation** if the **level is too high.** Side effects include **hirsutism, gingival hypertrophy,** allergic skin reactions, **Stevens–Johnson** syndrome, **osteoporosis.**

Causes fetal hydantoin syndrome if used during pregnancy

b. **Carbamazepine (Tegretol).** Diplopia, if level too high; may induce bone marrow suppression. *—must draw weekly CBC*

c. **Phenobarbital.** Sedation.

d. **Valproic acid (Depakene).** Possible **liver failure, fatal pancreatitis,** and **bone marrow suppression,** may help **atypical absence** spells.

e. **Primidone (Mysoline).** May cause sedation, **ataxia.**

f. **Ethosuximide (Zarontin).** ✱ **Drug of choice** for **absence** spells. ✱

g. **Adrenocorticotropic hormone (ACTH).** Used for **infantile spasms,** as is valproic acid and clonazepam.

2. **Treatment of focal seizures**—similar to that for generalized seizures; however, multiple medications may be needed.

w/u → find etiology of seizures : EEG (spikes on sharp waves)
Video EEG
MRI or other neuroimaging
r/o tumor, abscess, AVM, scar

IV. COMA

■ Description

Patient cannot be aroused, total unresponsiveness. Light coma may demonstrate response to noxious stimuli, whereas there is no response in deep coma.

Locked-in syndrome: quadriplegia and lower cranial nerve paralysis, but conscious with higher mental activity intact. **Akinetic mutism (coma vigile):** patient in coma, but appears awake. *→ vegetative state?*

■ Diagnosis

Physical exam. May have Battle's sign: blue mastoid area, suggesting basal skull fracture or temporal bone fracture. Breath odor fruity or acetone in ketoacidosis, musty in hepatic coma. Cheyne–Stokes respiration (hyperpnea alternating with apnea) noted with bilateral cerebral hemisphere damage. Apneustic respiration (long inspiration then pause): lower pontine lesions, as does ataxic (chaotic) breathing. See Chapter 12, Eyesigns.

Decerebrate posture. Midbrain lesion, extension/adduction of arms and legs.
Decorticate posture. Lower diencephalon lesion, flexion arms, wrists, and fingers.

Rx therapy → poorly controlled partial complex seizures temporal lobe resection

tPA for acute stroke (ischemic)
w/in 3hrs of onset
nonhemorrhagic (CT scan)

■ Pathology

Diffuse cerebral hemisphere dysfunction and/or involvement of the brain stem ascending reticular activating system.

1st LOC
→2nd lucid period
3rd LOC/coma

Trauma. History of injury. Epidural hematoma: lucid interval. Subdural: depressed consciousness, then focal findings.
Vascular disease. Sudden onset, nuchal rigidity, bloody cerebrospinal fluid (CSF).
Neoplasm. Focal signs, papilledema.
Infection. Cerebrospinal fluid increased protein normal or low CSF glucose.
Metabolic. Abnormal labs.

■ Treatment

Establish **airway**, and intravenous **(IV)** line, **determine cardiovascular status, history, and physical**. Obtain full lab, skull x-ray, CT and/or magnetic resonance imaging (MRI). May need lumbar puncture. Give thiamine, dextrose, and possibly naloxone. If **cerebral edema** or increased intracranial pressure, restrict fluids, hyperventilate, **mannitol,** and **steroids.**

blood in sulci →
SAH

ACA
MCA
PCA
embolic stroke
lacunar infarct

V. CEREBROVASCULAR DISEASE

■ Description

→ min/hrs

Stroke—sudden onset of a focal neurologic deficit due to cerebrovascular disease, lasting more than 24 hours

→ w/in vasc. distribution

Transient ischemic attack—focal, abrupt in onset. Same but fully resolved within 24 hours.

Two major types—**Ischemic** (embolic and thrombotic) and **hemorrhagic** (intraparenchymal and subarachnoid). **Stroke** is the third leading cause of death in the United States.

■ Diagnosis

Cerebral embolism—abrupt onset while active; most common source is the heart; rarely lose consciousness.

also lg arteries

younger pt
known embolic source (a fib)
(mitral stenosis)
s/p MI
endocarditis

Do TEE (echo)

Subarachnoid hemorrhage—abrupt onset while active from aneurysm at circle of Willis; may lose consciousness ~worst headache!

Intraparenchymatous hemorrhage—abrupt onset while active, may lose consciousness; CT positive for hematoma.

Thrombotic—often **preceded by transient ischemic attack (TIA)**, often **during sleep;** rarely lose consciousness. May have normal CT and lumbar puncture; rarely have headache. ~ *from atherosclerosis of carotid*

A. Ischemic Stroke (80%) ~85%

■ Symptoms

2nd atherosclerosis

1. **Middle cerebral artery**—embolism results in contralateral hemiplegia. **Nonfluent or Broca's aphasia** from upper-division occlusion. **Wernicke's (fluent)** aphasia from lower-division lesions. Most **common site for cerebral infarct is middle cerebral artery.**

2. **Anterior cerebral artery**—paralysis opposite leg.

3. **Carotid artery**—weakness, temporary unilateral loss of vision, speech disturbance, numbness. *amaurosis fugax*

4. **Posterior cerebral**—contralateral homonymous hemianopia.

5. **Vertebrobasilar**—ataxia, hemiplegia, horizontal gaze, palsy, nystagmus, vertigo, deafness, dizziness.

6. **Cerebellar**—ataxia, dizziness, nausea, vomiting.

7. **Lacunar infarct**—due to **lipohyalinosis,** may present with pure motor or sensory strokes, clumsy hand syndrome may be seen. *good prognosis*
   Rx → control HTN + ASA
   Small artery HTN occlusion of penetrating arteries

8. **Obtain CT**—(may not show acute bleed), **MRI.**

■ Treatment

Lower blood pressure (BP), avoid excess free water, anticoagulants.

Rx: carotid stenosis >70% do carotid endarterectomy ⊕ ASA

<70% c̄ ASA or antiplatelet meds (ticlid)

Rx: noninfectious cardiac emboli → full anticoagulation (heparin) (coumadin)

B. Hemorrhagic Stroke (20%)

■ Symptoms

1. **Hypertensive intracerebral hemor-rhage**—most common site is **puta-men**. Sudden onset **dizziness, vomiting**, inability to stand, ipsilateral facial paresis. **Unusual eye signs** may indicate **thalamic** hemorrhage. **Pontine** hemorrhage results in **pinpoint pupils**. **Cerebellar** bleed results in dizziness, vomiting, and ataxia.

petamen (BG)

Rx-surgical resection rx ↑ICP, HTN control

2. **Subarachnoid hemorrhage**—saccular aneurysm or vascular malformation. Sudden severe headache, meningeal irritation; exam may be normal.

D/D:- (trauma)
40-50s - ruptured berry aneurysm
- ruptured AVM (#1 in children)

rebleed risk
2° ischemia, vasospasm
→ Circle of Willis
"worst headache of my life"

MRI/MRA to r/o AVM vs aneurysm

3. **Test of choice—CT scan.** Do **lumbar puncture** only if CT not available.

→ fresh blood is white on CT
→ will get bloody tap ē blood in all 4 tubes (no clearing) or clear CSF then bloody
Xanthochromia → supernatant is yellow

■ Treatment

Control BP, steroids, **surgery**, antivasospasm agents.

↓ Nimodapine (Ca⁺⁺ channel blocker)
aneurysm → endovascular rx (newer) clipping

VI. DEMYELINATING DISEASE

A. Multiple Sclerosis (MS)

■ Description

Multiple areas of neurologic deficits, peak **age 24**. Increased incidence in **women** and **north temperate latitudes**, etiology unknown. Fewer exacerbations during pregnancy.

young ♀ from North ē strange neuro exam

Multiple focal deficits with relapse ē remission

■ Symptoms

Optic neuritis, **vertigo**, **paresthesias**, **incoordination**, bladder dysfunction, **nystagmus**, hearing loss in 50%, trigeminal neuralgia, diplopia, **internuclear opthalmoplegia** pathognomonic of MS if bilateral.

→ going gray/blind over hours or days +/- pain

b/l internuclear opthalmoplegia is pathognomonic

(tic delourexx)

AVM:
• artery-veins
• onset - rupt. SAH
- seizures
- throbbing HA (migraine-like)
• dx - MRA/MRI
• rx: focused RT surg. resection embolization

■ Diagnosis

Increased CSF **immunoglobulin G (IgG)**/lymphocytes and **positive oligoclonal bands** (cerebrospinal fluid pleocytosis), total protein normal or slightly up, increased latency in **visual evoked response (VER)** and brainstem auditory evoked response (BAER) studies.

also ⊕ myelin basic protein

- asymptomatic lesions

MRI shows focal demyelinized plaques in brain or spinal chord
often periventricular

■ Pathology

Plaques—areas of **myelin destruction** where lymphocytes and monocytes penetrate the white matter.

■ Treatment

Immunosuppressives, **ACTH**, **antivirals**. **Baclofen**: drug of choice for MS spasticity. **Carbamazepine** for neuritic pains.

few rx are very effective.

Rx: acute exacerb high dose IV steroid
Maintenance rx
1) β-interferon (Bseron avonex)
2) copolymer
3) IVIG

B. Optic Neuritis

■ Description

Visual loss of rapid onset from **optic nerve demyelination**. Episode of optic neuritis may precede MS. Papillitis is swelling of the optic nerve head.

■ Diagnosis

Abnormal VER, may have **increased CSF IgG and pleocytosis**; MRI and fluorescein angiography may be needed.

■ Treatment

Corticosteroids and ACTH.

C. Acute Disseminated Encephalomyelitis

■ Description

Self-limited, mostly **postinfectious** and **postvaccinal**.

■ **Symptoms**

Headache, stiff neck, confusion or coma, fever.

■ **Treatment**

Corticosteroids and ACTH.

D. **Guillain-Barré Syndrome—A Peripheral Neuropathy**

■ **Description**

Acute inflammatory polyradiculoneuropathy in young to middle-age adults.

■ **Symptoms**

Progressive ascending weakness, areflexia. *Following URI often or GI infection. Some association c̄ campylobacter jejuni*

■ **Diagnosis**

High CSF protein, short duration of progression; EMG.

■ **Pathology**

Proximally inflammatory segmental demyelination.

■ **Treatment**

Spontaneous recovery, plasmapheresis. *IVIG*

VII. **CNS INFECTIONS**

A. **Acute Meningitis**

■ **Symptoms**

Headache, fever, stiff neck. Minimal neurologic signs in viral meningitis, which is a benign self-limited disorder and also termed aseptic meningitis. Positive **Kernig** and **Brudzinski signs.** *(signs of meningeal irritation)*

■ **Diagnosis**

Gram stain and culture of CSF. Modest elevation in CSF protein. **Over 50, viral,**

in **bacterial** or **fungal** up to 400. **Hypoglycorrhachia** (CSF glucose less than 40% of serum level) **suggests bacterial** cause. **Tuberculous** (polymorphonuclear pleocytosis without pathogen isolated) active pulmonary disease is one third, positive purified protein derivative (PPD) in 50%.

■ **Pathology**

1. **Neonatal**—group B streptococcus, *Escherichia coli.*
2. **Early childhood**—*Haemophilus influenzae*[#2], *S. pneumoniae*[#1] and *Neisseria meningitidis.*
3. **Young adults**—*Neisseria meningitidis* (petechial or ecchymotic rash often).
4. **Nosocomial**—Gram-negative bacteria and *Staphylococcus aureus.*
5. **Immunosuppressed**—*Listeria monocytogenes.* *(also neonatal)*
6. **Human immunodeficiency virus (HIV) patients**—acute aseptic meningitis. *also get cryptococcus – india ink shows capsules*
7. **Viral meningitis**—most common agent is mumps; enterovirus is most common viral group.

■ **Treatment**

1. **Toxoplasma**—pyrimethamine plus sulfadiazine.
2. **Brucella**—tetracycline and aminoglycoside.
3. **Neonatal**—ampicillin and gentamicin.
4. **Adults**—ceftriaxone or ampicillin.
5. **Tuberculous**—isoniazid plus ethambutol.
6. **Fungal**—amphotericin B.

B. **Neurosyphilis**

■ **Symptoms**

→ dementia

Tabes dorsalis, general paresis, optic atrophy, cerebrovascular disease from invasion of leptomeninges with *Treponema*

Spinal chord ← post.columns? dorsal nerve roots
• ⊕ Romburg sign
• lighting pains
• charcot joints
• loss of position/ vibration

meningovascular (strokes) –ischemic
gumona – focal mass

CSF

	Viral	bacterial	fungal
glucose	2/3 serum	<40% serum	20-40 ~~100 mg/dL~~
protein	<50	50-1500	<500
WBC	10-500 lymphs	25-10,000 polys	10-500 lymph
gramstain	∅	bacteria	∅

pallidum. Neurosyphilis most often is asymptomatic.

■ Treatment

High-dose parenteral penicillin. **Jarisch–Herxheimer** reaction: hypotension, fever, headache, chills, and tachycardia in first 24 hours of treatment from release of treponemal products, not a penicillin reaction. ✗

C. Empyema (Subdural)

Infection spread from paranasal sinuses and middle ear, *Streptococcus* most often, marked peripheral leukocytosis.

D. Viral Encephalitis

■ Description

Mortality of 10%.

■ Symptoms

Focal signs and **acute febrile** illness, **seizures** and **coma**, or depressed state of consciousness. Headache, fever, and nuchal rigidity.

■ Diagnosis

Aseptic CSF, lymphocytic CSF with normal glucose.

■ Pathology

Caused by mumps, herpes simplex, and lymphocytic choriomeningitis. Mouse and hamster exposure linked to lymphocytic choriomeningitis.

■ Treatment

Treat edema and seizures.

Brain abscess: focal neurologic deficit
↑ICP (HA, N/V)
Sx of infection (fever/chills)

CT scan → ring enhancing lesions
Rx: surg. drainage + antibiotics

E. Other CNS Infections

1. **Rabies**—brain-stem encephalitis, incubation 30 to 60 days or more, dysphagia-hydrophobia, fatal in acute stage in 95%.

2. **Polio**—etiology: enteroviruses that damage anterior horn cells of spinal cord, an acute febrile illness with evidence of lower motor neuron paralysis.

3. **Toxoplasmosis**—intracellular parasite, **most common opportunistic CNS pathogen in acquired immunodeficiency syndrome (AIDS)** (cryptococcal is second most common).

4. **Slow viruses:**

   a. **Jacob–Creutzfeldt (JC), Kuru.** Ataxia and myoclonus, dementia.

   b. **Subacute sclerosing panencephalitis.** In childhood, mostly from post measles infection. Elevated gamma globulin and measles antibodies in CSF.

   c. **Progressive multifocal leukoencephalopathy (PML).** Due to SV40-PML or JC virus. *Immune suppressed oligodendrocytes—white matter disease*
   no effective rx

5. **AIDS**—see Infectious Disease section.

6. **Herpes simplex encephalitis**—treat with acyclovir. Diagnosis may be suggested by temporal lobe localization. ✗
   type I
   • Δ mental status over hrs/days
   • partial complex seizures
   MRI - Δ's in temp lobes
   PCR on CSF
   EEG - temp lobe

VIII. NEUROMUSCULAR DISEASE

A. Disorders of Muscle— Muscular Dystrophy

Weakness - proximal, diffuse, nl sensation

1. **Duchenne**—sex-linked recessive trait, **progressive muscle weakness** and **atrophy**, due to mutation on X chromosome, diagnosis by family history, weakness, muscle biopsy, probable death by age 20. Elevated creatine kinase (CK).
Calf pseudohypertrophy
→ ↓ dystro
rx: no effective rx

Polymyositis / Dermatomyositis: → *heliotropism (purple eyelids), red rash on knuckles*
autoimmune conditions   *rx: corticosteroids*
proximal weakness   *IVIG*
EMG- myopathic changes
↑CPK ; muscle bx- inflammatory cells

2. **Limb–girdle**—autosomal recessive.

3. **Myotonic**—thinning face muscles, electromyogram (EMG) shows a decremental pattern, and irregular afterpotentials. Autosomal dominant. Treat with phenytoin sodium (Dilantin).

4. **Fascioscapulohumeral**—autosomal dominant. No carriers.

B. **Disorders of Neuromuscular Junction** ← *fatigueable weakness*

1. *Myasthenia Gravis*

■ **Description**

Autoimmune defect of acetylcholine receptor. Associated with abnormalities of the thymus. Women more than men.   ↳ *hypertrophy or thymoma*

■ **Symptoms**

Weak with activity, fatigue, ocular symptoms, facial muscles, voice, and respiration can be affected.   *get better c̄ rest!*

edrophonium makes them stronger ←

■ **Diagnosis** → *decremental response*

Tensilon test, electromyogram, positive antibodies to acetylcholine receptor.

■ **Treatment**   *physostigmine* →

Thymectomy, **anticholinesterase** medication, steroids, plasmapheresis. → *brief help*
IVIG

2. *Eaton–Lambert Syndrome*

■ **Description**

Facilitating neuromuscular transmission disorder.

■ **Symptoms**

Limb weakness without cranial muscle weakness and absence of deep tendon reflexes. Found with **oat cell cancer (CA).**

■ **Diagnosis**

Response to repetitive stimulation (**increasing action potential).**

■ **Treatment**

Guanidine. Calcium channel antagonists are contraindicated.

3. *Botulism*

■ **Description**

Toxin of *Clostridium botulinum* blocks acetylcholine release.

■ **Symptoms**

Begin 12 to 36 hours after ingestion of exotoxin. **Dilated fixed pupil, flaccid quadriplegia,** blurred vision, dysphagia.

■ **Diagnosis**

Isolate toxin from stool, stomach, or food. **Spores** also found in **honey.**

■ **Treatment**

Cathartics, trivalent antitoxin (A, B, E), quinidine, and supportive therapy.

C. **Myotonia**

1. **Myotonia congenita**—impaired muscle relaxation, treat with phenytoin.

2. **Myotonic dystrophy—distal weakness,** cardiac conduction problems, increased sensitivity to medication with respiratory drive, ptosis, temporalis, and masseter muscle wasting.

D. **Trichinosis**

■ **Description**

Nematode *Trichinella spiralis* **infection, undercooked** pork most common source.

PN disease: motor & sensory disease.

polyneuropathy → stocking glove, distal weakness
radiculopathy → dermotome & myotome
mononeuropathy → trauma or compression

UMN	LMN
spinal chord or higher	*periph nerve or distal*
↑tone n/weakness	*↓tone atrophy fasciculations*
↑DTR	*↓DTR / absent DTR*
⊕ babinski	*silent babinski*

■ **Symptoms**

Eosinophilia, weakness, myalgia.

■ **Treatment**

Steroids, thiabendazole.

E. Tetanus

■ **Description**

Lockjaw, intense motor neuron activity.

■ **Symptoms**

Muscle rigidity, trismus, sneering *risus sardonicus*, opisthotonos, jaw and back discomfort.

hydrophobia!

■ **Diagnosis**

Clinical picture.

■ **Pathology**

Exotoxin from *Clostridium tetani*, a Gram-positive coccus.

■ **Treatment**

Cleaning and debridement of infected site. Antibiotics, antitoxin (human hyperimmune globulin).

F. Bell's Palsy

■ **Description**

Cranial nerve VII damage resulting in facial weakness.

■ **Symptoms**

Peripheral facial weakness, may have ipsilateral hyperacusis and decreased taste. *(chordae tympani effects)*

■ **Diagnosis**

Exam.

■ **Pathology**

Facial nerve anoxia.

■ **Treatment**

Steroids.

G. Motor Disease

1. **Amyotrophic lateral sclerosis (ALS)**—middle-age rapid progression of **weakness, atrophy, and spasticity**. **Is most common motor system disease.** Combination of both upper and lower motor neuron deficit is common.

2. **Werdnig–Hoffmann—floppy infant**, progressive, atrophy, fasiculations, respiratory and swallowing problems. Autosomal recessive. *→esp tongue*

3. **Kugelberg–Welander**—juvenile proximal motor weakness, autosomal recessive, atrophy, and fasiculations.

4. **Primary lateral sclerosis—progressive spasticity of extremities**, very rare.

5. **Polio**—febrile illness, meningeal irritation, and **flaccid motor paralysis**.

See CNS Infection section.

IX. MOVEMENT DISORDERS → *basal ganglia lesion*

A. Huntington's Disease

■ **Description**

Presents as **adult insidious onset of chorea** with mental deterioration, autosomal dominant with 100% penetrance, and positive family history, usually between ages 30 and 40.

CAG trinucleotide repeat (Chrom 4)

■ **Symptoms**

① **Progressive emotional or intellectual decline** associated with abnormalities in

② ⊕ *fam. hx*

③ *Chorea or other movement d/o*

gait, ocular motor function, and dexterity. Patients live an average of 15 years.

■ **Diagnosis**

Exam, family history.

■ **Pathology**

Caudate nucleus and cerebral cortex **atrophy,** neuronal loss and gliosis, and decreased γ-aminobenzoic acid (GABA) have been noted along with increased somatostatin levels.

■ **Treatment**

↓ chorea ← **No cure** but dopaminergic antagonists haloperidol (Haldol), cholinergic agonists, and GABA are possibly effective.

B. **Wilson's Disease (Hepatolenticular Degeneration)**

■ **Description**

Chromosome 13 autosomal recessive disorder of copper metabolism, characterized by **deficient ceruloplasmin.**

■ **Symptoms**

Neurologic—speech/extrapyramidal disorder is the most common presentation.
Hepatic—hepatitis, which may be acute or chronic; cirrhosis.
Ocular—Kayser–Fleischer ring in cornea noted (green-brown ring at limbus).
Psychiatric—variable presentation.

■ **Diagnosis**

Renal—renal tubular acidosis, high serum copper and high urine copper.
Slit lamp exam, low serum ceruloplasmin, and elevated 24-hour urine copper; liver biopsy and copper quantitation are also helpful; the disorder usually presents at age 18 to 20.

■ **Treatment**

D-penicillamine. Adverse effects of therapy include hypersensitivity, fever, nephrotic syndrome agranulocytosis, myasthenia gravis, Goodpasture syndrome, bone marrow suppression, and collagen vascular disorders. } result of rx!

C. **Parkinson's Disease**

■ **Description**

An **extrapyramidal movement disorder** affecting the elderly.

■ **Symptoms**

Characterized by **resting tremor,** *cogwheel rigidity,* **bradykinesia,** impaired postural reflexes, masked facies, simian posture, pill rolling, 5 to 7 cycle/second tremor, reptilian stare.

postural instability ←

■ **Diagnosis**   DD for 2° Parkinsonism ⇒
Clinical exam   1. Drug induced (neuroleptic

■ **Pathology** (Nigrostriatum)

Substantia nigra neurons undergo idiopathic **degenerative process** with loss of dopamine in corpus striatum. → caudate/putamen
Lewy bodies

■ **Treatment** Cogentin, Artane   prevents spread conversion of L-dopa
Anticholinergics, levodopa/carbidopa (Sinemet), toxicity with levodopa: dyskinesias have been observed, arrhythmia, hypotension. *Eldapril (Selegiline)* ? slow progression
Bromocriptine (dopamine agonists)
Amantidine

D. **Iatrogenic**

1. **Drug-induced parkinsonism—** methylphenyltetrahydropyridine (MPTP), neuroleptics block striatal dopamine receptor sites.
2. **Tardive dyskinesia—**linguofasciobuccal, choreiform. → 2° neuroleptic drug - worse c̄ anticholinergics

Hemiballism - contralateral subthalamic nucleus

3. <u>Dopamine agonist-induced chorea</u>—levodopa.

4. **Neuroleptic dystonia.**

E. Non-iatrogenic

1. **Dystonia**—a <u>twisting muscle contraction</u>, consisting of <u>repetitive movements</u>.

2. **Chorea**—<u>random, dancelike, excessive, involuntary, purposeless movements</u>.

3. **Blepharospasm**—<u>oromandibular dystonia (Meigs' syndrome).</u>

4. **Spasmodic torticollis**—most frequent <u>focal dystonia.</u>

5. **Essential tremor**—involves the <u>upper extremity, postural, is often progressive</u> and may be heredofamilial, the treatment is propranolol.

F. Tremor (Essential)   *arm, head, voice*

improves. c̄ EtOH

<u>Benign, heredofamilial</u> (<u>autosomal dominant</u>), and postural with early adult onset, of <u>unknown cause</u>; treatment with <u>propranolol may help</u>. Primidone and amantadine may be tried.

G. Myoclonus

<u>Rapid jerking movement</u>, treat primary cause when known. Clonazepam, 5-hydroxytryptophan (5-HTP) and valproic acid often used.

H. Asterixis — ~~Rapid flexion-extension of wrist~~ *hand flap*

X. DEMENTIA — *acquired intellectual loss - b/c brain dysfunction*

#1 Alzheimer
#2 Multiinfarct
also: HIV
Parkinson's
hydrocephalus
C-J disease

A. Alzheimer's Disease

■ **Description**

A **progressive dementia** (global cognitive decline) *- neurodegenerative d/o*

■ **Symptoms** — *Memory loss ⊕ any other deficit*

Memory loss, <u>confusion</u>, <u>speech difficulty</u>, and <u>difficulty with daily living activities</u> may present.

■ **Diagnosis**

55-65
40.

<u>Clinical</u>, by <u>dementia, abnormal mental status exam</u>, and <u>exclusion of other illnesses</u> (eg, <u>normal pressure, hydrocephalus, metabolic disease, multi-infarct dementia, tumor, and infections</u>). Etiology is unknown, but frequency increases with age, and a <u>genetic predisposition is</u> known.   ↳ *E4 allele of apolipoprotein E*

■ **Pathology**

large ventricles
& large sulci

<u>Senile plaques</u> and <u>neurofibrillary tangles</u> are prominent, associated with <u>cerebral atrophy</u> and enlargement of the cortical sulci.   *hippocampal involvement (memory)*
E4 allele of apolipoprotein E

■ **Treatment**

Symptoms such as <u>agitation and depression are treatable</u>, but Alzheimer's disease itself is not.

Cognex (tacrine HCl) - anticholinesterase ; Aricept (Donepa...)
3/d

B. Pick's Disease

■ **Description**

<u>Dementia similar to Alzheimer's.</u>

■ **Symptoms**

Same as Alzheimer's.
More prominent loss of social graces & personality Δ/o

■ **Diagnosis**

Occasionally familial.

■ **Pathology**

<u>Pick inclusion bodies</u> in *✗* frontal and temporal lobes. *✗*

■ **Treatment**

None, treat symptoms only.

C. Multi-infarct Dementia

■ **Description**

Gradual dementia.

■ **Symptoms**

Confusion, dementia.

■ **Diagnosis**

Gradual intellectual decline.

■ **Pathology**

Multiple strokes or infarctions.

■ **Treatment**

None. Treat hypertension, prevent emboli.

D. Hydrocephalus (Normal Pressure)

■ **Description**   ↳ no headaches, LP c̄ normal opening pressure

Progressive dementia.

■ **Symptoms**   ↗ usually mild

Incontinence, dementia, gait disturbance. (ataxia)

"wet, wild, wobbly"

■ **Diagnosis**

Exam. → CT scan

■ **Pathology**

Enlarged ventricles from blocked CSF.

↳ nl or sml sulci

■ **Treatment**

Shunt. → curative

usually VP shunt

E. Creutzfeldt–Jakob Disease

■ **Description**

Progressive dementia.

■ **Symptoms**

Subacute dementia, myoclonus.

↳ rapidly progressive

■ **Diagnosis**

Clinical, EEG high voltage, sharp activity on slow background.

■ **Pathology**

Slow virus, diffuse cerebral and spinal cord neuronal degeneration.

■ **Treatment**

None.

XI. NEUROLOGIC EYE SIGNS

A. Horner Syndrome

■ **Symptoms**

Ptosis, miosis, anhidrosis, enopthalmos, narrowing palpebral fissure, flushing on affected side of face.

■ **Pathology**

Interruption of the unilateral sympathetic system due to trauma, lung apex tumor, CNS lesions, vascular headache.

■ **Diagnosis**

Cocaine and *para*-OH-amphetamine tests.

B. Adie's Pupil

Symptoms

Unilaterally dilated pupil with slow response to light and accommodation; areflexia may be present.

■ **Pathology**

Postganglionic parasympathetic lesion.

■ **Diagnosis**

Weak pilocarpine solution results in Adie's pupil contraction.

C. **Argyll–Robertson Pupil**

■ **Symptoms**

Very small pupils that **fail to constrict to light** with accommodation preserved. One or both eyes affected.

■ **Diagnosis**

Argyll–Robertson pupil is a sign of **neurosyphilis.** Rule out CNS structural lesions.

D. **Uncal Herniation Syndrome**

■ **Symptoms**

Pupils fixed and **dilated,** ophthalmoplegia and contralateral hemiparesis.

E. **Marcus Gunn Pupil**

■ **Symptoms**

Defective light reflex with intact consensual reflex.

F. **Third Cranial Nerve Lesion**

■ **Symptoms**

Affects medial rectus, superior rectus, and inferior oblique paresis of contralateral eye elevation and ptosis.

G. **Fourth Cranial Nerve Lesion**

■ **Symptoms**

Superior oblique muscle affected; vertical diplopia.

H. **Sixth Cranial Nerve Lesion**

■ **Symptoms**

Weak lateral rectus, poor abduction, eye crossed.

I. **Pupil Signs in Examination**

Unreactive, midposition—midbrain lesion.
Pinpoint pupils—pontine lesion.
Unilaterally dilated and **unreactive—possible third nerve lesion.**

XII. SLEEP DISORDERS

A. **General Information**

Adults spend 20% of sleep in rapid eye movement **(REM)** sleep. Non-rapid eye movement sleep **(NREM) has four stages.** Three major disorders include **insomnia, hypersomnia,** and **parasomnia. Early morning awakening** is a **symptom of depression.**

Narcolepsy—**excessive daytime sleepiness** and **frequent early-onset REM pattern.**
Night terror—**arousal from NREM** sleep.
Nightmare—**awakening from REM** sleep.
Obstructive sleep apnea—**overweight,** hypertension, arrhythmias.
Central sleep apnea—older age, not overweight.

XIII. NEOPLASMS

A. **Gliomas (60% of CNS Tumors)**

1. **Astrocytoma**—most common of all gliomas, and **most common brain tumor in childhood.**

2. **Oligodendroglioma**—usually frontal lobe, slow growing, presents with headache, seizures, and the tumor may bleed.

[handwritten notes:]
glioblastoma multiforme → most common glioma bad prognosis
dx: MRI, bx
rx: corticosteroids (+edema) surg. resection RT & chemo rx
Adults → supratentorial
Children → infratentorial
multiple lesions → metastatic
Dx: neuroimaging (MRI c̄/s̄ contrast) contrast enhancing lesion (messy ring)

S&S: focal neurologic deficit → insidious onset, progressive sx (wk→months)
seizures → ↑↑ movement, cough, sneeze, valsalva
↑ICP (HA, N/V, papilledema)
hydrocephalus

← all brain tumors

1° CNS lymphoma - HIV pt
- multifocal lymphoma
- dx radiology + bx
- rx steroids, RT & chemorx (methotrexate)

3. **Medulloblastoma**—most **common posterior fossa tumor in children.**
✱ Fast growing, radiosensitive. ✱

4. Ependymoma.

B. **Meningiomas** - press into brain - attached to meninges

Usually benign, associated with **breast cancer** and **neurofibromatosis**, slow growing. - Rx: surgical resection Good prognosis

C. **Craniopharyngiomas**

Suprasellar, visual field defects often (bitemporal hemianopsia).

macro-

D. **Pituitary Tumors** → usually anterior lobe

→ pituitary adenoma

Secretory in 75%, **non-secretory** in 25%.
usually secretory ← Endocrine and visual symptoms. → macroadenoma
bitemporal hemianopsia ◑◐; hypopituitarism

Rx: transphenoidal hypophysectomy; chemorx (bromocriptine for prolactinoma)

8th nerve
cerebello-pontine angle

E. **Acoustic Schwannoma** (Vestibular schwannoma)
→ middle aged ♂

Unilateral hearing loss, facial numbness, **tinnitus,** unsteadiness. dx: BAER (brainstem auditory evoked response)
benign, slow growing tumor

Rx: surgical resection   Sx: wks, months, years   MRI

XIV. TRAUMA AND EMERGENCIES

A. **Epidural Hematoma**

■ **Symptoms**

tear of Middle meningeal artery

linear skull fx

Lucid interval after brief unconsciousness followed by increasing obtundation. Sometimes no lucid interval present. **Extreme headache, contralateral hemiparesis.**

■ **Diagnosis**

History and physical, CT scan.

B. **Subdural Hematoma**

■ **Symptoms**

Rupture of bridging veins

Acute, subacute, and **chronic** from cortical vein tear.

Acute—from high speed trauma, coma from impact; CT useful.

Subacute—several days of lethargy, then deterioration; MRI.

Chronic—minor trauma may cause gradual deterioration; MRI.

C. **Subarachnoid Hemorrhage**

■ **Symptoms**

Sudden-onset severe headache, may have **sentinel bleed** with minor symptoms. May have stiff neck, photophobia, nausea, and focal signs.

D. **Neuroleptic Malignant Syndrome**

■ **Symptoms**

High fever, muscular rigidity, extrapyramidal symptoms, all as a complication of antipsychotic medication.

■ **Treatment**

Includes **bromocriptine.**

E. **Myasthenic Crisis**

■ **Symptoms**

Muscle weakness affecting respiration in a patient with myasthenia gravis. 2 mg test done of edrophonium IV worsen the symptoms.

■ **Treatment**

Neostigmine (Prostigmin). There is approximately 10% need for assisted ventilation.

XV. TOXIC/METABOLIC DISEASE

A. **Uremic Encephalopathy**

■ **Symptoms**

Deterioration of cerebral functioning. Treat renal disease.

Spinal Chord compression:
- pt c any cancer c spinal chord sign - must r/o metastatic disease.
MRI spinal chord
rx: emergency → high dose steroids
radiation rx to lesion

B. Hyponatremia

■ **Symptoms**

Rx slow return to normal

Confusion, lethargy, headache, seizures. The more rapid the sodium drop, the more severe the symptoms. **Syndrome of inappropriate antidiuretic hormone (SIADH): treat with water restriction.**

C. Acute Intermittent Porphyria

■ **Symptoms**

Abdominal pain attacks, psychosis, confusion, seizures, neuropathy.

■ **Diagnosis**

Watson–Schwartz test for **elevated aminolevulinic acid.**

■ **Pathology**

Deficiency of porphobilinogen deaminase.

■ **Treatment**

Hematin and high-carbohydrate diet.

D. Lead Toxicity

■ **Symptoms**

Anemia, abdominal colic, encephalopathy, peripheral neuropathy (called **plumbism**), ataxia, seizures, **wrist drop.**

■ **Diagnosis**

Basophilic stippling, lead line on x-ray. **Lead colic is most frequent sign in adults.** Screen with lead level, ethylenediaminetetraacetic acid (EDTA) test if lead level not over 80.

■ **Pathology**

Neuropathy from segmental demyelination.

■ **Treatment**

Chelation with EDTA and dimercaprol (BAL).

E. Liver Disease—Hepatic Encephalopathy

■ **Symptoms**

Asterixis, slow EEG, depressed mental status, elevated blood ammonia. Give protein-free diet, neomycin, or lactulose.

F. Arsenic Toxicity

■ **Symptoms**

Nausea, vomiting, abdominal pain, renal failure, neuropathy, encephalopathy.

■ **Diagnosis**

History, exam, Mees' lines (transverse lines in nails).

■ **Treatment**

Use BAL.

G. Carbon Monoxide Toxicity

■ **Symptoms**

Cherry-red color, lethargy, hypoxia without cyanosis.

■ **Diagnosis**

History.

■ **Treatment**

Remove from source; 100% oxygen.

Sometimes hyperbaric

H. Vitamin Disorders

1. **Thiamine (B$_1$) deficiency—**(*Wernicke's encephalopathy*), nystagmus, ataxia, confusion.

2. **Cobalamin (B₁₂) deficiency**—*(pernicious anemia)*, megaloblastic anemia, subacute combined spinal cord degeneration.
3. **Pyridoxine (B₆)**—*excess can produce sensory neuropathy.*

I. Salicylate Toxicity

■ **Symptoms**

Tinnitus, hearing loss, delirium, coma, seizures.

■ **Diagnosis**

History, respiratory alkalosis, serum salicylate level, rapid screen: ferric chloride test.

■ **Treatment**

Treat shock, protect airway, routine drug intoxication measures.

J. Reye Syndrome

■ **Symptoms**

Vomiting, lethargy, and delirium after a viral illness with abnormal liver functions, hypoglycemia, and respiratory alkalosis. Liver shows **microvesicular fatty infiltration.**

XVI. GENETIC DISORDERS

A. Gaucher's Disease

■ **Description**

Cerebroside lipidosis.

■ **Symptoms**

Progressive loss of motor skills, anemia, protuberant abdomen, seizures.

■ **Diagnosis**

Bone marrow may contain Gaucher cells.

■ **Pathology**

Deficiency of glucocerebrosidase. Autosomal recessive.

B. Fabry's Disease

■ **Description**

Sphingolipidosis.

■ **Symptoms**

Abnormalities in cardiac and renal function, aphasia, cerebellar signs.

■ **Diagnosis**

Ophthalmologic exam.

■ **Pathology**

Deficiency of galactosidase A, sex-linked recessive.

C. Tay–Sachs Disease

■ **Description**

Infantile cerebromacular degeneration.

■ **Symptoms**

Progressive visual impairment, muscle weakness, clonus, spasticity, seizures.

■ **Diagnosis**

Cherry-red spot in the fovea.

■ **Pathology**

Accumulation of gangliosides in retina and CNS neurons. Autosomal recessive.

D. McArdle's Disease

■ **Description**

A glycogen-storage disorder.

■ **Symptoms**

Pain and stiffness on exertion.

■ **Diagnosis**

Elevated muscle glycogen on biopsy.

■ **Pathology**

Deficient muscle phosphorylase.

■ **Treatment**

Glucose and reduce exercise.

E. Pompe's Disease

Acid maltase deficiency.

F. Episodic Muscle Weakness

1. **Familial hypokalemic periodic paralysis**—autosomal dominant, weakness, low potassium.
2. **Familial hyperkalemic periodic paralysis**—autosomal dominant, shorter weakness attacks, elevated potassium.

G. Pick's Disease

See Section X, Dementia.

H. Huntington's Disease

See Section IX, Movement Disorders.

I. Laurence–Moon–Biedl Syndrome

Obesity, mental retardation, retinitis pigmentosa, hypogonadism, polydactyly, autosomal recessive.

J. Shy–Drager Syndrome

Orthostatic hypotension and CNS degeneration.

K. Friedreich's Ataxia

Most common spinocerebellar degeneration, onset childhood.

L. Charcot–Marie–Tooth Disease

Polyneuropathy, slowly progressive, peroneal muscle atrophy.

M. Amino Acid Metabolism Disorders

Maple syrup urine. Hartnup disease.

N. Neurofibromatosis

Pigmented skin lesions, spinal and cranial nerve tumors, gliomas. Café au lait spots of more than six of 1.5-cm size. Multiple cranial nerves affected. Autosomal dominant trait.

O. Tuberous Sclerosis

Autosomal dominant trait, mental retardation, epilepsy, cutaneous facial lesions.

P. Hippel–Lindau Disease

Simple autosomal disorder, retina angiomas, cysts in kidney and pancreas, cerebellar hemangioblastomas.

Q. Ataxia Telangiectasia

XVII. OTHER DISORDERS

A. Cerebral Palsy

■ **Description**

Neonatal brain pathology, most often affecting motor function.

■ **Symptoms**

Motor and **coordination abnormality,** may show seizures, delay in reaching milestones, spasticity, and mental retardation.

■ Diagnosis

History and physical examination, skull x-ray, CT of the head, EEG, and psychological testing.

■ Pathology

Etiology includes **infection (TORCH:** toxoplasmosis, rubella, cytomegalovirus [CMV], herpes simplex), **medication, and anoxia.** Other conditions include meningitis, trauma, kernicterus, toxemia, fever.

■ Treatment

Control seizures, physical/occupational therapy.

Additional Information. **Most common type of cerebral palsy (CP): spastic CP** of **hemiplegic variety,** presenting with **hyperreflexia, seizures, and hemiplegia.**

B. Attention-Deficit Disorder

■ Description

Hyperkinetic, hyperactive syndrome.

■ Symptoms

Increased impulsive behavior, motor activity, and impatience, along with **learning disorder.**

■ Diagnosis

History and physical examination, psychological evaluation, neurologic evaluation.

■ Pathology

Unclear, may involve multiple environmental and organic factors.

■ Treatment

Parental/child counseling, medication with methylphenidate hydrochloride (Ritalin).

C. Febrile Seizures

■ Description

Seizure in child age 3 months to 5 years, **associated with fever/infection.**

■ Symptoms

Febrile seizure (short seizure without focal features).

■ Diagnosis

History and physical exam; rule out meningitis, septicemia. Hospital admission, including routine lab, lumbar tap.

■ Pathology

Unknown.

■ Treatment

Temperature reduction (tub bath, acetaminophen [Tylenol]), medication (diazepam [Valium] 0.2 mg/kg rectally or IV).

XVIII. OPHTHALMIC DISORDERS

A. Glaucoma

■ Description

Ophthalmic disorder of elevated intraocular pressure, which is etiology of 10% of blindness in the United States.

■ Symptoms

Asymptomatic, or may demonstrate **pain, red eye,** and **vision loss. May note halos around lights.**

■ **Diagnosis**

History and physical examination, elevated intraocular pressure (**over 22 mm Hg** by Schiøtz'tonometry).

■ **Pathology**

Primary angle-closure, open-angle, secondary, and congenital types; may be of sudden obstructive (primary angle-closure) etiology, or chronic obstruction (open-angle).

■ **Treatment**

Primary angle-closure—surgical iridectomy, with acetazolamide (Diamox) and beta-blockers preop.
Primary open angle—medication.

Additional Information

Primary angle-closure—pain, vomiting, vision loss, sudden onset.
Primary open-angle—vision field defects, disc cupping, no pain!

B. **Papilledema**

■ **Description**

Elevation/swelling of optic nerve head.

■ **Symptoms**

Narrowed visual field; larger blind spot, vision may be normal or impaired. Papilledema may cause optic atrophy.

■ **Diagnosis**

Fundoscopic exam (disc swelled, associated hemorrhages/exudates).

■ **Pathology**

Secondary to elevated CSF pressure, and a result of infection, optic neuritis, metabolic disease, CNS lesions.

■ **Treatment**

Treat primary cause.

Additional Information. **Consider optic atrophy, if disc is pale.** Etiology of optic atrophy: demyelinating disease, drugs, glaucoma, familial.

C. **Cataract**

■ **Description**

Lens opacity (nuclear, cortical, and subcapsular).

■ **Symptoms**

Progressive painless visual loss, or asymptomatic.

■ **Diagnosis**

Ophthalmoscopic examination.

■ **Pathology**

Age related; ultraviolet light exposure association, and may also relate to trauma, corticosteroids, and diabetes.

■ **Treatment**

Cataract removal and intraocular lens implantation.

Additional Information. **Corticosteriods—posterior subcapsular cataract inducing.**

D. **Other Items of Interest**

1. Retinal detachment—light flashes, retinal degeneration or trauma induced.
2. Constricted pupil—iritis, drugs, Horner's.
3. Dilated pupil—Adie's, glaucoma, drugs, third nerve lesion.
4. Pinguecula—thickened conjunctiva.

5. Pterygium—pinguecula encroaching on cornea.

6. Most frequent etiology of bacterial conjunctivitis—*Staphylococcus aureus.*

7. Iritis—small pupil, ciliary injection (treat with cycloplegics and steroids); glaucoma: large pupil, diffuse injection (treat with pilocarpine, acetazolamide [Diamox], etc).

8. Hyphema—trauma induced, anterior chamber blood.

9. Chalazion—blocked meibomian gland duct.

10. Sudden vision loss—rule out artery (secondary to emboli, retina white), or vein occlusion.

BIBLIOGRAPHY

Adams RD. *Principles of Neurology.* 5th ed. New York: McGraw-Hill; 1993.

Aminoff MJ. *Neurology and General Medicine.* New York: Churchill Livingstone; 1989.

Glaser JS. *Neuroophthalmology.* 2nd ed. Philadelphia, Pa: JB Lippincott; 1990.

Pryse-Phillips W. *Essential Neurology.* 4th ed. New York: Medical Examination Publishing Co; 1992.

Rowland LP. *Meritt's Textbook of Neurology.* 8th ed. Philadelphia, Pa: Lea & Febiger; 1989.

Samuels MA. *Manual of Neurology.* 4th ed. Boston, Mass: Little, Brown and Co; 1991.

Smith DB. *Epilepsy: Current Approaches to Diagnosis and Treatment.* New York: Raven Press; 1991.

Weiner WJ. *Neurology for the Non-Neurologist.* 2nd ed. Philadelphia, Pa: JB Lippincott; 1989.

Weiner WJ. *Emergent and Urgent Neurology.* Philadelphia, Pa: JB Lippincott; 1992.

Woodley M. *Manual of Medical Therapeutics .* 27th ed. Boston, Mass: Little, Brown and Co; 1992.

Polyneuropathy

- Diabetes mellitus - #1
- EtOH
- toxic/drugs

dx: EMG- conduction study
- demyelinating ⟹ slow NCS velocity

Guillane-Barré

acute, inflammatory demyelinating polyneuropathy   autoimmune

URI or GI infections preceeds neuropathy
- campylobacter jejuni

Mostly motor findings → legs to arms over hours or days
also face
respiratory involvement

EMG → slowed nerve conductions
LP → ↑ protein, few WBC

Rx: plasmaphoresis (or)
IVIG

Amyotrophic Lateral Sclerosis

middle aged
motor system: both UMN/LMN
tongue atrophy ↑↓ DTR
normal sensory exam
exclude spinal chord lesion

Rx: rilusole

CHAPTER 12

Normal Growth and Development and General Principles of Care

JOEL S. GOLDBERG, DO

I. REPRODUCTION—PHYSIOLOGIC AND ENDOCRINE ASPECTS

A. Reproductive Anatomy

■ **Description**

1. **Male**—sperm are formed in the **seminiferous** tubules of the testis, then travel to the **epididymis,** and then to the **vas deferens.** The **vas enters the prostate gland,** via the ejaculatory duct, on the way to the urethra. The **seminal vesicle** also empties into the ampulla of the vas, and ejaculatory duct.

2. **Female**—midcycle release of ovum, which travels via the fallopian tube to the uterus. Ovarian function depends on **anterior pituitary** release of follicle-stimulating hormone (FSH) and luteinizing hormone (LH).

Genetics—ovum and spermatozoon nuclei divide (meiosis), reducing the 46 chromosomes in each to 23. Fertilization brings the number back to 46. Core to heredity and present on chromosomes are genes. Alleles (genes from one parent) are dominant or recessive.

Dominant inheritance—parent-to-child transmission with 50% of male or female offspring affected. Trait on dominant allele is always displayed in the carrier.

Recessive inheritance—need both genes at locus to produce trait. Offspring have 25% chance of being affected.

Sex-linked—sex chromosome (XX female, XY male) transmit trait. Single gene will produce trait. Female carrier will result in 50% of male offspring having trait (hemophilia: sex-linked recessive)

B. Menstruation

■ **Description**

Cyclic monthly flow.

1. **Follicular phase**—lasts 14 days, with **primordial follicle** enlarging. **Graafian** follicle is the resulting

maturing follicle. **Main estrogen source** is the **theca interna cells** of this follicle. Follicular phase ends with ovulation.

   a. **Corpus hemorrhagicum** is the blood-filled ruptured follicle.
   b. **Mittelschmerz** is midcycle abdominal pain secondary to peritoneal irritation from release of small amounts of this blood in the abdomen.
   c. **Ovulation** is preceded by a **LH surge** following an estradiol surge, and the mature follicle becomes the **corpus luteum.**
   d. **At ovulation, positive ferning and greatest spinnbarkeit** is noted.

   Cervical mucus most conducive to fertilization

   e. **Ferning**—palm-leaf cervical mucus pattern.
   f. **Spinnbarkeit**—elastic cervical mucus.

2. **Luteal phase**—from ovulation to menses, lasting 14 days. **Progesterone** is **produced by the corpus luteum,** resulting in increased tortuosity and coiled gland appearance. **Cervical mucus is thick without ferning or spinnbarkeit.**

   this part does not vary
   follicular phase varies 14d is avg

C. Intercourse and Conception

■ **Description**

Ovum will survive 72 hours after release from the follicle. **Sperm will survive 48 hours.** Autonomically controlled contractions of the vaginal wall and bulbocavernosus muscles (orgasm) is not necessary for fertilization.

Sexual response cycle includes four phases: excitement, plateau, orgasm, and resolution (Masters and Johnson).

D. Pregnancy—Physiologic Changes

■ **Description**

Increased cardiac output, heart rate, blood volume (50%), appetite, salivation, and gum fragility, glomerular filtration rate (GFR) (50%).

Decreased gastrointestinal (GI) motility—pregnancy testing detects elevated β-hCG levels produced by the placenta.

Physical changes include breast tenderness, purple cervical color (**Chadwick's** sign), softening uterine isthmus (**Hegar's sign**), urinary frequency.

Gestational age—fundus palpable above the pubic symphysis (14 weeks), umbilicus (20 weeks), xiphoid process (38 weeks). Sensation of fetal movements noted by the mother at 16 to 18 weeks is termed **quickening.**

E. Labor and Delivery

■ **Description**

Exact physiologic triggers are unknown, but prostaglandin release may stimulate uterine contractions, and oxytocin levels increase during labor.

First stage—from start of labor to full dilation (10 cm) lasting 8 to 12 hours in a primigravida, 6 to 8 hours in a multipara, includes latent and active phases.

Second stage—includes full dilation to infant delivery, primigravida duration 1 hour, multipara one half hour.

Third stage—includes infant birth to placenta delivery.

F. The Puerperium

Puerperium means postpartum. Most common postpartal time of maternal hemorrhage is shortly after placenta delivery, due to uterine relaxation. Later hemorrhage may result from infection (number one cause) or a retained placenta (number two cause). Physiologic changes include **uterine involution** with **lochia rubra** (bloody tissue discharge), **lochia serosa** (lighter color), and **lochia alba** (thicker yellow for several weeks postpartum). Water loss is associated

with elevated serum sodium and diminished progesterone levels.

G. Lactation and Breast-Feeding

■ **Description**

Estrogen produces **mammary duct tissue growth**. **Progesterone** stimulates **alveolar glands.** Postpartum, estrogen/progesterone levels drop, and **prolactin increase** is needed for milk formation. **Oxytocin is responsible for "milk letdown."** **Nipple stimulation** results in **oxytocin release** and increased prolactin secretion by the anterior pituitary.

Prolactin inhibits ovulation and is a 90% effective contraceptive (breast-feeding). ⤷ *if mom breast feeds Q4°!*

H. Fetus, Placenta, and Newborn

■ **Description**

Fetal-placental unit secretes human chorionic gonadotropin (hCG), progesterone, estriol, thyroid hormone, and adrenocorticotropic hormone (ACTH). Placenta utilizes oxygen and glucose to supply nutrition to the fetus and remove byproducts.

Cord contains two **umbilical arteries** and one **vein.**

Wharton's jelly is **umbilical** cord **connective tissue.**

Large placenta noted in diabetes, erythroblastosis, and syphilis.

Small placenta with hypertension.

Nuchal cord found at delivery in 25%, without consequence.

Absence of an **umbilical artery** may reflect multiple anomalies. *most often is nl, tho*

Hydatidiform mole—**vesicular grape-like placental villi** with elevated hCG and metastases.

Short cord may result from reduced amniotic fluid in early pregnancy.

Velamentous insertion—**umbilical cord travels in placental membranes** before reaching the fetal surface.

Vasa praevia describes membranes with fetal vessels covering the cervical os. → can get fetal bradycardia c̄ what seems to be minimal blood loss

Check painless vaginal bleeding for fetal hemoglobin to detect **hemoglobin F**, which is the **major fetal hemoglobin.**

I. Obstetric Care

■ Description

1. Pregnancy diagnosis:
   a. Presumptive signs and symptoms—nausea, amenorrhea, urinary frequency, **chloasma** (mask of pregnancy, increased facial pigmentation), **linea nigra** (nipples and linea alba darkening), **quickening** (fetal movement).
   b. Probable signs—**Chadwick's** (blue cervix), **Hegar's** (enlarged soft isthmus), **Braxton Hicks** (false) **contractions,** uterine souffle (auscultated blood-flowing sound from the placenta), **Ladin's sign** (anterior midline uterine softening).
   c. Positive signs—x-ray/ultrasound, fetal heart tones, palpated fetal movement.

2. Pregnancy age:
   a. *Gestational age* by ultrasound. Uterus at 8 weeks is at the pubic symphysis; 20 weeks, at the umbilicus. >14 wks passes pubic symphysis
   b. *Quickening* at 17 to 18 weeks.
   c. *Nagele's Rule*—estimated date of conception (EDC) = last known menstrual period (LNMP) month minus 3, then add 7 to the first day of the LNMP. **Fetal maturation** best determined by **amniocentesis.**

3. Prenatal care:
   a. *Prenatal care* will identify the high-risk patient, and address the need to avoid drugs, alcohol, smoking and toxin exposure.

   b. *Contractions* are effective when regular and strong and produce cervical effacement and dilation.
   c. *False labor* contractions are irregular without cervical change; discomfort is abdominal.
   d. *Bloody show* is the passage of a **bloody cervical mucus plug** from cervical dilation.

4. **Fetal position:**
   a. *Fetal presentation.* Vertex, 95%; breech, 5%. Palpate abdomen **(Leopold maneuver).**

5. **Fetal station:**
   a. *Presenting part* at ischial spines is **zero,** above the spines in centimeters is minus, below the spines in centimeters is plus.
   b. *Pelvic inlet* should be 12 cm or greater; **midpelvis,** 9 cm or longer.
   c. *Pelvic types*—android, gynecoid, anthropoid, and platypelloid.
   d. *Midpelvis* is smallest pelvic measurement.

6. **Monitoring of labor**—frequent exam, fetal internal or external monitoring. Observe fetal **rate, variability,** and **effect under contractions. Normal fetal rate** 110 to 150, some beat-to-beat variability is normal. Small dips that recover with contraction end are OK; if severe, get scalp pH, (from vagal response of uterine pressure on baby's head). *Late decelerations* after uterine relaxation may indicate fetal distress. *Fetal scalp* pH 7.25 to 7.45 is OK. ↳chord compression
   variable decels = fetaluteroplacental insufficiency

7. **Puerperium**—check for blood loss, infection, mastitis (breast infection, *Staphylococcus aureus* usually), endometritis (bleeding, fever), anesthetic complications, cardiomyopathy, psychosis.

8. **Breast-feeding**—baby should nurse at both breasts at each feeding, on demand. Mother needs to be relaxed and rested. To stop lactation, dis-

continue nursing, bind breasts, ice if needed.

9. **Newborn care**—clear and suction airway, dry and warm infant, apply antibiotic eye drops, give vitamin K, 1 mg, intramuscularly (IM), check hemoglobin and glucose if indicated, check **Apgar** score. **Newborn examination notes:**

Caput succedaneum is scalp edema, trauma, or vacuum extractor use, **which will cross the suture line.**

Cephalohematoma is scalp hematoma not crossing suture line.

Mongolian spot is bluish low-back non-significant discoloration.

Vernix caseosa is filmy material covering newborn.

Omphalocele is intestine or abdominal contents protruding through umbilicus (versus gastroschisis, or abdominal wall absence/fissure). [handwritten: > c̄ peritoneal lining] [handwritten: no peritoneum ←]

Acrocyanosis is bluish hands and feet color, normal if lasting short time.

Moro reflex is embracing/startle reaction to slightly lifting infant's upper torso by the hands, and suddenly releasing.

Rooting reflex (stroke infant's cheek and infant turns toward your finger), **sucking** reflex and **grasp** reflex present, positive Babinski reflex is normal. [handwritten: (up to ~12 mo!)]

Also check for red reflex in eye (rule out retinoblastoma, congenital cataracts), Ortolani and Barlow maneuvers (to recognize dislocated hips), and abdomen for masses (polycystic kidneys, Wilms' tumor, neuroblastoma, hernia, etc).

II. INFANCY AND CHILDHOOD

A. Physical Growth and Development

■ **Description**

Evaluate growth and development at each visit. Monitor blood pressure (BP) and advise dental evaluation after age of 3 years. Discuss accident prevention, drowning, fire, and automobile safety.

1. **Development:**

One month—positive head lag, prone may lift head above surface.

Three months—some head lag, prone may raise head/chest.

Six months—rolls over both ways, sits alone.

Nine months—creeps or crawls, may take steps if hands held, says ba-ba, da-da.

Twelve months—walks if one hand held, speech of three words.

Fifteen months—walks, builds two-block tower. [handwritten: one word sentences]

Twenty-four months—six-cube tower, talks, [handwritten: 2 word phrase] checks everything out. Poison-proof home!

2. **Infant size**—infants double weight by 6 months and triple weight by 1 year. **Anterior fontanel** closes 9 to 18 months. **Posterior by 3 to 4 months.**

3. **Teeth**—**lower central incisors** are **first** at 6 to 9 months, followed by upper central incisors. **Six or more teeth** present **by age 1.**

B. Psychosocial Development

■ **Description**

Social smile at 3 to 5 weeks. Laughs at 4 months, possible stranger anxiety at 6 months, less dependent on mother at 12 months. ✖ **Second-year play is solitary, third-year involves other children.** ✖

C. Well-Baby Care

■ **Description**

Monitor physical development, orthopedic development, dental, hearing and vision screening, hemoglobin and tuberculosis (TB) screening. Provide routine immunizations and lead screening. **Child abuse** may present as failure to thrive, emotional or physical deprivation. High frequency of parents having been abused.

III. ADOLESCENCE

A. Puberty

■ **Description**

Adolescent sexual maturity.

■ **Symptoms**

Onset of secondary sexual characteristics (growth spurt, genital development, pubic hair, menarch).

■ **Diagnosis**

Tanner stages 1 to 5: 1 = preadolescent, 5 = maturity.

■ **Physiology**

1. **Females**—estrogen secreted by the ovary in response to FSH results in breast development. Adrenal androgens produced result in axillary and pubic hair. **Female sequence: ovary growth, breast bud, growth spurt, then pubic hair.**

2. **Males**—testicular enlargement from testosterone. Adrenal androgens for pubic and axillary hair also. **Male sequence: testicular growth, followed by growth spurt, then pubic**

hair, then facial hair and voice change.

B. Nutrition and Growth

■ **Description**

Rapid growth at a time of increased activity is present. Poor dietary planning is common. Anemia and/or iron deficiency may be present, as well as dental caries and obesity.

C. Emotional and Cultural Adaptations

■ **Description**

Quest for independence and concern with peer group, self-image anxiety, and possible conflicts may take place. Increasing interest in peer group and attempt at separation from parental control. Increasing interest in sex, and reduced impulse control may be noted. Dangers of risk-taking behavior may be of concern. Acceptance of body, parents, needs, and trials of adolescence are noted in later stages of adolescence.

D. Adolescent Sexuality

■ **Description**

Increasing sexual energy and interest. Guilt over masturbation or sexual fantasies may be present. Peer and media pressure may play a role. Sex education for sexually transmitted disease (STD) prevention and guidance, as lack of knowledge is common.

E. Physician–Parent–Patient Communication

■ **Description**

Need to recognize both parental concerns and adolescent's privacy. Need to discuss with adolescent concerns regarding confidentiality and privacy. Importance of discussion regarding **drugs, alcohol, and birth control (including safe sex).**

IV. ADULTHOOD

A. General Checkups

■ **Description**

Routine evaluation to include review of systems, physical examination, preventive care and instruction, and screening testing and/or procedures where indicated. Key aspects may include alcohol and smoking cessation, cancer screening (breast, colon/rectal, prostate), immunization review, and cholesterol/lipid evaluation. Additional evaluations indicated in high-risk individuals may include glucose, TB testing, human immunodeficiency virus (HIV) testing, STD screening, dermatologic and audiometric examination.

B. Contraception

■ **Description**

Abstinence remains difficult; peer pressure not helpful.

Vaginal spermicides are safe and more effective if a condom is used in addition.

Condoms are safe and effective if correctly used.

Diaphragms are safe, but preparation may inhibit use.

Oral contraceptives are safe and effective with proper instruction and medical follow-up. May aggravate migraine. Contraindicated with prior thromboembolic disease, coronary artery disease, pregnancy, liver tumors, breast malignancy, vaginal bleeding of unknown etiology, or hypertension.

Estrogen excess—nausea, headache, hypermenorrhea, bloating.

Estrogen shortage—amenorrhea, reduced libido, early-cycle spotting.

Oral contraceptive use and cancer—reduced endometrial and ovarian cancer.

Intrauterine device (IUD)—will not protect against STDs, and infertility complication is present.

C. Stress Management

■ **Description**

Increasing and **frequent stress** may result in **increased illness. Most stressful event is death of a spouse. Holmes and Rahe** scale of life stress events **ranks divorce** number two.

■ **Treatment**

Support of family and friends, exercise, hobbies, biofeedback, counseling, medication when indicated, remove source of stress, relaxation techniques.

D. Menopause

■ **Description**

Cessation of menses.

■ **Symptoms**

Increasing irregularity of menstrual cycle, average age 51. Anxiety, depression, hot flushes (or flashes, due to estrogen withdrawal), dyspareunia, bone loss.

■ **Diagnosis**

Elevated FSH and LH.

■ **Pathology**

Decreasing ovarian function.

■ **Treatment**

Estrogen replacement.

E. Osteoporosis

■ **Description**

Bone demineralization.

■ **Symptoms**

Back pain, spontaneous fractures, "dowager's hump."

■ **Diagnosis**

X-ray, normal labs, symptoms, **rule out multiple myeloma** (serum/urine electrophoresis).

■ **Pathology**

Estrogen loss, inactivity, malabsorption, endocrine disease.

■ **Treatment**

Vitamin D, estrogen, calcium, anabolic steroids.

■ **Prevention**

Identify risk factors (smoking, early menopause, small size/weight, inadequate calcium intake, inactivity).

Estrogen replacement as soon after menopause as possible.

F.   Male and Female Climacteric

■ **Description**

Female—menopause.

Male—diminished sexual activity.

■ **Symptoms**

Reduced sexual frequency and/or reduced libido.

■ **Diagnosis**

Sexual history, physical examination, rule out other physical disorders.

■ **Pathology**

Female—lack of estrogen.

Male—reduced testosterone.

■ **Treatment**

Hormone replacement(?), office discussion/counseling.

V. SENESCENCE

A.   Physical/Mental Aging Changes

■ **Description**

1. **Cardiac**—decreased output.
2. **Musculoskeletal**—reduced bone mass.
3. **Pulmonary**—decreased muscle strength and chest wall compliance.
4. **Immune system—thymus involution.**
5. **Senses**—decreased visual, auditory, tactile, and taste sensation.
6. **Endocrine**—reduced insulin-secreting cells, glucose intolerance.
7. **Mental**—reduced memory, learning ability, and calculation speed.

■ **Treatment**

Adequate nutrition, exercise, mental stimulation, preventive medical evaluations.

B.   Nutrition in the Elderly

■ **Description**

Often inadequate; psychosocial problems may exist.

■ **Symptoms**

Inadequate diet may present with **weight loss, cognitive impairment** from vitamin deficiency.

Protein-calorie malnutrition—depression, mental changes, anorexia, and weight loss.

■ **Diagnosis**

Patient examination and physician–patient, physician–family discussion. Careful history.

■ **Treatment**

Encourage family support and psychosocial health. Periodic evaluations to prevent potential problems. Treat other medical problems (poor dentition, depression), monitor medications for side effects and discuss nutrition. Evaluate for alcohol abuse.

C. Social Adaptation

- **Description**

Ability to accept aging process and cope with physical and mental changes and illness. Sleep disturbances and depression are common.

D. Death and Dying

- **Description**

Honest physician–patient discussion is essential. Common patient reaction is **denial.**

- **Treatment**

Importance of support system for patients and their ability to maintain control must be stressed. Pain medication to effect comfort is essential. Hospice to support patient and family.

VI. GENERAL PRINCIPLES OF MEDICAL CARE

A. Informed Consent

- **Description**

If the patient is competent, the physician must obtain patient consent prior to medical treatment, when the patient is not coerced and full disclosure of the procedure is given.

Exceptions—emergency treatment to save the patient when consent cannot be obtained. If attempt to obtain consent would harm the patient due to the nature of the needed discussion, consent need not be obtained.

Incompetent patient—obtain from closest family member or legal guardian.

Minors—need only the minors' consent in cases of STD, contraception, pregnancy, drug addiction.

B. Confidentiality

- **Description**

Physician is obligated to maintain patient confidentiality (found in the Hippocratic oath). Family members of competent adult patients may receive information on the patient's approval only.

C. Mental Competency

- **Description**

Patient must possess adequate mental status to interpret and evaluate information, and make decisions.

D. Use of Controlled Substances

- **Description**

Limit prescribing to clearly indicated cases, for needed time only. Exercise caution in patients requesting medication by name.

- **Symptoms**

  1. **Psychedelics**—wild behavior, hallucinations.
  2. **PCP**—phencyclidine (angel dust), ataxia, disorientation, blank stare, psychotic reactions.
  3. **Cocaine**—purer free-base called "crack," nose bleeds, septal perforation, insomnia, arrhythmias, psychosis, myocardial infarction, death.
  4. **Opiates**—lethargy, nausea, miosis, reverse with naloxone (Narcan).

E. Medication Compliance

- **Description**

Adherence to physician instruction and/or medication directions. **Compliance decreases** with longer courses of therapy, more frequent dosing, and increasing number of prescriptions.

■ Symptoms

Missed appointments and poor response to therapy may indicate poor compliance.

■ Treatment

Physician intervention to prescribe only indicated medications at least complicated dosing intervals, with instruction given to the patient and their concerns discussed. Special instruction and care for children and the elderly.

F. Preoperative Assessment

■ Description

Evaluation of preoperative patient, including current health and operative risk factors, and use of prophylactic measures where indicated.
   Surgical risk factors: diabetes, cardiac status, pulmonary function, weight, age, nutritional status.

G. General Surgical Care Principles

■ Description

See Chapter 18.

H. Selection of Anesthetic Agents

■ Description

1. **Inhalational agents**—depress myocardial contractility, respiration, and renal blood flow. Relax skeletal muscle.

   Halothane is inexpensive, may cause hepatic necrosis.
   Nitrous oxide results in **minimal cardiorespiratory depression.**
   Enflurane/isoflurane relax muscles and have **strong odor.**

2. **Barbiturates**—act fast with short duration (sodium thiopental). Re-

duced cardiac output and blood pressure.
   Thiopental extravasation results in **pain** and **possible skin necrosis.** Thiopental has a negative inotropic effect.

3. **Narcotics**—may induce hypotension and respiratory depression.
   Opioids cause miosis.

4. **Ketamine**—related to PCP, and will increase blood pressure and intracranial pressure. Patient will have **no recall of procedure. Dose-related respiratory depression.**
   May have vivid dreams or nightmares

I. Anesthetic Complications

■ Description

Malignant hyperthermia—elevated temperature from overactive muscle metabolic response to anesthetic agent.

■ Symptoms

Elevated pulse and respiration, fever, and cyanosis.

■ Treatment

Dantrolene.
   Other anesthetic complications: prolonged neuromuscular blockade, respiratory depression, nausea, urinary retention, hypoventilation, delayed awakening.

J. Medical Ethics

■ Description

The physician is trained to practice to the best of his ability with concern for patient care and confidentiality. The physician must obtain informed consent where indicated and accept both the patient's decision and input into their treatment plan. "Quality of life" must be considered in medical decisions.

K. Medical Jurisprudence

■ **Description**

Patient care in 1993 remains strongly centered on the practice of **defensive medicine,** in an effort to avoid lawsuits. Result is increase in health care costs. Doctrines of informed consent, accurate record-keeping, and patient education are receiving increased emphasis. Communication with your patients and exhibiting genuine interest in their cases reduces frequency of litigation. **Duty, injury, proximate cause, and negligence** are **needed for a patient to win a malpractice case.**

L. Disability Assessment and Compensation

■ **Description**

Accurate assessment and documentation required to protect both the patient and physician. **Worker's compensation** laws will provide the patient with lost wages and medical costs for injuries sustained at work. Physician needs to be alert for patients attempting to have unnecessary time away from the job, and fabrication of symptoms. Physician must protect patient from returning to work (if reinjury is likely) as well.

VII. QUANTITATIVE METHODS

A. Concepts of Measurement

1. Central Tendency

■ **Description**

A measure of the "average" in a set of frequency distributions.

Mean is the **average, the sum of the data divided by their number.**
Median is the **middle number** where half fall at or above, and half fall at or below. **Median is the 50th percentile. The median is insensitive to extreme scores,** whereas the mean is sensitive to extreme scores. *Mode* **is the value that occurs most often.**

2. Variability, Probability, and Distribution

■ **Description**

Variability is concerned with the range of the most frequent values and their relation to the center. **Variability** may also refer to inconsistencies found in any study. **Standard deviation** is used to define data variability.
Probability is the number of times an event occurs, divided by the total number of events.
Distribution as a graphic picture will aid in interpretation of information, the value of an item, and frequency of its occurrence.

3. Tables and Graphs

■ **Description**

Collection and display of data in multiple types of formats. Need to be aware of ability to mislead and misrepresent information in graphing technique.

Line graph—two points are plotted with connecting line drawn.
Histogram—like line graph, but rectangle instead of points.
Bar graph—like histogram, but bar thickness is of no significance.

4. Disease Frequency

■ **Description**

The number of times a disease occurs.

5. Prognosis

■ **Description**

Measurements of prognosis include case fatality studies and survivorship studies. Duration of the study is of importance.

6. Associations

■ **Description**

Odds ratio represents patient odds of risk-factor exposure divided by control exposure odds.

Relative risk ratio is frequency of disease in exposed versus non-exposed persons.

Standardized mortality ratio is observed deaths divided by expected deaths.

7. Health Impact

■ **Description**

Risk differences and attributable risk.

B. Concepts of Statistical Inference

1. Hypothesis Generation and Testing

■ **Description**

Hypothesis generation and **testing** extrapolates from a small sample to a larger group of which the sample is a small part, and confirms the validity of the test by statistical methods.

2. Type 1 Error

■ **Description**

Rejecting the null hypothesis (null hypothesis is the hypothesis you are testing) **when it is true.**

3. Type 2 Error

■ **Description**

Not rejecting a false null hypothesis. **Power** is the chance of rejecting a false null hypothesis, or accepting the true alternative hypothesis.

4. Confidence Intervals

■ **Description**

Range estimates with upper and lower limits, linked to a probability.

5. Inference

■ **Description**

Reaching conclusions about events from a sample of events.

C. Study Design

1. Experimental Studies

■ **Description**

Clinical trials, community intervention trials, controlled and non-controlled trials.

2. Observational Studies

■ **Description**

Case-control, case-series, cross-sectional, and cohort.

1. Case-control—**start with** outcome, **then check backwards to evaluate risk or cause.**
2. Case-series—features noted **in a group of patients are reviewed.**
3. Cross-sectional—**evaluate data on a group of patients at one point in time.**
4. Cohort—**a group with a common factor observed over a period of time.**

3. Exposure Allocation

■ **Description**

Allocation on the basis of randomization, self-selection, and systematic assignment.

4. Advantages and Disadvantages of Different Designs

■ **Description**

1. **Case-control**—may have elements of bias, and difficulty establishing causality, but are less expensive and quicker to perform. Good for conditions that develop over long periods.
2. **Case-series**—simple but **subject to bias.**
3. **Cross-sectional**—quick and inexpensive. Good for evaluation of a condition in a population base. Disadvantage is that the study observes conditions only at one instant.
4. **Cohort studies**—establish hypothesis better, but causation difficult to prove. More costly as requires more time.

VIII. EPIDEMIOLOGY OF HEALTH AND DISEASE

A. Patterns of Disease Occurrence

1. Demographic Characteristics

■ **Description**

Age, race, gender, socioeconomic features. Different socioeconomic environments result in very different disease patterns.

2. Geographic Distribution

■ **Description**

Consider national, international, and regional variations.

3. Temporal Trends

■ **Description**

Consider sporadic, seasonal, secular, and birth cohort patterns.

4. Disease Surveillance

■ **Description**

Observe and compare frequency of events.

Prevalence = mean duration incidence—incidence is the amount of events during a certain time, divided by the total number at risk.

5. Excess Disease Occurrence

■ **Description**

1. **Epidemic**—may be point (one source, many cases in short time), or may be contact (slower person-to-person spread).
2. **Endemic**—disease in small numbers in a given area or group.
3. **Pandemic**—disease in many numbers in many areas at once.

6. Outbreak Investigation

■ **Description**

Key concerns are evaluation of the source, host, and environment. Necessary next step is a plan to control the outbreak.

7. Etiology of Death and Disability

■ **Description**

Epidemiologic study obtained from death certificates, where the cause of death and the contributing causes are listed.

B. Natural History and Prognosis

1. Modes of Disease Transmission

■ **Description**

Primary as by person-to-person, secondary via vectors.

2. Incubation Periods

■ **Description**

Longer incubation period may allow increased disease transmission by infected, but still asymptomatic individuals (as in HIV infection).

3. Early-Detection Methods

■ **Description**

Patient education and screening.

4. Disease Manifestation

■ **Description**

Disease produced when an **agent** (bacteria, virus, etc), via a **transmission vehicle** (insect, food, etc), finds a **reservoir** (person or animal) who is a **susceptible host.**

5. Treatment Efficacy Evaluation

■ **Description**

Perform an experimental study to compare outcome in both treated and control group.

6. Disease Progression Determination

■ **Description**

Measure rate of disease in terms of incidence and prevalence (defined in Section 2).

C. Risk Factors for Disease Occurrence

1. Hereditary/Genetic Traits

■ **Description**

Genetic disorders resulting in reduced defense mechanisms (neuromuscular disorder resulting in poor cough reflex, for example).

2. Personal Characteristics

■ **Description**

Age, race, gender, socioeconomic status, heredity, immunization programs, habits (cleanliness, food selection), and customs.

3. Lifestyle and Behavioral Aspects

■ **Description**

Habits including alcohol and tobacco use, drug abuse, exercise, sexual behavior, religion (avoiding blood transfusions for reduced hepatitis and HIV exposure, for example).

4. Occupational Exposure

■ **Description**

Chemical agents including chemicals, pollution.
Infectious or biologic agents such as bacteria, fungi, viruses, protozoa, insects.
Mechanical agents as in equipment at work.

5. Environmental Aspects

■ **Description**

Food, air, and water purity. Exposure to hazardous materials. Temperature and humidity, sanitation conditions.

6. Nutritional Aspects

■ **Description**

Vitamin, mineral, and nutritional excess and deficiency in adults, infants, and during pregnancy.

7. Iatrogenic Exposure

■ **Description**

Medications, risky behavior, toxins.

8. Prenatal Exposure

■ **Description**

Tobacco, alcohol, drugs, chemicals, toxins.

9. Abnormal Physiologic or Metabolic States

■ **Description**

Multiple medical conditions (hypertension, diabetes, hyperlipidemia, etc).

IX. HEALTH SERVICES—ORGANIZATION AND DELIVERY

A. Health Care Policy and Planning

■ **Description**

Quality assurance is often judged by medical audits and peer review process, and may help to determine health care policy.

Other determinants include United States Medical Licensing Examination (USMLE)-listed fiscal issues, health care gaps, medical education, and health manpower.

B. General Aspects of Health Care System Structure

■ **Description**

Be aware of programs available including USMLE-listed community preventive medicine service programs, health education, community nursing, chronic and infectious disease control, consulting services, immunization, school and occupational health programs, and programs for the elderly and industry.

C. Health Care Financing and Programs

■ **Description**

Health care costs have risen dramatically, partly due to new and costly technology, and the practice of defensive medicine. Increase in illness rises with advancing age and poor socioeconomic class (groups often unable to pay for health care). Insurance may be traditional or prepaid health maintenance organizations (HMO). State taxes support state health departments.

Social Security Act of 1935 brought the government into health care, to help states develop public health services.

Medicare Act of 1965 provided hospital/health insurance for those older than 65.

Hill Burton Act was to help supply funds for hospital construction and renovation.

Kerr–Mills Bill developed the **Medicaid** program for indigent persons.

Sheppard–Tower Act was to supply funds for maternal and child health concerns.

X. COMMUNITY DIMENSIONS OF MEDICAL PRACTICE

A. General Aspects of Community Organization

■ **Description**

Population health assessment. Health surveys and vital statistics are produced by the State Health Department. Disease reporting systems allow monitoring of reportable diseases, which may result in earlier detection and treatment.

B. Public Health Issues

■ **Description**

Public health programs need to be available to all, and comprehensive in scope.

C. Environmental and Occupational Health

■ **Description**

1. **Environmental control**—multiple aspects including providing community education (to prevent lead poisoning, for example), and acci-

dents. Insect vector education and control (mosquito: encephalitis).

2. **Air and water quality**—impure water may result in cholera, typhoid, and *Salmonella* transmission. Air pollution could predispose to chronic obstructive lung disease, allergic reactions.

3. **Occupational health**—caution with machinery, radiation, toxin exposure, noise exposure, and accident prevention. Exposure to inhalants (miners: silicosis, asbestosis, etc). Occupational health also includes treatment and rehabilitation of employees injured at work, and acute emergency care.

BIBLIOGRAPHY

Dawson-Saunders B. *Basic and Clinical Biostatistics.* Norwalk, Conn: Appleton & Lange; 1990.

Farrow JA. *Medical Clinics of North America—Adolescent Medicine.* Philadelphia, Pa: WB Saunders; 1990.

Feldstein PJ. *Health Care Economics.* 3rd ed. New York: John Wiley and Sons; 1988.

Grant M. *Handbook of Community Health.* 4th ed. Philadelphia, Pa: Lea & Febiger; 1987.

Hanlon JJ. *Public Health: Administration and Practice.* 8th ed. St Louis, Mo: CV Mosby Co, Inc; 1983.

Illingworth RS. *The Normal Child.* 10th ed. New York: Churchill Livingstone; 1991.

Longnecker DE. *Introduction to Anesthesia.* 8th ed. Philadelphia, Pa: WB Saunders; 1992.

Maxcy-Rosenau. *Public Health and Preventive Medicine.* 12th ed. New York: Appleton-Century-Crofts; 1986.

Milio N. *The Care of Health in Communities.* New York: Macmillan Publishing Co, Inc; 1975.

Pernoll ML. *Obstetric and Gynecologic Diagnosis and Treatment.* 7th ed. Norwalk, Conn: Appleton & Lange; 1991.

Rakel RE. *Textbook of Family Practice.* 4th ed. Philadelphia, Pa: WB Saunders; 1990.

Smith LH. *Pathophysiology: The Biologic Principles of Disease.* Philadelphia, Pa: WB Saunders; 1985.

CHAPTER 13

Obstetrics and Gynecology

JOEL S. GOLDBERG, DO

I. HEALTH AND HEALTH MAINTENANCE— OBSTETRICS

A. Prenatal Care

■ Description

Determine health condition of both mother and fetus, evaluate and monitor risk factors, determine pelvic measurements, lab screening. Ensure adequate nutrition, and prevent vitamin and/or iron deficiency. Increased protein and calcium is needed.

1. Rh Immunoglobin Prophylaxis

■ Description

Erythroblastosis fetalis is fetal red blood cell hemolysis from maternal antibodies produced in response to fetal cells getting into maternal blood (where the fetus may have a different blood group from the mother). Incompatibility of Rh or ABO.

■ Symptoms

Fetal hemolytic anemia, heart failure, acidosis.

■ Diagnosis

History, elevated bilirubin (jaundice).

■ Pathology

Kernicterus—elevated bilirubin deposition in the brain; antibodies cause hemolysis, high output failure, edema, ascites.

■ Treatment

Delivery, transfusion. **Prevention**—give Rh-negative mother Rh immune globulin (Rh IgG) at 28 weeks, or any episode of bleeding, amniocentesis, or trauma.

2. Prenatal Diagnosis

Amniocentesis is performed between 16 and 18 weeks. Pedigree and history.

Chorionic villus sampling is performed at about 10 weeks.
Alpha-fetoprotein level helps to detect neural tube defects.
Triple screen—AFP, hCG, estriol.
Teratology—teratogens include isotretinoin (Accutane), lithium, tetracycline, diethylstilbestrol (DES), antithyroid medications (propylthiouracil [PTU], methimazole [Tapazole]), alcohol, coumadin, anticonvulsants, environmental, toxins, chemicals (lead, insecticides).

B. Assessment of the At-Risk Pregnancy

■ Description

Detailed history and physical.

Non-stress test if non-reactive, indicates a problem. Should have two accelerations (every 20 minutes) of 15 seconds or longer, at 15 beats above baseline.
Stress test involves testing uteroplacental/fetal well-being by inducing uterine contractions with oxytocin or nipple stimulation.
Pulmonary maturity evaluation performed by amniotic fluid analysis for **lecithin/sphingomyelin ratio.** Ratio of 2 or greater is preferred.
Ultrasound—amniotic fluid volume, biophysical profile.

C. Intrapartum Care

■ Description

Monitor mother, fetus, and stages of labor. Fetal monitoring to identify problems early.

D. Newborn Care

Description

Suctioning, laryngoscopic exam if meconium is thick, clamp cord, dry, and position infant in Trendelenberg position in warmer. Mother–infant bonding if infant stable. Physical examination, *Neisseria gonorrheae* conjunctivitis prophylaxis and vitamin K. Hepatitis B vaccine now indicated for newborn. PKU test.

CHECK APGAR SCORE:

Heart rate	None, 0	Below 100, 1	Over 100, 2
Respiration	None, 0	Weak, 1	Good cry, 2
Muscle tone	None, 0	Slight, 1	Active, 2
Irritability	None, 0	Grimace, 1	Strong, 2
Color	All blue, 0	Body pink, 1	All pink, 2

E. Postpartum Mother Care

■ Description

Relieve episiotomy pain, observe for infection, hemorrhage, anesthetic complications.

F. Community and Social Dimensions

■ Description

Maternal mortality most commonly is due to hemorrhage. Mortality is greater with advancing age.

Neonatal mortality and morbidity most often is due to low birth weight secondary to prematurity.

Teenage pregnancy has increased due to multiple factors including increased adolescent sexual activity, and earlier menarche. Maternal mortality, infant mortality, and frequency of low birth weight are all increased in teenage pregnancy.

G. Contraception and Sterilization

■ Description

Oral contraceptives—increased risk of deep-vein thrombosis (DVT) and myocardial infarction (MI), decreased risk of endometrial and ovarian cancer. Absolute contraindications include liver tumor, pregnancy, breast cancer, heart disease, thromboembolism, cerebrovascular disease, genital bleeding of unknown cause, estrogen-dependent tumor.

Other methods include diaphragm, rhythm, cervical cap, intrauterine device (IUD), condoms and spermicides, abstinence, sponge, Norplant, Deprovera, vaginal condom.

Sterilization—tubal ligation is effective, but not 100%. Vasectomy is effective (also not 100%), but semen analysis should be performed to confirm sperm absence.

II. MECHANISMS OF DISEASE AND DIAGNOSIS—OBSTETRICS

A. Obstetric Complications of Pregnancy

1. Ectopic Pregnancy

■ Description

Implantation of the ovum outside of the endometrial cavity. **Most common site of ectopic—ampullary portion of tube.**

■ Symptoms

Symptom triad of **abdominal/pelvic pain, adnexal mass, missed period/spotting.** Also syncope, shoulder pain, and symptoms of early pregnancy.

■ Diagnosis

Ultrasound, culdocentesis, beta hCG, laparoscopy.

■ Pathology

Extrauterine pregnancy. Enlarging ovum may cause bleeding. **Arias–Stella reaction** is abnormal hypersecretory glands in endometrium.

■ Treatment

Fluids and surgery (pelviscopy with salpingectomy or salpingostomy).

2. Spontaneous Abortion

■ Description

Pregnancy termination before 20 weeks, includes embryo demise, under 9 weeks or fetal demise after 10 weeks. In missed abortion, the fetus dies before 20 weeks, but it is retained in the uterus for 8 weeks or longer. **Septic abortion** may present with discharge, pain, fever, and peritonitis; treat with antibiotics, dilatation and curettage (D and C), and possibly hysterectomy.

■ Symptoms

Vaginal bleeding and cramping.

■ Diagnosis

Physical examination, beta-human chorionic gonadotropin (hCG), ultrasound. Differential diagnosis includes ectopic pregnancy, mole, tumor, anovulatory bleeding.

■ Pathology

Uterine contractions expel detached products of conception.

■ Treatment

Oxytocin, D and C, progesterone suppository.

3. Hypertension

■ Description

Pre-eclampsia is **hypertension, edema,** and **proteinuria after 20 weeks. Eclampsia** is **seizures** in a patient with pre-eclampsia. The HELLP syndrome is hemolysis, liver abnormality, low platelets; occurs in hypertensive pregnancy disease.

■ Symptoms

Edema of **face** and **hands,** rapid weight gain, **elevated blood pressure (BP) more than** 15 mm **diastolic** or 30 mm **systolic.** Proteinuria.

■ Diagnosis

See preceding.

■ Pathology

Typical kidney lesion: glomeruloendotheliosis.

■ Treatment

Bed rest, antihypertensive medications, delivery. Magnesium sulphate for seizure prevention. Monitor patient for deep tendon reflexes, urinary output, and respirations. **For elevated BP, drug of choice is hydralazine.**

4. Third-Trimester Bleeding

■ Description

Abruptio placenta involves placenta separation after 20 weeks.
Placenta previa is implantation of part of the placenta in the lower uterine segment (marginal, partial, or total covering cervix).

■ **Symptoms**

Abruptio placenta presents with vaginal bleeding **(hemorrhage may be concealed),** shock, poor fetal heart tones, tetanic uterine contractions, pain, expanding uterus.

Placenta previa associated with **painless hemorrhage.**

[margin handwritten note: Vasa previa → fetal vessel that ruptures - small bleeding ≈ big fetal prob. decels or bradycardia]

■ **Diagnosis**

Ultrasound, coagulation studies (PT, PTT, FIBRINOGEN, FSP).

■ **Pathology**

Abruptio placenta results in hemorrhage between uterine wall and placenta.

■ **Treatment**

Abruptio placenta—delivery, treat shock and possible coagulopathy.

Placenta previa—delivery if possible. —C-section!

May observe in mild cases of abruption and previa.

5. Preterm Labor

■ **Description**

Premature labor (between 20 and 36 weeks), includes regular, painful, contractions and intact membranes.

■ **Symptoms**

Cervical dilation and effacement with regular contractions.

■ **Diagnosis**

History and physical exam, with findings in Symptoms.

■ **Pathology**

PGF$_2$-α(?) and PGE$_2$ prostaglandin release, resulting in increased uterine muscle contractility.

■ **Treatment**

Tocolytic medications (Ritodrine), magnesium sulfate, and terbutaline, if fluids and bed rest fail. Also consider steroids and tocolytic medications (Indocin, niphedipine).

With **premature rupture of membranes (PROM),** perform sterile exam and check fluid with nitrazine test (amniotic fluid pH 7.0 to 7.25, blue/green color is positive for amniotic fluid), cervical culture. Check for L/S ratio, obtain cultures (watch for amnionitis [fever, uterine tenderness, elevated white blood count [WBC]), stop labor (but if PROM at term, induce labor). Multiple factors interplay, and treatment/management decisions in preterm PROM may vary.

6. Hydramnios - *polyhydramnios*

■ **Description**

Increased amniotic fluid over 2000 mL.

■ **Symptoms**

Excessive uterine size.

■ **Diagnosis**

Ultrasound.

■ **Pathology**

Excess amniotic fluid, cause unknown. Positive association with fetal anomalies.

[margin handwritten note: duodenal atresia or other GI problem]

■ **Treatment**

Bed rest and observe, amniocentesis if necessary.

7. Rh Isoimmunization

■ **Description**

See Section IA.

8. Multiple Gestation

■ **Description**

More than one fetus.

■ **Symptoms**

Size greater than dates, two or more heartbeats, increased weight gain.

■ **Diagnosis**

Ultrasound.

■ **Pathology**

Family/genetic female tendency, race, medication (clomiphene citrate [Clomid]), and good luck!

■ **Treatment**

Complex management protocol depending on fetal weight, position, and results of external version attempt, if not vertex.

9. Intrapartum Fetal Distress/Death

■ **Description**

Pattern of failing fetal response to stress.

■ **Symptoms**

Abnormal stress test, or non-stress test, abnormal fetal monitor pattern or scalp pH. Decreasing variability, prolonged/late decelerations.
See Section IB.

■ **Diagnosis**

See Section IB, also Ultrasound.

■ **Pathology**

Uteroplacental insufficiency, with multiple possible etiologies.

■ **Treatment**

Reposition patient, oxygen, stop oxytocin, elevate legs, delivery, amnioinfusion.

10. Anxiety/Depression

■ **Description**

Postpartum depression may be mild to severe in intensity. Temporary "baby blues" may occur and require only supportive treatment. With more severe depression, antidepressant medication and psychologic evaluation may be necessary.

Postpartum psychosis is less common and may require both medication and inpatient management.

Anxiety disorders are treated with counseling and medication as necessary.

11. Maternal Mortality

■ **Description**

Maternal mortality has been decreasing.

■ **Pathology**

Hemorrhage, infection, and hypertension.

12. Fetal Growth and Congenital Abnormalities

■ **Description**

See Chapter 14.

Screen with amniocentesis if mother is older than 35, or has prior history of giving birth to child with neural tube defect, or chromosome abnormality. Consider targeted level II ultrasound, triple screen. May also screen when positive history for multiple miscarriages, and if the mother is diabetic.

13. Gestational Trophoblastic Disease

■ Description

Trophoblastic placental growth presenting as hydatidiform mole, invasive mole, or choriocarcinoma.

■ Symptoms

Large uterus, first trimester bleeding, very elevated beta-hCG, passing vesicles, ovarian cysts, no fetal heart tones, theca lutein cysts on ultrasound. *hyperemesis gravidarum*

■ Diagnosis

Symptoms as stated including early toxemia, and **ultrasound.** *(snowstorm pattern)*

■ Pathology

Complete mole
46XX-paternal
Partial mole
47XXY- may have fetus

1. **Hydatidiform mole**—villous stroma edema, avascular villi, syncytiotrophoblastic groups near the villi.
2. **Invasive mole**—invades myometrium.
3. **Choriocarcinoma**—epithelial tumor. → *worse prognosis if occurs related to pregnancy*

■ Treatment

Cure rate 90%, so obtain beta-hCG to diagnose. Hydatidiform mole: **suction curettage is method of choice.** Invasive mole, and choriocarcinoma: chemotherapy.

B. Non-obstetric Complications of Pregnancy

1. Major Medical Complications

■ Description

Most important **non-obstetric complication** is cardiovascular disease.

Most important postanesthetic cause of death is gastric aspiration. All other systems may be affected by pregnancy with potential problems including renal, hematologic, endocrine, pulmonary, gastrointestinal, dermatologic.

2. Surgical Complications

■ Description

Appendicitis is the **most common surgical condition** during pregnancy. Cholecystitis is the second. Need to ensure adequate fetal oxygenation, and be aware of fetal risk with anesthesia.

3. Hyperemesis Gravidarum

■ Description

Persisting nausea and vomiting.

■ Symptoms

As described.

■ Diagnosis

Nausea and vomiting, may be worse in the AM, possibly associated with metabolic abnormalities.

■ Pathology

Uncertain.

■ Treatment

History, physical, and lab evaluation. Correction of dehydration and electrolyte abnormalities, psychological support, hospital care, and hyperalimentation if necessary, medication.

4. Abnormal Labor

■ Description

Breech, face, and other abnormal presentations. Breech is treated with possible external version attempt, labor trial, possible cesarean section (c-section).

Uterine dysfunction—including prolonged latent and second stages, secondary arrest, and protraction disorder. Treat prolonged latent phase with sedation. Protraction and arrest disorders: oxytocin(✹), ambulation, amniotomy, c-section.

Cephalopelvic disproportion (CPD) —perform c-section.

Use of forceps—

Outlet scalp at introitus.

Low forceps skull +2 or more.

Midforceps head engaged but skull above +2.

C. Complications of the Puerperium

1. Breast-Feeding and Mastitis

■ Description

Mastitis is most often due to *Staphylococcus aureas*. Occurs after several weeks, often from infant's germs. Breast is red and tender, patient with chills or fever. Treat with warm soaks and antibiotics. Prevent by good hygiene and infant care. *Galactocele* is milk excess from blocked duct.

Painful nipples often during early days of breast-feeding. Treat with local measures.

Engorgement treated with analgesics, breast-feeding, cool compress.

→ may continue to breast feed!

2. Postpartum Hemorrhage

■ Description

Blood loss over 500 mL after delivery.

■ Symptoms

Hemorrhage, hypotension.

■ Diagnosis

Examination. If uterus firm, look for laceration.

■ Pathology

Lacerations, retained placenta, atonic uterus, coagulation abnormalities, uterine eversion.

■ Treatment

Prevent if possible by patient evaluation and risk screening. Remove placenta if still in uterus. Control atony **(postpartum hemorrhage: atony most common cause).**

Sheehan's syndrome may follow hemorrhage/hypotension (**anterior pituitary gland necrosis** with amenorrhea, reduced breast size and pubic/axillary hair).

3. Postpartum Sepsis

■ Description

Endometritis most common. Presents with fever, uterine tenderness, discharge may be foul, elevated WBC.

■ Symptoms

As described.

■ Diagnosis

As described; cultures.

■ Pathology

Infection by germs normally present in the urogenital tract. Elevated incidence with more frequent exams, prolonged PROM, scalp monitor use, obesity, c-section, prior infections.

Mixed flora infection

■ Treatment

Give IV antibiotics. Other potential infections include wound, urinary tract, mastitis (see Section II, C, 1), and septic thrombophlebitis.

4. Postpartum Depression and Psychosis

■ Description

See Section II, A, 10.

III. PRINCIPLES OF MANAGEMENT—OBSTETRICS

A. Intrapartum Care

1. Anesthesia and Analgesia

■ Description

During active labor, meperidine hydrochloride (Demerol) may be given in small doses. Morphine, Nubaine, and Stadol are used. Nitrous oxide infrequently used and will provide analgesia but **not true anesthesia.** If general anesthesia used, precautions must be taken against aspiration (number 1 cause of anesthetic death), including fasting, intubation with cricoid pressure, antacids. Other methods include pudendal block (second-stage labor), paracervical block (for first-stage labor, complications include fetal bradycardia), spinal and epidural blocks, and saddle block. Complications of spinal/epidural block include hypotension, whereas contraindications include hypertension?, hemorrhage, and infection near needle-insertion location. **Most prevalent second-stage method is epidural.** Spinal virtually not used except for c-sections with intrathecal narcotic (phentanyl, Duramorf).

Early labor: uterine pain. Later labor: lower tract pain via **pudendal** nerve.

2. Induction of Labor

■ Description

Use of medication or other means to stimulate uterine contraction and bring on labor. Oxytocin commonly used. Also amniotomy, laminaria, and stimulation of the breast.

1. **Indications**—pre-eclampsia, PROM, prolonged pregnancy, diabetes, and others.
2. **Contraindications**—cephalopelvic disproportion is a relative contraindication (CPD), and placenta previa.
3. **Complications**—uterine rupture, hemorrhage, infection, amniotic fluid embolism.

3. Episiotomy

■ Description

Mediolateral:

Median is more simple to repair and less bloody/painful.

Lateral results in increased problems, more pain.

Repair under local anesthesia.

4. Forceps Delivery

■ Description

Each forcep consists of a blade, shank, lock, and handle. Low forceps (outlet) are applied with the fetal head at the perineal/pelvic floor. If head is higher, it is termed midforceps.

Indications—any problem affecting mother or fetus that would be resolved by delivery. This includes uterine inertia, maternal illness/exhaustion, prophylactic. **High forceps never to be performed.**

Conditions required—membrane rupture, empty bladder, known position, anesthesia, cervical dilation, no CPD present, head vertex (or face with anterior chin) and engaged.

Tucker–McLane for outlet forceps where little or no traction needed. **Simpson** for molded heads.

5. Emergency Problems and Cesarean Delivery

■ **Description**

Indications for cesarean include CPD, placentia previa, abruptio placenta, failure to progress, fetal distress, preeclampsia/eclampsia, cord prolapse, and others.

6. Vaginal Birth after Cesarean Delivery

■ **Description**

Vaginal birth after cesarean (VBAC) is possible in about 75% of patients if given a trial of labor.

Indicated with a non-complicated pregnancy and one or two prior c-sections with a low transverse incision.

Contraindications include classic c-section incision previously. Complications include uterine rupture.

7. Vacuum-Assisted Delivery

■ **Description**

Traction is applied to a suction cup attached to the baby's head. Pull is maintained during contractions. Cephalhematoma is common.

B. Postpartum/Immediate Newborn Care

1. Immediate Action Situations

■ **Description**

Hemorrhage, thromboembolism, amniotic fluid embolism (hypotension, cardiorespiratory collapse, treat with CPR, pressors, fluids, oxygen), newborn resuscitation if indicated.

Routine newborn care see I, D in this chapter.

2. Postpartum Contraception

■ **Description**

Amenorrhea by breast-feeding. Other methods as in section I, G in this chapter.

C. Abortion: Elective and Therapeutic Indications

■ **Description**

Therapeutic abortion is medically necessary pregnancy termination.

Indications—breast and cervical cancer, severe hypertensive and cardiovascular disease, and other medical disorders affecting the life of the mother.

Methods—suction curettage and D and E (dilation and evacuation), up to 20 weeks. Intra-amniotic saline has been used at 14 to 24 weeks, but complications include disseminated intravascular coagulation (DIC), renal failure, seizures, and hypernatremia. Hyperosmotic urea and prostaglandins have been employed.

IV. HEALTH AND HEALTH MAINTENANCE—GYNECOLOGY

A. Annual Pelvic Examination

■ **Description**

Important for patient screening, education, and disease prevention/treatment. Must include breast, abdomen, pelvic, and rectal examination.

B. Sexually Transmitted Diseases

■ **Description**

Epidemiology/transmission involves close contact and/or intercourse. **Impact** may mean death from human immunodeficiency virus (HIV), infertility (gonorrhea), increased cancer risk human papillomavirus (HPV). **Screening/prevention** should involve evaluation of high-risk patients and their partners. Role of patient/community education to be noted.

C. Cervical and Uterine Cancer

■ Description

Screening by the Pap test has reduced the frequency of invasive cancer. **Epidemiology**—early intercourse age and increased sexual activity raise the risk of cervical cancer, as does HPV 16 and 18. Reduced rate in Jewish women. For uterine cancer, risk elevated with infertile, nulliparous, obese patients, and estrogen increase. Importance of **screening** and **prevention** by Pap test and endometrial tissue exam in high-risk individuals.

D. Breast Cancer

■ Description

Epidemiologic evidence demonstrates higher incidence in patients with family history of breast cancer, and those who had children later in life. One of the leading causes of cancer and cancer death in women. Importance of **screening** and patient education should be noted. Between age 40 and 50, every two years; after age 50, yearly.

Mammogram Breast exam

E. Osteoporosis

■ Description

Epidemiology—increased in fair, thin, smokers. Other risk factors include lack of exercise, early menopause, and steroids. Significant impact in multiple areas including hip fractures and increased morbidity/mortality. **Prevention** via screening, patient education, diet, exercise, calcium and institution of calcium/estrogen replacement.

V. MECHANISMS OF DISEASE AND DIAGNOSIS—GYNECOLOGY

A. Infections

1. *Vulvovaginitis*

■ Description

Vulvar/vaginal irritation and/or infection/inflammation.

■ Symptoms

Itching, discharge (leukorrhea), burning, swelling, dysuria.

■ Diagnosis

Physical and microscopic specimen examination including KOH and saline wet mount slides, culture.

1. *Candida*—thick white discharge, itching, hyphae on wet mount exam, no odor.
2. *Trichomoniasis*—**may be asymptomatic,** irritating gray discharge, **punctate cervical hemorrhages (strawberry cervix),** trichomonads on microscopic exam.
3. *Gardnerella*—previously termed non-specific or *Hemophilus,* thin discharge with fishy odor (especially on 10% KOH slide prep), **clue cells on microscopic exam.**

■ Pathology

Organisms as described, but also may include foreign body, pinworms, atrophic, viral (herpes, condylomata), chemical, and others.

■ Treatment

Candida—clotrimazole, miconazole, terconazole. *diflucan 2nd line*
Trichomonas—metronidazole or Metrogel.

Gardnerella—metronidazole, Cleocin vaginal cream.

Additional Information

Behçet's syndrome—**oral** and **genital ulcers.**

Molluscum contagiosum—**viral umbilicated lesions,** curette, or try tretinoin (Retin-A).

Lichen sclerosus et atrophicus—**vulvar atrophic dystrophy,** unknown cause.

Hidradenitis suppurativa—**apocrine sweat gland infection.**

2. Salpingitis, Pelvic Inflammatory Disease, and Toxic Shock

■ **Description**

Salpingitis—tube infection/inflammation.

Endometritis—endometrial infection/inflammation.

Pelvic inflammatory disease (PID)—consists of salpingitis and/or endometritis.

Toxic shock syndrome—acute multisystem failure illness.

■ **Symptoms**

PID—pelvic pain and fever. *adnexal tenderness*

Toxic shock—fever, rash, hypotension, vomiting. (*desquamation*)

■ **Diagnosis**

PID—tender abdominal and adnexal/cervical discharge and pain with motion, fever, leukocytosis, ultrasound.

Toxic shock—presentation, cultures.

■ **Pathology**

PID—pelvic spread of infection, *Chlamydia and Neisseria gonorrhoeae* often.

Toxic shock—*Staphylococcus aureus*.

■ **Treatment**

Antibiotics as per culture and degree of infection.

Additional Information. **Fitz-Hugh–Curtis** syndrome may be **seen in PID,** as **perihepatitis** (abnormal liver functions, abdominal, shoulder pain). **Complications of PID: infertility, tubo-ovarian abscess,** elevated ectopic pregnancy risk.

3. Sexually Transmitted Diseases

■ **Description**

Genital herpes, gonorrhea, syphilis, chlamydia, chancroid, human papillomavirus (HPV), scabies, lice, molluscum contagiosum, hepatitis B, vaginitis, HIV, granuloma inguinale, lymphogranuloma venereum (LGV).

■ **Symptoms**

Herpes—inguinal nodes, fever, crop of tender vesicles.

Gonorrhea—discharge, abdominal pain, or asymptomatic.

Syphilis—chancre, fever, secondary skin rash, condyloma lata—tertiary syphilis.

Chlamydia—endocervicitis or asymptomatic.

Chancroid—soft painful ulcer.

Human papillomavirus—multiple fleshy warts.

Lymphogranuloma venereum—groove sign (line between lymph nodes), buboes.

■ **Diagnosis**

Herpes—clinical, viral culture.

Gonorrhea—culture on Thayer–Martin plate.

Syphilis—RPR, Venereal Disease Research Laboratory (VDRL), fluorescent treponexral antibody absorption (FTA-ABS).

Chlamydia—culture.

Chancroid—biopsy.

Granuloma inguinale—Donovan bodies.

■ **Pathology**

Herpes—herpesvirus.

Gonorrheae—*Neisseria gonorrhoea.*

Syphilis—*Treponema pallidum.*

Chlamydia—*Chlamydia trachomatis.*

Chancroid—*Hemophilus ducreyi.*

Lymphogranuloma venereum—*Chlamydia trachomatis.*

Granuloma inguinale—*Calymmatobacterium granulomatis.*

■ **Treatment**

Herpes—acyclovir. —does not cure infection ↓ duration of outbreak

Gonorrhea—tetracycline, amoxicillin/probenecid, cefoxitin, Rocephin, Azithromycin, Cipro and others.

Syphilis—benzathine penicillin intramuscular (IM).

Chlamydia, LGV, and granuloma inguinale—tetracycline.

Chancroid—sulfamethoxazole-trimethoprim (Bactrim) or erythromycin.

4. **Endometritis**

■ **Description**

Endometrial infection.

■ **Symptoms**

Fever, tender uterus, pain, discharge possible.

■ **Diagnosis**

History and physical, elevated WBC, ultrasound to rake out retained products of conception.

■ **Pathology**

Enterococci and strep. Bacteroides.

■ **Treatment**

Antibiotics IV.

5. **Urethritis**

■ **Description**

Urinary tract infection at the urethra.

■ **Symptoms**

Dysuria, frequency, and urgency.

■ **Diagnosis**

Urine analysis and culture, history and physical exam.

■ **Pathology**

Ascent of vaginal/rectal bacteria, increased risk with poor hygiene, catheter use, reflux, short urethra. *Escherichia coli* most common cause.

■ **Treatment**

Antibiotics. —Short course! 1–3d.

6. **Bartholin's Gland Abscess**

■ **Description**

Bartholin's gland duct obstruction, resulting in cyst, which becomes infected.

■ **Symptoms**

Enlarging mass, pain, dyspareunia, fever.

■ **Diagnosis**

History and physical examination. **Tender mass at posterior fourchette, to the side.**

■ **Pathology**

Duct obstruction by mucous or infection.

■ **Treatment**

Incision and drainage (I and D), Ward catheter, marsupialization.

7. *Breast Abscess/Mastitis*

■ **Description**

Mastitis—see Section II, C, 1 in this chapter.
Breast abscess—local infection.

■ **Symptoms**

Pain, erythema, fever, induration.

■ **Diagnosis**

History and physical, culture.

■ **Pathology**

Infection, rule out **cancer (especially if not lactating).** Rule out abscess.

■ **Treatment**

Antibiotics, drain local abscess.

B. **Urinary Incontinence: Infection**

■ **Description**

See Section V, A, 5. May be a sign of urethritis.

C. **Uterovaginal Prolapse**

■ **Description**

Cystocele, rectocele, urethrocele, pelvic relaxation.

Cystocele—bladder wall/trigone drops into the vagina.
Rectocele—rectum prolapse into vagina.
Enterocele—rectouterine pouch of Douglas herniation.
Urethrocele—urethral wall protrusion.

■ **Symptoms**

Stress incontinence, difficulty with defecation, vaginal fullness sensation, and mass.

■ **Diagnosis**

History and physical, cystoscopy (cystocele), barium enema (rectocele).

■ **Pathology**

Pelvic support relaxation, postpartum.

■ **Treatment**

Cystocele treated by observation if minimal symptoms. Otherwise pessary, Kegel exercises, estrogen if postmenopausal, surgery. Rectocele treated by a pessary, surgery.

D. **Endometriosis and Adenomyosis**

■ **Description**

Endometriosis—functioning ectopic endometrial tissue.
Adenomyosis—endometrial glands and stroma in the myometrium.

■ **Symptoms**

Endometriosis—symptoms include **dysmenorrhea, infertility, pelvic/ low back pain and dyspareunia.** *also pain on defecation*
Adenomyosis—symptoms include **hypermenorrhea and dysmenorrhea.**

■ **Diagnosis**

Endometriosis—history and physical. Posterior fornix nodules. **Fixed retroverted uterus. Laparoscopy.**
Adenomyosis—"nutmeg" tender uterus, microscopic diagnosis. Rule out leiomyomas, cancer, and pelvic congestion syndrome.

■ **Pathology**

Endometriosis—endometrial stroma, glands and hemorrhage. Cause unknown. — *Reflux theory*
Adenomyosis—stroma and glands in muscular wall.

■ **Treatment**

Endometriosis—**Danazol,** Leupron, Synaral and surgery. Will regress with **menopause.** Observation if minimal symptoms.
Adenomyosis—surgery.

E. **Neoplasms**

1. *Cervical Dysplasia and Cancer*

   ■ **Description**

   Dysplasia is cells of disordered growth, which if untreated may turn into cancer in situ, then invasive.

   ■ **Symptoms**

   None.

■ **Diagnosis**

Papanicolaou (Pap) smear—colposcopic exam.
Positive Schiller test—(non-staining iodine area), biopsy.

■ **Pathology**

Human papillomavirus 16 and 18, herpesvirus 2 all increase the risk of cancer.

■ **Treatment**

Mild dysplasia (CIN 1), recheck in 6 months, treat infection, colposcopy.

Moderate (CIN 2), colposcopy with biopsy, cryosurgery, LEEP.
Severe (CIN 3, CA in situ), conization with biopsy, laser cone.

Cervical cancer is third most common female cancer, **most common metastatis site: liver. Most common type: squamous cell.** Treatments include radiation and surgery.

Additional Information. Abnormal colposcopic findings include mosaicism and white epithelium. Normal findings include original squamous and columnar epithelium. If entire lesion and transformation zone not seen, perform conization.

2. *Uterine Myoma*

   ■ **Description**

   Benign uterine smooth muscle growth. **Most frequent gyn pelvic neoplasm.**

   ■ **Symptoms**

   Hypermenorrhea, enlarging uterus, pain, irregular menses.

   ■ **Diagnosis**

   History and physical, ultrasound.

■ **Pathology**

Smooth muscle submucous, intramural, or subserous tumors.

■ **Treatment**

Observation, myomectomy, hysterectomy.

Additional Information. **More common in blacks,** **Cause unknown.** **Decrease with menopause.**

[handwritten: most common degeneration → hyaline]

[handwritten: during pregnancy may undergo cavernous degen.]

3. **Cancer of the Endometrium**

■ **Description**

Endometrial cancer.

■ **Symptoms**

Abnormal bleeding. Postmenopausal vaginal bleeding.

■ **Diagnosis**

History and physical exam. **Ultrasound and dilation and fractional curettage.** Endometrial biopsy.

■ **Pathology**

Usually **adenocarcinoma.**
   Uterus (stage 1), cervix (stage 2), still in true pelvis (stage 3), bladder/rectum or out of pelvis (stage 4).
   Risk factors: obesity, diabetes, estrogen use, nulliparous, infertile.

■ **Treatment**

Total hysterectomy (TAH) and bilateral salpingo-oophorectomy (BSO; ovaries/tubes removed). Adjuvant radiation.

Additional Information. Most tumors are stage 1 at time of diagnosis. Three types: adenocarcinoma, adenoacanthoma, adenosquamous carcinoma.

4. **Ovarian Carcinoma**

■ **Description**

Ovarian cancer.

■ **Symptoms**

Pain, weight loss.

■ **Diagnosis**

Diagnosis is difficult. Marker CA-125 of limited use. Ultrasound. Doppler flow. Adnexal mass, ascites.

■ **Pathology**

Children: germ cell. Adults: epithelial.

■ **Treatment**

Total hysterectomy, BSO, and omentectomy. Adjunctive chemotherapy.

Additional Information. Higher frequency where spontaneous abortions and infertility are noted.
   Peritoneum and **omentum** are most common epithelial **metastatic sites.**

5. **Neoplastic Breast Disorders**

■ **Description**

Intraductal papilloma, fibroadenoma, carcinoma.

■ **Symptoms**

a. **Carcinoma**—breast mass. Nipple retraction, erythema and/or discharge. Breast asymmetry.

b. **Fibrocystic disease**—tender lumps, may change size during cycle.

c. **Papilloma**—bloody discharge.

d. **Fibroadenoma**—smooth non-tender mass.

■ **Diagnosis**

History, physical examination, mammography, ultrasound, biopsy.

■ **Pathology**

Breast cancer most often infiltrating ductal (indians in a line!)

■ **Treatment**

Obtain estrogen receptor assay. Treatments include surgery and/or radiation, adjuvant chemotherapy. Consult current journals for latest treatment options at each stage.

Fibroadenoma treatment is excision.

Additional Information. **Risk factors** for cancer include **maternal breast cancer, prior breast cancer, nulliparity, and early menarche.** Prevention via breast self-exam, radiologic screening (mammography), patient education.

Paget's carcinoma—mostly infiltrating intraductal, **may appear harmless.**

Cystosarcoma phyllodes—large fibroadenoma.

Most common breast tumor—fibroadenoma.

Intraductal papilloma—most frequent cause of bloody nipple discharge; treat by excision.

6. *Vulvar Neoplasms*

■ **Description**

Malignant vulvar neoplasms.

■ **Symptoms**

Discharge, mass, dysuria.

pruritis

■ **Diagnosis**

History and physical, biopsy.

■ **Pathology**

Squamous cell, Paget's, adenocarcinoma, sarcoma, melanoma. **More common in the aged. Spreads to Cloquet's (deep femoral) node. Epidermoid cancer most common.**

■ **Treatment**

Surgery and radiation if unresectable.

F. Fibrocystic Breast Disease

■ **Description**

Common cystic breast disorder.

■ **Symptoms**

Multiple lumps of changing size, tender.

May vary with cycle

■ **Diagnosis**

History and physical, biopsy, mammography, and ultrasound.

■ **Pathology**

Benign papillomatosis, fibrosis, cysts. Ductal and fibrous tissue hyperplasia.

■ **Treatment**

Biopsy, cyst aspiration, support bra. Danazol.

G. Menstrual and Endocrinologic Disorders

1. *Amenorrhea*

■ **Description**

Primary is defined as **no menses by age 16.**

Secondary is 3 months or longer amenorrhea in a normal-cycle individual.

■ **Symptoms**

Amenorrhea.

- **Diagnosis**

  Primary—history and physical exam, ultrasound, buccal smear and karyotype, follicle-stimulating hormone (FSH) (if not sexually developed). If normal development, follow as per secondary amenorrhea.

  Secondary—obtain history and physical examination, prolactin, FSH, testosterone, and progesterone withdrawal test.

  Elevated FSH—ovarian failure.

  Elevated testosterone—rule out **hyperandrogenism** and **adrenal hyperplasia.**

  Elevated prolactin—rule out **hypothyroid,** computed tomography (CT) pituitary to rule out tumor.

- **Pathology**

  Primary—genetic/congenital anomaly etiology (Turner's as example), may have endocrine/nutritional cause.

  Secondary—**most common cause is pregnancy.** If not pregnant, **next common cause hypothalamic etiology** (weight loss, anorexia, running/exercise, stress, or hypothalamic disease).

- **Treatment**

  Treat specific etiology. Hormone replacement, ovulation induction, surgery if tumor.

  Additional Information. Amenorrhea is physiologic after birth, with lactation.

  Empty sella—possible hypopituitarism/amenorrhea.

  Sheehan syndrome—**postpartum pituitary necrosis.**

  Premature ovarian failure—ovaries fail before age 40 (often genetic cause).

  *Asherman syndrome—*intrauterine scars, posttraumatic, amenorrhea not responsive to estrogen/progesterone cycle.

  *Kallmann syndrome—***gonadotropic deficiency,** amenorrhea, eunuchoid.

  Galactorrhea–amenorrhea syndrome—elevated prolactin/amenorrhea. Treat with bromocriptine.

  In amenorrhea, check for use of antihypertensive and psychiatric medications. Common cause of secondary amenorrhea with high estrogen is **polycystic ovary disease.**

2. Abnormal Uterine Bleeding

- **Description**

  Hypermenorrhea or menorrhagia—increased amount/length of flow.

  Oligomenorrhea—increased length between menses.

  Metrorrhagia—bleeding outside of normal menses.

- **Symptoms**

  Abnormal bleeding as described.

- **Diagnosis**

  History and physical. Cytology, lab, and pregnancy testing. Possible D and C, endometrial sampling.

- **Pathology**

  Most common cause is **dysfunctional uterine bleeding.** Infrequent etiology is organic (trauma, foreign body, tumor, hormonal, coagulopathy, etc). In child, usually due to infection; in teenager, usually anovulatory cycle.

- **Treatment**

  Hormones.

Additional Information. **Hartman's sign is bleeding at ovulation.**

3. Dysmenorrhea

- **Description**

Painful menstruation.

- **Symptoms**

Pain, cramping, nausea, bloating.

- **Diagnosis**

History and physical, laparoscopy possibly.

Primary or idiopathic, is without pathology.
Secondary is due to pathology (multiple etiologies such as endometriosis, fibroids, infection, cancer).

- **Pathology**

Primary cause uncertain, prostaglandin excess (?).
Secondary as per individual disorder.

- **Treatment**

Primary is treated with prostaglandin synthetase inhibitor (ibuprofen [Motrin], naproxen sodium [Anaprox]). Also birth control pills and vitamin B_6 (?).
Secondary treatment as per individual etiology.

4. Postmenopausal Disorders

- **Description**

Atrophic cystitis, hot flash, thinning skin, osteoporosis, and others.

- **Diagnosis**

Pap smear/maturation index to evaluate estrogen effect, serum FSH and luteinizing hormone (LH), history and physical.

- **Treatment**

Estrogen.

Additional Information. Rule out other causes of amenorrhea; rule out other causes of hot flash (pheochromocytoma, carcinoid, etc).

5. Premenstrual Syndrome (PMS)

- **Description**

Multiple symptoms prior to menses.

- **Symptoms**

Anxiety, bloating, headache, depression, acne, breast tenderness, aggression.

- **Diagnosis**

History and physical.

- **Pathology**

Uncertain.

- **Treatment**

Counseling, diet (reduce sugar, salt, alcohol, caffeine), vitamin B_6, progesterone, diuretics.

6. Virilization and Hirsutism

- **Description**

Hirsutism is **excessive sexual hair**.
Virilization is **excessive androgenic influence** (acne, balding, deep voice, increased strength, etc).

- **Symptoms**

As described.

■ Diagnosis

History and physical. Serum testosterone, dihydroepiandrosterone (DHEAS) level, and other testing including **dexamethasone-suppression test** to rule out **Cushing's disease**, ultrasound.

■ Pathology

Medication, ovarian/adrenal disorders.

■ Treatment

As per individual cause.

Additional Information. **Hypertrichosis** is **excessive non-sexual hair, may be** drug or hereditary etiology.

7. Infertility

■ Description

Attempts at conception without success for 1 year unless over age 35 (then 6 months).

■ Symptoms

As described.

■ Diagnosis

History and physical (both partners). Complex protocol for work-up including semen analysis, basal body temperature, hysterosalpingogram, laparoscopy.

■ Pathology

Multiple causes including infection, anovulation, structural lesions, and others.

■ Treatment

As individual condition dictates.

8. Ovarian Disorders

■ Description

Includes hyperestrogenism, ovarian failure, and polycystic ovarian disease.

Ovarian failure may be genetic or due to disease.

Polycystic ovary syndrome (Stein–Leventhal syndrome), presents with **hirsuitism, obesity, amenorrhea, infertility.** Diagnosis by history and physical, elevated testosterone, family history, large ovaries, ultrasound, and laparoscopy. Treat with clomiphene, wedge resection.

BIBLIOGRAPHY

Burrow GN. *Medical Complications during Pregnancy.* Philadelphia, Pa: WB Saunders; 1988.

Clark-Pearson DL. *Green's Gynecology: Essentials of Clinical Practice.* 4th ed. Boston, Mass: Little, Brown and Company; 1990.

Green R. *Human Sexuality—A Health Practitioner's Text.* Baltimore, Md: Williams & Wilkins Co; 1975.

Havens C. *Manual of Outpatient Gynecology.* Boston, Mass: Little, Brown and Company; 1986.

Martin DH. *The Medical Clinics of North America: Sexually Transmitted Diseases.* Philadelphia, Pa: WB Saunders; November 1990.

Newton ER. *Medical Clinics of North America: Medical Problems in Pregnancy.* Philadelphia, Pa: WB Saunders; May 1989.

Niswander KR. *Manual of Obstetrics, Diagnosis and Therapy.* 4th ed. Boston, Mass: Little, Brown and Company; 1991.

Pernoll ML. *Current Obstetric and Gynecologic Diagnosis and Treatment.* 7th ed. Norwalk, Conn: Appleton & Lange; 1991.

Pritchard JA. *Williams Obstetrics.* 17th ed. Norwalk, Conn: Appleton-Century-Crofts; 1985.

Ryan KJ. *Kistner's Gynecology Principles and Practice.* 5th ed. Chicago, Ill: Year Book Medical Publishers, Inc; 1986.

Sweet RL. *Infectious Disease of the Female Genital Tract.* 2nd ed. Baltimore, Md: Williams & Wilkins; 1990.

CHAPTER 14

Congenital Anomalies and Perinatal Medicine

ROBERT S. WALTER, MD

CHARLES POHL, MD

I. MALFORMATIONS—GENETIC FACTORS

Malformations are primary structural defects of development affecting 5% (**2% major**) of all newborns, causing 9% of perinatal deaths and 20 to 50% of spontaneous abortions. Causes include genetic, environmental, and unknown.

A. Down Syndrome (Trisomy 21)

■ **Description**

Most common autosomal chromosome abnormality with a characteristic appearance. A common cause of **mental retardation** (1/700 live births).

■ **Symptoms**

Epicanthal folds, simian creases (50%), flat occiput, upslanting palpebral fissures, 40% with **cardiac anomalies** (ventricular septal defect [VSD], atrioventricular [AV] canal), small stature, leukemia (1%), **duodenal atresia** (4 to 7%), atlantoaxial instability (12%), thyroid disease, sterility in males, early Alzheimer's disease.

■ **Diagnosis**

Clinical with chromosome confirmation: classic trisomy 95% (sporadic), 4% translocation, 1% mosaic.

■ **Prevention**

Maternal risk factor: advanced maternal age. Prenatal diagnosis: amniocentesis, chorionic villus sampling. **Most mortality from heart disease.** Family genetic counseling required (**especially translocations**), optimal potential in home setting (versus institution), **special education.** Life span to fourth decade.

B. Trisomy 18

■ **Description**

Second most frequent autosomal disorder (1/5000) with severe malformations.

■ **Symptoms**

Intrauterine growth retardation, micrognathia, **clenched hand,** overlapping fingers, **rocker-bottom feet, congenital heart disease** (VSD, patent ductus arteriosus [PDA]), mental retardation, central nervous system (CNS) malformation.

■ **Diagnosis**

Clinical with chromosome confirmation. Translocations rare.

■ **Treatment**

Poor prognosis. Aggressive treatment usually not indicated. Most die within 3 months. Grief and genetic counseling needed, recurrence < 1%.

C. Trisomy 13

■ **Description**

Third most common autosomal disorder (1/10,000) with severe malformations.

■ **Symptoms**

Cleft lip and/or **palate** (60 to 80%), CNS malformation **(holoprosencephaly),** microcephaly, **urinary tract** malformations, **ocular** malformations, polydactyly.

■ **Diagnosis**

Clinical with chromosome confirmation.

■ **Treatment**

Aggressive treatment usually not indicated. Most die within 3 months of cardiac or CNS malformation. Grief and genetic counseling needed, recurrence < 1%.

D. 5p-Syndrome (Cri du Chat Syndrome)

■ **Description**

Chromosome deletion syndrome named for the characteristic **cat-like cry**.

■ **Symptoms**

Mental retardation, **microcephaly**, congenital heart disease.

■ **Diagnosis**

Clinical, chromosome confirmation.

■ **Prognosis**

Variable life span, some to adulthood.

E. Gonadal Dysgenesis 45,XO (Turner Syndrome)

■ **Description**

Most common female sex chromosome disorder in which there is only one X chromosome (1/2500 newborn girls).

■ **Symptoms**

Most are spontaneously aborted in early pregnancy (95%), **transient lymphedema** feet and hands at birth (80 to 90%), **short webbed neck**, short fourth metacarpal, renal anomalies **(horseshoe kidney)**, cardiac defects **(coarctation of aorta)**, **short stature**, lack of secondary sex characteristics with **primary amenorrhea** (due to **gonadal dysgenesis**), normal intelligence.

■ **Diagnosis**

Clinical with chromosome confirmation (60% chromatin negative 45,XO, 40% mosaic).

■ **Treatment**

Correct anomalies, estrogen replacement at puberty, growth hormone therapy. Psychosocial counseling.

F. Seminiferous Tubule Dysgenesis 47,XXY (Klinefelter Syndrome)

■ **Description**

Male sex chromosome abnormality with extra X chromosome (1/1000 newborn boys).

■ **Symptoms**

Hypogonadism (number 1 cause in males), infertility, gynecomastia, tall stature, behavior problems.

■ **Diagnosis**

Chromosomes.

■ **Treatment**

Testosterone replacement at puberty, counseling.

G. Fragile-X Syndrome

■ **Description**

Abnormality of X chromosome and common cause of mental retardation in males (1/1000); can also affect females.

■ **Symptoms**

Prominent ears, long face, **macro-orchidism**, **mental retardation**, seizures, hyperactivity.

■ **Diagnosis**

Chromosomes with fragile-X study.

■ **Treatment**

Genetic counseling, multidisciplinary approach.

H. Achondroplasia

■ **Description**

The most common genetic skeletal dysplasia (1/25,000) with characteristic features. **Autosomal dominant,** 80% new mutations.

■ **Symptoms**

Short limbs (especially proximally), low nasal bridge, large head and forehead, small foramen magnum, kyphosis, **hydrocephalus,** severe otitis media.

■ **Diagnosis**

Clinical.

■ **Treatment**

Watch closely for hydrocephalus. Treat spine complications. Life span usually normal, as is intelligence. Genetic counseling.

I. Xeroderma Pigmentosa

■ **Description**

Defect in DNA repair mechanism of ultraviolet radiation-induced lesions, causing **skin scarring** and **malignancy.**

■ **Features**

Sunlight sensitivity (from first exposure), skin atrophy, **basal** and squamous cell carcinomas, melanomas, conjunctivitis leading to scarring and **blindness.**

■ **Diagnosis**

Autosomal recessive. Clinical diagnosis plus characteristic biopsy. Often fatal before adulthood due to malignancies.

II. MALFORMATIONS—MATERNAL/ ENVIRONMENTAL FACTORS

A. Fetal Alcohol Effects/Syndrome

■ **Description**

Results from fetal exposure through maternal alcohol use. Fetal alcohol exposure is **the most common teratogen** and a leading cause of mental retardation.

■ **Symptoms**

Intrauterine growth retardation, **mental retardation,** microcephaly, flattened philtrum, thin upper lip, upturned nose, cardiac defects (septal).

■ **Diagnosis**

Clinical.

■ **Prevention**

Education programs and **prenatal care** important. Greatest damage in first trimester but maternal alcohol use is **never safe.**

B. Tobacco

Considered a common cause of intrauterine **growth retardation.**

C. Cocaine

Maternal use during pregnancy can cause CNS damage, low birth weight, urinary tract abnormalities in newborns.

D. Coumadin Derivatives

Fetal warfarin syndrome: typical facial features, auditory and ocular defects, CNS malformations, mental retardation, perinatal hemorrhage.

E. Thalidomide

A popular antiemetic for pregnant women in the 1960s, caused **phocomelia** (absence of long bones in extremities).

F. Fetal Hydantoin Syndrome

Maternal use of this antiseizure medication causes congenital heart defects, nail hypoplasia, growth retardation.

G. Tetracycline

Maternal use in second and third trimester causes **tooth enamel** hypoplasia and staining.

H. Maternal Diabetes (Infant of Diabetic Mother)

Increases risk of congenital anomalies **threefold:** congenital heart defects, sacral agenesis, anencephaly, small left colon, and caudal regression syndrome.

I. Maternal Phenylketonuria

If mother **not** controlled with diet, infant with increased risk for **mental retardation,** microcephaly, heart defects.

J. Congenital Syphilis

■ **Description**

Congenital infection caused by **spirochete** *(Treponema pallidum)* with multiorgan involvement and variable severity, usually transmitted in later pregnancy.

■ **Symptoms**

Early—rash **(palms and soles), snuffles** (blood-tinged nasal discharge), hepatosplenomegaly, jaundice, pseudoparalysis of Parrot (periostitis), anemia, often asymptomatic early.

Late—frontal bossing, saber shins, Hutchinson (peg) teeth, **saddle nose.**

■ **Diagnosis**

Serology (rapid plasma reagin [RPR], fluorescent treponemal antibody absorption [FTA-ABS]), dark-field examination.

■ **Treatment**

Screen all pregnant women and treat all mothers/infants who are serology positive (with penicillin) who do not have documented adequate treatment.

K. Congenital Cytomegalovirus Infection

■ **Description**

A herpes virus, the most common cause of congenital infections, especially severe fetal effects in early pregnancy.

■ **Symptoms**

Majority are asymptomatic. Hepatosplenomegaly, jaundice, chorioretinitis, **deafness, microcephaly,** petechial rash, developmental delay, periventricular **CNS calcifications.**

■ **Diagnosis**

Urine isolation, serology.

■ **Treatment**

Difficult to prevent due to ubiquitous nature. Transmitted with **primary or recurrent maternal infection.** No proven antiviral treatment. Multidisciplinary approach.

L. Congenital Toxoplasmosis Infection

■ **Description**

Intracellular protozoan parasite *(Toxoplasma gondii)*, which affects fetus in all trimesters (usually the third).

■ **Symptoms**

Hydrocephalus, chorioretinitis (99%), microcephaly, scattered CNS calcifications, developmental delay.

■ **Diagnosis**

Serology, parasites in cerebrospinal fluid (CSF).

■ **Treatment**

Harmful to fetus only if new **(primary)** maternal infection. Pregnant women should avoid cat litter and undercooked meat (sources for toxoplasma oocysts). Shunt for hydrocephalus. **Pyrimethamine** has variable effectiveness.

M. Congenital Rubella Infection (German Measles)

■ **Description**

Virus occurring in epidemics that causes multiple congenital anomalies, especially in first trimester exposure.

■ **Symptoms**

Hepatosplenomegaly, **"blueberry muffin"** lesions, anemia with extramedullary hematopoiesis, thrombocytopenia, **cardiac lesions** (patent ductus arteriosus [PDA], ventricular septal defect [VSD]), **cataracts,** mental retardation.

■ **Diagnosis**

Serology, virus isolation (pharyngeal, urine, CSF).

■ **Treatment**

Incidence decreased with immunization of children and prenatal serologic screening. No specific treatment.

N. Herpes Simplex Virus (HSV)

■ **Description**

Neonatal HSV infection affects 1 of 5000 deliveries, occasionally by in utero transmission (10%) but usually at delivery. Most common HSV-2 (70%), highest transmission during **primary maternal infection.**

■ **Symptoms**

Intrauterine—**seizures,** microcephaly, chorioretinitis, CNS calcifications. Neonatal acquired—**encephalitis, skin vesicular lesions** (also eye and mouth).

■ **Treatment**

Acyclovir, supportive.

O. Human Immunodeficiency Virus (HIV)

Retrovirus causing immune defects in those infected. One of three infants of HIV-positive mothers will later develop acquired immunodeficiency syndrome (AIDS). Diagnosis by traditional serology useless in the first year (maternal IgG present in infant). Culture isolation, rising titers, and immune markers most accurate. Children with AIDS have more bacterial infections than do adults. Developmental delay, failure to thrive common. **Antiretroviral therapy to pregnant woman reduces perinatal transmission.** Prognosis poor.

III. RENAL AND URINARY SYSTEM DISORDERS

Of all newborn abdominal masses, 60% are renal in origin, and ultrasound is the imaging modality of choice.

A. Hypospadias

■ Description

Anomaly of penile urethra that opens on ventral glans, shaft, or perineum.

■ Symptoms

Hooded prepuce, chordee (ventral curving of penis), undescended testis (10%), **if severe,** consider ambiguous genitalia.

■ Treatment

Avoid circumcision; save foreskin for surgical reconstruction in first year.

B. Bladder Exstrophy

■ Description

Uncommon (1/20,000 births) congenital absence of anterior wall of bladder and abdomen, with exposure of bladder mucosa.

■ Symptoms

Pubic rami and rectus muscles widely separated, males with **epispadias** (urethra opens on dorsum of penis), undescended testes, inguinal hernia.

■ Treatment

Closure in first 48 hours, severe genitourinary (GU) reflux common.

C. Prune-Belly Syndrome (Eagle–Barrett Syndome)

Triad of **deficient abdominal muscles, undescended testes,** and **urinary tract abnormalities**. Prognosis based on degree of renal and pulmonary dysplasia.

D. Posterior Urethral Valves

■ Description

Congenitally abnormal sail-like valves in male posterior urethra causing variable degrees of obstruction.

■ Symptoms

If severe, may be stillborn with **Potter syndrome** due to severe oligohydramnios (lung hypoplasia, fetal compression: **flat nose, recessed chin, low-set ears**). Milder cases may present with abdominal masses (hydronephrosis), urinary tract infections (UTIs) or a **weak urinary stream.**

■ Diagnosis

Voiding cystourethrography.

■ Treatment

Transurethral ablation of valve. Prognosis depends on renal/pulmonary damage.

E. Ureteropelvic Junction (UPJ) Obstruction

Common cause of congenital renal obstruction, usually unilateral (80%).

F. Unilateral Renal Agenesis

Usually seen on left, often with single umbilical artery (1/1000 births).

G. Multicystic Kidney

Non-functioning, unilateral cystic flank mass with little or no identifiable renal tissue. Usually excised due to possible risk of later malignancy or infection.

H. Polycystic Diseases of the Kidney

1. Infantile

Autosomal recessive inheritance presenting at birth with severe oligohydramnios/Potter syndrome or bilateral flank masses and hypertension. Multiple small renal cysts. Congenital hepatic fibrosis. Poor prognosis.

2. Adult

Autosomal dominant, cause of **renal failure in adults**, presents in the fourth or fifth decades. Variable number of renal cysts, **may** have some cysts beginning in childhood.

I. Undescended Testicle (Cryptorchidism)

■ Description

Failure of location of testes in scrotum. Location may be intra-abdominal, inguinal canal, ectopic, or absent. Incidence in preterm infants 17%, newborns 3%, adults 0.7%. Testis rarely spontaneously descends after 1 year of life.

■ Diagnosis

Clinical, must differentiate from **retractable testis.** Ultrasound helpful if testis not palpable.

■ Treatment

Due to increased risk of **testicular malignancy** and **infertility,** must do **orchiopexy** (preferred) or **orchiectomy.** Can try human chorionic gonadotropin (hCG) treatment in newborn when bilateral.

J. Pseudohermaphroditism

■ Description

A state in which an individual is distinctly one sex or another with somatic characteristics of both sexes.

1. Female

Genotype XX, ovaries and uterus with virilized genitalia due to androgen exposure.

a. **Congenital adrenal hyperplasia (adrenogenital syndrome [CAH])** —disorder of steroidogenesis, 95% caused by **21 hydroxylase deficiency** with **ambiguous genitalia, 50 to 75% salt losing** with severe life-threatening **hyperkalemia.**

   ■ Diagnosis

   Elevated serum 17-OH-progesterone. **Newborn screening** program in some states.

   ■ Treatment

   Glucocorticoid and mineralocorticoid replacement.

b. **Maternal use of androgens in pregnancy.**

2. Male

Genotype XY, lack of virilization. Testicular feminization (TF): phenotypic female with blind vaginal pouch due to **lack of testosterone receptors;** X-linked recessive. Typically presents in later childhood with inguinal masses (testes) or amenorrhea. Raise as female, orchiectomy, and careful psychosocial counseling indicated.

IV. RESPIRATORY SYSTEM DISORDERS

A. Pierre Robin Anomaly

Severe **micrognathia** (hypoplastic mandible) plus glossoptosis (displacement of tongue downward) causing variable degrees of respiratory distress.

B. Choanal Atresia

■ **Description**

Unilateral or bilateral bony or membranous septum between nose and pharynx.

■ **Symptoms**

Respiratory distress/cyanosis **relieved by crying** (bilateral); unilateral discharge (unilateral). Up to 50% with associated anomalies. **Charge syndrome** (Coloboma of eye, *h*eart defects, *a*tresia of choanae, *g*enital hypoplasia/cryptorchidism, *e*ar anomalies).

[handwritten margin note: Coloboma of eye / heart defects / atresia of choanae / genital hypoplasia / ear anomalies]

■ **Diagnosis**

Inability to pass catheter through nostril to pharynx, confirm with computed tomography (CT) scan.

■ **Treatment**

Oral airway, eventual surgical correction.

C. Congenital Laryngeal Stridor (Laryngomalacia)

■ **Description**

Common condition of delayed maturation of newborn larynx with increased flexibility causing noisy "crowing" respirations. Diagnose clinically by radiograph or direct visualization. Self-limited but consider vocal cord paralysis and true airway lesions (hemangiomas, papillomas, webs).

D. Vascular Rings and Slings

Anomalous thoracic vessels compressing the airway causing wheezing or stridor. Examples include double aortic arch, right aortic arch with either aberrant subclavian artery or ligamentum arterosum (PDA remnant).

E. Congenital Lobar Emphysema

■ **Description**

Number 1 congenital lung lesion, usually unilateral lobar hyperinflation (often left upper lobe) due to early in utero bronchial obstruction with **normal alveolar** histology.

■ **Symptoms**

Newborn respiratory distress, mediastinal shift.

■ **Diagnosis**

Chest radiograph with hyperinflation (must distinguish from pneumothorax).

■ **Treatment**

Surgical resection.

F. Cystic Adenomatoid Malformation

■ **Description**

Number 2 congenital lung lesion, single enlarged lobe due to early **embryonic** insult with **little normal lung tissue** seen in the cystic structures.

■ **Symptoms**

Newborn respiratory distress, mediastinal shift.

■ **Diagnosis**

Chest radiographic variable with opaque or multiple cystic areas (must distinguish from diaphragmatic hernia).

■ **Treatment**

Surgical resection.

G. Pulmonary Sequestration

■ Description

Segments of embryonic lung tissue that is non-functional and nourished by anomalous systemic vessels.

1. **Intralobar**—within normal visceral pleura, 2/3 left-sided; arterial supply, aorta. Venous drainage, pulmonary veins.

2. **Extralobar**—separate visceral pleural covering, 90% left-sided, arterial supply, pulmonary artery or systemic artery. Venous drainage, azygos or portal vein.

■ Diagnosis

Infection, incidental chest x-ray (CXR) finding.

■ Treatment

Surgery as indicated.

H. Diaphragmatic Hernia

■ Description

Disorder of fetal diaphragm development with intrusion of abdominal contents into the thorax (1/2000 births).

■ Symptoms

Foramen of Bochdalek hernia—left-sided 90%, severe newborn respiratory distress, scaphoid abdomen, mediastinal shift, pulmonary hypoplasia.

Foramen of Morgagni hernia—often presents later as a bowel obstruction.

■ Diagnosis

Clinical, CXR shows bowel in thorax. Often diagnosed at prenatal ultrasound.

■ Treatment

Prompt, emergent surgical repair. Survival depends on degree of pulmonary hypoplasia. Possible role for extracorporeal membrane oxygenation (ECMO).

V. CARDIOVASCULAR SYSTEM DISORDERS

Congenital heart disease (CHD) is present in 8 of 1000 live births; 50% present in first month, most multifactorial inheritance.

Cyanotic lesions—right (R)-to-left (L) shunt. Acyanotic lesions—obstructive or L-to-R shunt.

Eisenmenger syndrome—longstanding L-to-R shunt causing pulmonary hypertension and reversal to R-to-L (cyanotic) flow.

Common presentations of congestive heart failure (CHF) in infants include **feeding difficulties, sweating, failure to thrive, tachycardia, hepatomegaly, respiratory distress.**

A. Coarctation of the Aorta

■ Description

Constriction of an aortic segment, usually in descending aorta opposite ligamentum arterosum (8% of all CHD).

■ Features

If severe constriction, presents as CHF in infancy, ductal dependent. **Most asymptomatic. Decreased femoral pulses, hypertension upper extremity (UE) >> lower extremity (LE).** Associated with Turner syndrome, **10% CNS berry aneurysms, 50% bicuspid aortic valve.**

- **Diagnosis**

  Clinical. Systolic ejection murmur at back, four extremity blood pressure UE > LE

  CXR. Inferior **rib notching** (erosions from interostal collaterals—older than age 5)

  ECG. Normal or left ventricular hypertrophy (LVH); echocardiogram or catheterization diagnostic.

- **Treatment**

  Balloon angioplasty or open surgical repair.

B. Patent Ductus Arteriosus (PDA)

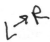

- **Description**

  Failure of the normal closure of ductus arterosus, the fetal connection between the pulmonary artery and aorta producing a left-to-right shunt, especially common in **premature** babies and in congenital rubella.

- **Symptoms**

  Congestive heart failure if large. Hypoxia, acidosis, and prostaglandin E keeps the PDA patent.

- **Diagnosis**

  Clinical—continuous "machinery murmur," bounding pulses (wide pulse pressure).

  CXR—normal or cardiomegaly with increased vascularity.

  ECG—normal or LVH.

  Echocardiogram—diagnostic.

- **Treatment**

  Spontaneous closure after infancy rare. Indomethacin sometimes used in premature babies. Usually requires surgical division or ligation.

C. Ventricular Septal Defect (VSD)

- **Description**

  L→R Most common cardiac malformation (25% of CHD). It is a persistent patency in the interventricular septum (**membranous** > muscular) causing a L-to-R shunt due to the **pressure gradient.**

- **Symptoms**

  Congenital heart failure from L-to-R shunt. Murmur often first detected at 1 to 2 months when pulmonary resistance lowers enough for shunting. Small defects loudest.

- **Diagnosis**

  Clinical—holosystolic murmur left sternal border.

  CXR—normal or slight cardiomegaly/increased vascularity.

  ECG—normal or left ventricular hypertrophy (LVH).

  Echocardiogram—diagnostic.

- **Treatment**

  Often closes on own. Medical treatment for CHF. Subacute bacterial endocarditis (SBE) prophylaxis. If large shunting, surgical repair indicated to prevent Eisenmenger syndrome. ↑ pulmon. pressure → R→L shunt

D. Atrial Septal Defect (ASD)

⤷ most common CHD in adults

- **Description**

  L→R Defect in midportion of atrial septum (ostium secundum) causing a L-to-R shunt due to the lower compliance of the right ventricle compared to the left.

- **Symptoms**

  Usually asymptomatic.

- **Diagnosis**

Clinical—systolic ejection murmur LUSB, wide fixed split of S_2 heart sound from increased flow to R heart.
CXR—increased vascularity.
ECG—right axis.
Echocardiogram—diagnostic.

- **Treatment**

Surgical repair as early as possible to prevent pulmonary hypertension and Eisenmenger's. No SBE prophylaxis needed.

E. Endocardial Cushion Defect/Ostium Primum (AV Canal)

- **Description**

Spectrum of abnormalities with lower atrial septal and contiguous interventricular defects, often with a single common atrioventricular (AV) valve.

- **Symptoms**

Commonly seen in **Down syndrome.** Recurrent pulmonary infections, CHF.

- **Treatment**

Medical management of CHF. Early surgical repair.

F. Hypoplastic Left Heart Syndrome

- **Description**

Underdeveloped left ventricle and ascending aorta often with mitral valve abnormalities or AV canal. Responsible for up to 20% CHD neonatal deaths.

- **Symptoms**

Ductal-dependent lesion: when PDA closes in first 2 weeks, get sudden cyanosis, respiratory distress, **acidosis,** and CHF with **vascular collapse.**

- **Diagnosis**

Echocardiogram diagnostic.

- **Treatment**

Palliative medical management, prostaglandin E to keep PDA open. Surgical correction (Norwood procedure or heart transplant) has high morbidity/mortality.

G. Tetralogy of Fallot

- **Description**

Most common cyanotic CHD (6%); classic tetrad of

1. **Right ventricular outflow obstruction.**
2. **Ventricular septal defect** (VSD).
3. **Dextroposition of aorta** (overriding ventricular septum).
4. **Right ventricular hypertrophy.**

- **Symptoms**

Timing and severity of presentation signs/symptoms depends on degree of RV outlet obstruction.

 Cyanosis (may begin later infancy), **clubbing of** digits, **squatting position** (increases systemic resistance, thus decreasing R-to-L shunt). **"Tet spells"**—paroxysmal cyanotic spells due to sudden pulmonary infundibular spasm/obstruction.

- **Diagnosis**

Clinical—single S_2 with right ventricular heave.
CXR—right aortic arch 25%, boot-shaped heart.
ECG—right axis and RVH.
Echocardiogram—diagnostic.

■ **Treatment**

Palliative surgical shunt (Blalock–Taussig shunt: subclavian artery to pulmonary artery). Definitive surgical correction when possible.

H. Transposition of the Great Vessels (TGV)

■ **Description**

Defect in which the aorta arises from right ventricle (RV) and pulmonary artery from left ventricle (LV), usually with mixing through VSD, ASD, or PDA (5% of all CHD).

■ **Symptoms**

Cyanosis from birth, CHF. Later clubbing.

■ **Diagnosis**

Clinical—RV heave with loud S_2.
CXR—**narrow cardiac waist.**
ECG—normal as newborn.
Echocardiogram—diagnostic.

■ **Treatment**

Balloon atrial septostomy (Rashkind procedure) for early palliation to increase mixing. Mustard (atrial switch) procedure now replaced with definitive arterial switch with coronary reimplantation when possible.

I. Truncus Arteriosus

■ **Description**

A single great artery arising from the base of the heart giving origin to the coronary, pulmonary, and systemic arteries, usually with VSD (2% of all CHD).

■ **Symptoms**

Presentation dependent on degree of pulmonary flow. Increased flow: get severe CHF in early months. Decreased flow: cyanosis predominates.

■ **Diagnosis**

May hear ejection click of truncal valve.

CXR—right aortic arch 33%.
ECG—RVH.
Echocardiogram—diagnostic.

■ **Treatment**

Treat CHF medically. Surgical correction when possible.

J. Anomalous Pulmonary Venous Return

Anomalous pulmonary veins drain **partially or totally** into systemic venous circulation. (RA, superior vena cava; SVC, inferior vena cava; IVC, portal veins) instead of left atrium. May have **cyanosis, often with ASD.** Heart may have "snowman" appearance on CXR.

■ **Treatment**

Surgical correction when possible.

VI. NERVOUS SYSTEM AND SPECIAL SENSES

A. Hydrocephalus

■ **Description**

Condition of impaired circulation, absorption, or overproduction of CSF leading to **increased intracranial pressure (ICP)** and risk of brain herniation.

1. *Communicating Hydrocephalus*

Blockage of CSF outside the ventricular system or its exit foramina or an overproduction of CSF. Commonly from subarachnoid hemorrhage as seen in premature infants and post-meningitis, causing obstruction of arachnoid villi with decreased CSF resorption.

2. Non-communicating Hydrocephalus

Ventricular system obstruction including

a. **Aqueductal stenosis**—congenital, postinfectious.

b. **Chiari malformation**—low cerebellar tonsils.

c. Dandy–Walker cyst of fourth ventricle.

■ **Symptoms**

Rapid increase in head circumference, split sutures, bulging anterior fontanelle, setting-sun sign (of eyes), irritability, lethargy, vomiting, *sixth nerve palsy, papilledema, long tract signs*

■ **Diagnosis**

Clinical plus CT scan. **Avoid lumbar puncture: risk of herniation.**

■ **Treatment**

Usually ventriculoperitoneal (VP) shunt.

B. Congenital Cataract

■ **Description**

Any opacity of the lens, requires early intervention to prevent permanent visual impairment.

■ **Pathology**

[margin note: rubella CMV galactosemia hypocalcemia prematurity]

Hereditary (autosomal dominant/recessive, X-linked), chromosomal abnormalities (trisomies), congenital infection (**rubella**, cytomegalovirus [CMV], toxoplasmosis), metabolic (**galactosemia**, hypocalcemia), prematurity (usually resolves spontaneously).

■ **Treatment**

Surgical removal of lens.

C. Congenital Glaucoma

■ **Description**

[margin note: Infant ē tearing & clouded cornea must r/o glaucoma]

Abnormal elevation of intraocular pressure causing eye damage and visual impairment. May present with **tearing,** photophobia, **corneal clouding,** eye enlargement, conjunctivitis. Seen in Sturge–Weber syndrome (facial port-wine stain, seizures, CNS calcifications), neurofibromatosis, congenital rubella, and retinopathy of prematurity. Treatment is surgical.

D. Congenital Deafness

■ **Description**

Conductive (abnormal sound transmission up to middle ear) or **sensorineural** (disorder of inner ear or auditory nerve) hearing disorder. Hearing loss often manifested by delay in language skills.

■ **Pathology**

Syndromes:

Waardenburg (autosomal dominant, **white forelock**).

Alport (X-linked dominant, **nephritis**).

Familial (70% recessive).

Craniofacial anomaly/syndrome (Pierre Robin, Treacher–Collins, Crouzon's).

Isolated ear malformations.

Congenital infection (CMV, rubella).

Maternal ototoxic drugs.

Prematurity.

■ **Diagnosis**

[margin note: white forelock, nephritis, cranio-facial anomalies]

Clinical suspicion (especially by caretaker). Screen high-risk newborns (family history, ear anomalies, congenital infections, prematurity) with auditory-evoked brain stem response test, audiology assessment.

■ **Treatment**

Early amplification, surgical implants, sign language, social support.

E. Neural Tube Defects (Spina Bifida)

Failure of neural tube closure in utero (normally closes by 26 days).

1. Spina Bifida Occulta

Failure of posterior lumbosacral spinal canal closure. May be completely benign or have associated bowel/bladder or motor disorders. May have **hair tuft, dimple** or **birthmark** over spine. Rule out tethered spinal cord, syringomyelia (fluid in central spinal cord), diastematomyelia (spinal cord cleft).

2. Meningocele

Meninges herniate through spinal canal defect without neural tissue.

3. Encephalocele

Meninges and brain substance herniate through bony skull defect.

4. Myelomeningocele

Severe spinal dysraphism (1/1000 births) with herniation of meninges and spinal cord, 75% **lumbosacral.** Multifactorial inheritance, possible decreased risk with maternal folate supplements. More than 80% **Chiari II** malformation with hydrocephalus requiring VP shunt. Neurogenic bowel/bladder dysfunction, variable paralysis below lesion. Treatment is multidisciplinary; 70% normal intelligence. Prenatal screen: fetal ultrasound. Maternal alpha-fetoprotein (increased).

5. Anencephaly

Congenital absence of cranial vault and cerebral hemispheres; **75% stillborn,** most others die soon after birth; 50% polyhydramnios.

VII. MUSCULOSKELETAL AND SKIN DISORDERS

A. Osteogenesis Imperfecta

■ **Description**

Inherited disorder of collagen characterized by variable bone fragility.

■ **Symptoms**

There are four types with variable severity. Severe form (type III) = early death. **Blue sclera**, hearing loss, **osteoporosis, multiple fractures.** Autosomal dominant or recessive.

■ **Diagnosis**

Child abuse a common differential diagnosis when multiple fractures. Triad of positive family history, frequent fractures, or blue sclera not 100% sensitive. Need skin biopsy for definitive diagnosis.

■ **Treatment**

Supportive, depending on severity. Genetic counseling needed.

B. Developmental (Congenital) Dysplasia of the Hip (DDH)

■ **Description**

Spectrum of hip dysplasia ranging from mild subluxation to total dislocation of the femoral head from the acetabulum, due to multifactorial genetic plus environmental factors (1 to 2/1000 births).

■ **Symptoms**

Risk factors include **female, breech** presentation, positive family history.

■ **Diagnosis**

Clinical: decreased hip abduction, positive Ortalani or Barlow hip maneuvers, asymmetric folds. Late diagnosis: limp. *(but still >6 mo.)* Hip ultrasound most accurate in early infancy, hip radiographs later.

■ **Treatment**

Early diagnosis: best chance for satisfactory treatment. Harness treatment, closed casting, or open surgical reduction.

C. **Talipes Equinovarus (Clubfoot)**

Complex foot deformity with plantar flexion, medial rotation, varus angulation, and metatarsal adduction (1/1000 births). Diagnosed by characteristic appearance, treatment is early casting and eventual surgical correction. Increased risk of DDH.

D. **Congenital Torticollis (Wryneck)**

Characterized by head tilting to affected side and chin rotation to opposite side. Usually due to sternocleidomastoid fibrosis with palpable subcutaneous mass over muscle. Typically resolves in 2 to 6 months with stretching; differentiate from **Klippel–Feil syndrome** (cervical spine anomalies, renal, genital, cardiac, nervous system anomalies) and isolated hemivertebra.

E. **Cerebral Palsy**

■ **Description**

Collective term for non-progressive disorders of posture and movement, often (but not always) associated with seizures, abnormal speech, and mental deficiency. *not always assoc. c̄ mental retardation* Usually due to **prenatal factors,** fewer than 10% from perinatal or postnatal asphyxia or trauma.
    Types:
✓*Spastic hemiplegic*
✓*Quadriplegic*
✓*Diplegic* (legs more involved than arms)

✓*Athetoid* (rare now, was classically seen with kernicterus of hyperbilirubinemia).

■ **Diagnosis**

Clinical: usually in first 2 years with motor delay, increased tone with scissoring of lower extremities, increased reflexes.

■ **Treatment**

Multidisciplinary including orthopedics, physical therapy, social work, pediatrics.

F. **Albinism**

Defect in the formation of the pigment melanin. Multiple variants, tyrosinase + or −. Autosomal recessive oculocutaneous forms common with numerous ocular abnormalities. Treatment is sun protection, ophthalmologic follow-up, genetic counseling, and psychosocial support.

G. **Epidermolysis Bullosa**

Heterogeneous group of congenital hereditary blistering disorders with lesions often produced by mechanical trauma. Range from mild simplex form to life-threatening fetalis form. Characteristic **mitten hand** deformities in severe cases. Autosomal dominant or recessive. Treatment is supportive; infection causes most morbidity/mortality.

VIII. GASTROINTESTINAL SYSTEM DISORDERS

A. **Cleft Lip/Palate**

Common defects (2/1000 live births) with classic **multifactorial inheritance** (recurrence 3 to 5% with affected parent or sibling, 10% if two parents/siblings. **Feeding problems, otitis media,** speech problems. Linked with many syndromic disorders. Treatment is surgical repair.

B. Tracheoesophageal Fistula (TEF)

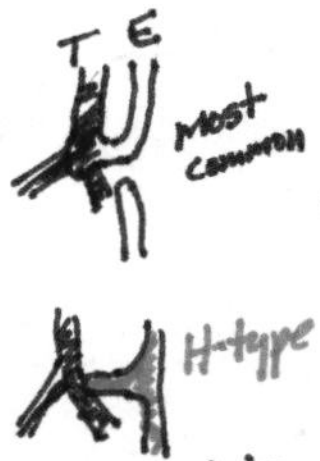

■ Description

Failure of division of trachea and esophagus most commonly (85%) resulting in proximal esophageal atresia plus tracheal to distal esophageal fistula. Also H-type (TE fistula with patent esophagus) and isolated esophageal atresia.

[handwritten: T E, most common, H-type, presents later & repeated pneumonia]

■ Symptoms

Maternal polyhydramnios, excessive oral secretions.

■ Diagnosis

Failure to pass nasal catheter to stomach, air-distended proximal esophageal pouch on radiograph. Barium studies rarely needed.

■ Treatment

Surgical in stages, usually initial gastrostomy tube. Search for VATER or VACTERL association: **V**ertebral defects, **A**nal atresia, **C**ardiac anomalies, **T**racheoE**s**ophageal fistula, **R**enal anomalies, **L**imb abnormalities.

C. Duodenal Atresia

Complete obstruction of duodenal lumen, classically seen in **Down syndrome.** **Double bubble** on abdominal study (air-distended stomach and proximal duodenum). Associated with malrotation. Treatment surgical.

D. Pyloric Stenosis

■ Description

Mechanical gastric outlet obstruction due to hypertrophied pylorus, increased in **males/first born** (1/250 births).

■ Symptoms

Progressive **non-bilious emesis (projectile).** Palpable right upper quadrant (RUQ) mass (OLIVE). Dehydration with hypochloremic alkalosis.

■ Diagnosis

Clinical. Can confirm with ultrasound or barium study if necessary.

[handwritten: donut or target sign]

■ Treatment

Correction of fluid and electrolyte abnormality then **pyloromyotomy.**

E. Malrotation of Small Intestine

■ Description

Potentially life-threatening gastrointestinal (GI) malformation due to incomplete rotation of bowel leading to **Ladd's bands** obstructing the duodenum and **midgut volvulus.**

■ Symptoms

Neonatal bilious emesis **(think malrotation with volvulus),** abdominal distention. Malrotation may be asymptomatic, found incidentally.

■ Diagnosis

Barium study: locate ligament of Treitz and cecum.

■ Treatment

Surgical.

F. Meckel's Diverticulum

■ Description

Anomalous outpouching in distal ileum 50 to 100 cm from ileocecal junction in 2%

of population, 35% with ectopic gastric tissue.

■ **Symptoms**

Most common presentation is **painless rectal bleeding** (peak at 2 years). Also can present as abdominal pain, intussusception.

■ **Diagnosis**
→ for gastric mucosa

Clinical plus technetium-labeled nuclear scan, barium study.

■ **Treatment**

Surgical excision of the diverticulum.

G. Congenital Megacolon (Hirschsprung's Disease)

Functional obstruction of colon due to absence of normal innervation (aganglionosis) of distal colon.

■ **Symptoms**

Presents as intestinal obstruction (with risk of enterocolitis), failure to pass meconium in first week, emesis, long-term constipation.

■ **Diagnosis**

Barium enema with **transition zone** (not always reliable). **Rectal biopsy** to detect ganglion cells for definitive diagnosis (80% involves rectum only; 20%, longer segment).

■ **Treatment**

Surgical excision of aganglionic segment.

H. Imperforate Anus

Failure of anal development with bowel ending in pelvis with various fistulas. Associated with VACTERL anomalies.

■ **Treatment**

Surgical.

IX. HEMORRHAGIC AND HEMOLYTIC DISEASES

A. Hemorrhagic Disease of Newborn

■ **Description**

Vitamin K deficiency causing decreased production of clotting factors II, VII, IX, X. Usually presents in first week of life. A delayed form due to malabsorption of vitamin K can occur at 4 to 12 weeks (ie, cystic fibrosis).

■ **Symptoms**

Bleeding from **GI tract**, nose, intracranium or **circumcision site.** Increased risk with **prematurity**, breast-feeding (poor source of vitamin K), or prenatal maternal drug use (**phenytoin,** phenobarbital, **salicylates,** coumadin).

■ **Diagnosis**

Suspect with bleeding in infants who have not received vitamin K. **Prolonged** prothrombin time (PT)/partial thromboplastin time (PTT), low serum clotting factors, presence of serum PIVKA (protein produced in vitamin K absence). **Normal bleeding time. Normal platelet count. Hemophilia usually presents later.**

■ **Treatment**

Vitamin K injection, intramuscular (IM) for all newborns is key to prevention. In acute bleeding, give vitamin K and consider fresh frozen plasma.

B. **Hemolytic Disease**

1. *Rh Incompatibility*

■ **Description**

Hemolytic process of infant red blood corpuscles (RBCs) due to transplacental passage of maternal antibody against Rh D antigen from Rh-negative mother to Rh-positive infant.

■ **Symptoms**

Wide spectrum of presentation from mild anemia and jaundice to profound anemia, extreme jaundice leading to **kernicterus** (neurotoxicity), **hydrops fetalis (hepatosplenomegaly, respiratory distress, massive anasarca and circulatory collapse)** often causing death. Hemolysis worsens with each subsequent pregnancy or fetal blood exposure. Thus previously affected infant, stillborn, transplacental hemorrhage (abortion), or previous maternal blood transfusions are risk factors.

■ **Diagnosis**

Clinical picture, blood typing, positive direct Coombs' test, high maternal anti-D antibodies, smear (nucleated RBCs, cells of hemolysis), reticulocytosis, indirect hyperbilirubinemia. Prenatal ultrasound diagnosis of hydrops shows skin/scalp edema, ascites, pleural/pericordial effusions. Prenatal confirmation by spectophotometric **analysis** of **amniotic fluid.**

■ **Treatment**

Rhogam (anti-D gamma globulin) injection to all Rh-negative women with possible fetal blood exposure within 72 hours to prevent sensitization is essential. Monitor maternal anti-D antibodies in pregnant women at risk. In utero transfusion (intraperitoneal or umbilical vein) and/or early delivery (32 to 34 weeks) if severe; in liveborns consider **exchange transfusion and** supportive care.

2. *ABO Incompatibility*

■ **Description**

Infant hemolytic process due to major blood group incompatibility between mother (type O) and infant (type A or *more common* B). Milder than Rh incompatibility.

■ **Presentation**

Usually mild with **jaundice** as only manifestations. Rarely severe anemia, hydrops.

■ **Diagnosis**

Suspect with type O mother and jaundice. Positive direct Coombs', indirect hyperbilirubinemia, mild anemia, and spherocytosis and hemolysis on blood smear.

■ **Treatment**

Phototherapy for jaundice. Rarely exchange transfusion for anemia or hyperbilirubinemia (**bilirubin level for exchange is controversial**).

X. FETAL GROWTH AND MONITORING

A. Fetal Growth

■ Description

Minimal growth in first half of pregnancy (5 g/day at week 14 to 15 gestation). Peak growth rate at week 33 to 36 gestation (30 to 35 g/day).

B. Categories of Intrauterine Growth Retardation

1. Early Onset (Symmetric)

Fetal insult in early pregnancy (less than 28 weeks' gestation). **Proportional head:body size.** Causes include maternal vascular disease (hypertension [HTN], renal disease), congenital malformation, chromosome abnormalities (trisomies).

2. Late Onset (Asymmetric, Head Sparing)

Fetal insult in later pregnancy (more than 28 weeks' gestation). Head size relatively large for body size. Causes include milder maternal diseases (including HTN), poor maternal weight gain/nutrition.

C. Fetal Monitoring

1. Non-stress Test (NST)

Monitors fetus by skin surface electrodes or Doppler ultrasonic device on maternal abdomen. Reliable and harmless. At 32 weeks' gestation, **reflex acceleration** of fetal heart rate (FHR) normally occurs with fetal activity. If a repeated NST is non-reactive, contraction stress test or delivery is indicated.

2. Contraction Stress Test (CST)

Monitors uterine contraction in relation to fetal heart rate (FHR usually increases 15 to 30 seconds after onset of maternal contractions). Abnormal study is associated with higher mortality (88/1000 deaths versus 0.4/1000 deaths if normal response).

3. Intrapartum Continuous

Electronic monitor (FHR and uterine activity during labor).

1. **Baseline pattern (normally 120 to 160 beats/min)**—bradycardia may suggest congenital heart block (fetal congenital heart defect, maternal systemic lupus erythematosus [SLE]). Tachycardia reflects maternal fever, chorioamnionitis, fetal dysrhythmia.

2. **Beat-to-beat variability (usually 5 to 10 beats/min fluctuation in FHR)**—loss of variability is associated with autonomic nervous system, fetal sleep, fetal immaturity, maternal narcotic or sedative use, fetal CNS depression.

3. **Deceleration pattern**

   a. **Type I (early deceleration, head compression)**—asymmetric fetal heart pattern that closely mirrors uterine contraction. **Benign pattern**—often due to fetal head compression against maternal bony pelvis.

   b. **Type II (late decelerations, uteroplacental insufficiency)**—asymmetric fetal heart pattern associated with a prolonged deceleration phase and shorter return to baseline. Suggestive of **fetal hypoxia.** Management consists of mother repositioning, intravenous fluids, oxygen and/or prompt delivery.

   c. **Type III (variable, cord patterns)**—variable shape and timing of FHR in relation to uterine contraction. Associated with **cord compression.**

Worrisome if severe pattern (<< 60 beats/min, lasting more than 60 seconds) or if associated with late decelerations or poor beat-to-beat variability. Management includes maternal and/or fetal repositioning.

4. Fetal Scalp Blood Sample

pH under 7.20 suggests fetal hypoxia and requires prompt attention.

5. Maternal Serum Alpha-Fetoprotein (AFP)

Elevated with **neural tube defects** (80 to 85%), omphalocele defect, multiple gestation, intrauterine fetal demise. Low AFP with fetal chromosome anomalies such as Down syndrome, trisomy 13 and 18, and Turner syndrome.

6. Amniocentesis

Measures karyotype, biochemical or enzyme assays. Performed at **15 to 16 weeks' gestation.** Procedure associated with small risk of spontaneous abortion. (1%)

7. Chorionic Villus Sampling

Placental tissue sampling. Similar study as aminocentesis, but **earlier results** (first trimester).

D. Fetal Positioning

1. Breech Presentation

Of all deliveries 3 to 4% incidence **(incidence inversely proportional to gestational age).** Higher neonatal **morbidity and mortality** than with cephalic presentation at all gestational ages and birth weight. Delivery problems result from umbilical cord prolapse, cephalopelvic disproportion, trauma. Management includes early diagnosis, preparation, external ver-

sion maneuver, vaginal delivery (assuming frank breech position, fetal weight 2,000 to 3,800 g, normal gynecoid pelvis), and/or cesarean section (c-section).

2. Transverse Lie (Shoulder Presentation)

One in 300 deliveries. Associated with **prematurity, increased parity,** premature rupture of membrane, placenta previa. Management depends on fetal size, gestational age, and placental position. External version attempts if gestation age over 37 weeks, membranes intact, no cephalopelvic disproportion (CPD), no placenta previa. Cesarean section unless no chance of fetal survival.

3. Deflexion Abnormality (Brow and Face Presentation)

One in 500 deliveries. **Spontaneous correction** often results as labor progresses. Associated with CPD, increased parity, prematurity, premature rupture of membranes, fetal anomaly (anencephaly). Higher perinatal mortality related to fetal abnormality, prematurity, trauma, asphyxia.

XI. PERINATAL ASPHYXIA

■ Description

Inadequate oxygenation and/or perfusion of visceral tissue leading to tissue hypoxia, hypercapnia, and acidosis. Incidence 1.0 to 1.5% in newborns (related to gestational age and birth weight).

■ Symptoms

Fetal and/or neonatal distress, depending on the severity as well as the timing of the insult. Often **multiorgan involvement.** The presentation of hypoxic-**ischemic brain injury** depends on which area of the CNS is involved. Diffuse hypoperfusion of the brain results in mental retardation, seizures, motor deficits, and/or spastic diplegias. Hypoxia to the brain stem or thalamus results in cranial nerve palsy, reflex disorders, or problems with breathing and temperature regulation. Watershed infarcts result in auditory/visual deficits or motor weakness. Impaired ventricular function or congestive heart failure usually resolves over 1 to 3 months. Newborns rarely present with thrombocytopenia, bleeding (secondary to impaired clotting factor production), or disseminated intravascular coagulation (DIC). Risk factors include intrauterine growth retardation (IUGR), breech presentation, prematurity, placental abnormalities, or systemic maternal insult (diabetes, drugs, infection).

[handwritten: b/k ↑ risk in labor?]

■ Treatment

Treatment is **supportive.** Mortality 10 to 20% for full-term infant. Of the survivors 20 to 45% have **neurologic sequelae.** Preterm newborns have worse mortality and morbidity. Worse outcome: associated with prolonged asphyxia, severe encephalopathy, poorly controlled seizures, persistent abnormal CT scan, elevated serum creatine kinase (CK)-BB, or absent heart beat for 5 minutes. Survivors have subsequent epilepsy (20 to 30%); (50% risk if presence of neurologic deficit). If infant survives, organ systems excluding the nervous system usually resolve spontaneously.

XII. PREMATURITY

■ Description

[handwritten: #1 cause of perinatal death]

Delivery **prior to 37 weeks' gestation.** Incidence 4 to 8% in United States. Number 1 cause of perinatal death in non-anomalous newborns.

■ Symptoms

Multisystem involvement depending on gestational age, birth weight, and etiology. Acute

problems include **respiratory distress, apnea, intraventricular hemorrhage,** hypoxic-ischemic encephalopathy, feeding dysfunction, necrotizing enterocolitis (NEC), PDA, cardiovascular compromise, and temperature instability. Long-term problems include CNS dysfunction (intellectual, motor, visual, auditory), chronic lung disease, poor growth, metabolic problems, retinopathy of prematurity (ROP).

■ Risk Factors

Lower socioeconomic status, black race, maternal age (under age 16 years; over age 35 years), maternal history of preterm labor, pregnancy complications (infections, fetal anomaly, antepartum hemorrhage, pre-eclampsia, first trimester bleeding), multiple gestation, maternal smoking, uterine anomalies (incomplete septae, bicollis bicornuate), uterine trauma.

■ Treatment

[handwritten: ✱] **Prenatal care/counseling** is the key to prevention. Early identification. Bed rest (before 25 weeks' gestation). Consider pharmacologic intervention to prolong pregnancy (beta-adrenergic agonist, ritodrine, or terbutaline (?); magnesium sulfate). Steroids ± to mature fetal lung. High-risk perinatal center. Marked increase in mortality/morbidity < 26 weeks' gestation and < 500 grams.

XIII. MULTIPLE GESTATION

■ Description

Monozygous: identical twinning. **Dizygous:** fraternal twinning. Twins 1 in 80 incidence (851 monozygous; 852 dizygous). Pregnancies 1 in 86 are triplets.

■ Symptoms

Problems include abortions, congenital anomalies, severe pregnancy-induced HTN, preterm delivery, intrauterine growth retardation, fetal malpresentation, cord prolapse, cord entrapment, and **twin–twin tranfusion syndrome (donor [arterial] twin** is associated with oligohydramnia, growth retardation, anemia, hypovolemia, and microcardia. **Recipient [venous] twin** is associated with polyhydramnia, large size, polycythemia, hypervolemia, and cardiac hypertrophy).

■ **Diagnosis**

Antepartum **sonogram.** Elevated maternal serum AFP. Zygosity determination is aided by sex (different sex = dizygous), placenta (monochorion = monozygous) blood or tissue typing, DNA fingerprinting. Suspect if family history, fertility hormonal treatment, in vitro fertilization.

■ **Treatment**

Early detection and **careful antepartum monitoring.** Early intervention for potential complications. Mortality rates: 65 to 120 of 1000 births (twins) and 250 to 310 of 1,000 births (triplets). Increased mortality: if monozygotic twins (versus dizygotic), under 32 weeks' gestation, under 1500 g body weight, discordancy of fetal size, late detection of monozygosity, malpresentation, labor outside high-risk center.

XIV. RESPIRATORY DISTRESS SYNDROME (HYALINE MEMBRANE DISEASE)

■ **Description**

Pulmonary disease in newborns is responsible for the majority of neonatal deaths. Incidence is inversely proportional to newborn's gestational age and birth weight (60 to 80% < 28 weeks, 10 to 15% < 2500 g).

■ **Symptoms**

Early onset (hours after delivery). Present with respiratory distress (tachypnea, grunting, nasal flaring, retractions). **Early problems**

include breathing problems/asphyxia, metabolic disturbances, anemia, infection, cardiovascular compromise. **Long-term complications** include **bronchopulmonary dysplasia** (BPD), cor pulmonale, ROP, poor growth, tracheal/glottic damage, persistent PDA. In mild cases, the severity of symptoms peaks by day 2 to 3. **Risk factors** include prematurity, maternal diabetes, multiple pregnancy, precipitous delivery.

■ **Diagnosis**

Clinical presentation. CXR: fine reticular [ground glass] granularity of lung fields, air bronchograms. Prenatal lung maturity tests include amniotic fluid's **lecithin/sphingomyelin ratio > 2:1 and** (> 34 wks) positive **phosphatidyl glycerol.** Must differentiate from sepsis, congenital heart disease, hypothermia, congenital lung anomaly (diaphragmatic eventration, cystic malformation), central nervous system disorder.

■ **Pathology**

Lung immaturity is due to **surfactant deficiency,** incomplete structural development of lung, and highly compliant chest wall. These factors result in atelectasis, hyaline membrane formation, retractions, and pulmonary edema. Surfactant reduces surface tension of alveoli (prevents collapse). Synthesized and stored in **type II pneumocytes** of fetal lung. Composed of phospholipids (77%), protein (11%), cholesterol (8%). **Dypalmitoyl phosphatidycholine** is major ingredient.

■ **Treatment**

Prevention of prematurity is goal (see Prematurity section). Consider **maternal steroid** administration 48 to 72 hours prior to delivery to stimulate fetal surfactant production if less than 34 weeks' gestation (exception: maternal toxemia, diabetes, renal disease). Neonatal **surfactant** administration (via endotracheal tube) at delivery. Known benefits of early surfactant therapy include improved initial respiratory status, decreased incidence of pneumothorax and pulmonary interstitial emphysema, decreased mortality incidence. Surfactants theoretical risk is IVH, pneumonia, sepsis, pulmonary hemorrhage, allergic reaction. Correction of acidosis, hypoxia, hypercapnia, hypotension, hypothermia, anemia. Maximize air exchange. Avoid unnecessary pulmonary barotrauma or oxygen toxicity. Survival rate 95% if birth weight more than 2500 g; 65% survival if birth weight less than 1000 g.

XV. PERINATAL BACTERIAL INFECTIONS

A. *Chlamydia*

■ Description

Chlamydia trachomatis. Most common sexually transmitted infection in United States. Transmission 50% from infected mother.

■ Symptoms

Conjunctivitis; afebrile pneumonia **(repetitive staccato cough).**

■ Diagnosis

Organism isolation, monoclonal antibody, enzyme-linked immunoassay.

■ Treatment

Erythromycin. Appropriate isolation.

B. Gonococcal Infections

■ Description

Neisseria gonorrhoeae. Concurrent infection with chlamydia is common.

■ Symptoms

Ophthalmia conjunctivitis, disseminated infection (bacteremia, arthritis, meningitis, endocarditis), scalp abscess.

■ Diagnosis

Organism isolation (chocolate agar in 10% CO_2 ; Thayer–Martin media).

■ Treatment

Parenteral antibiotics (pending sensitivity). Appropriate isolation.

C. Gram-Negative Bacilli (GNB)

■ Description

Escherichia coli, Klebsiella, Enterobacter, Proteus, citrobacter, *Salmonella.*

■ Symptoms

[handwritten: meningitis sepsis] Neonatal distress. Increased risk with maternal perinatal infection, low birth weight, prolonged rupture of membranes, traumatic delivery, underlying immunologic or metabolic abnormalities.

■ Diagnosis

Bacterial isolation. Bacterial antigen test (*E. coli* K1 only).

■ Treatment

Broad antibiotics pending sensitivity. Isolation for *Salmonella* meningitis. *[handwritten: amp i gent]*

D. Group B Streptococcal Infection

■ Description

One to 5 cases per 1,000 live births.

■ Symptoms

1. **Early onset** (first 3 days of life)—respiratory distress, apnea, pneumonia, meningitis, cardiovascular compromise.
2. **Late onset** (7 days to 3 months of age)—meningitis, osteomyelitis, septic arthritis.

■ **Diagnosis**

Bacteria isolation.

■ **Treatment**

Antibiotics similar to those for GNB. *amp ē gent*

E. **Tetanus**

■ **Description**

Clostridium tetani spores. Contamination of umbilical stump.

■ **Symptoms**

Marked dysphagia, respiratory distress, high fever, ± seizure, continuous crying. **High mortality rate.**

■ **Diagnosis**

Organism isolation, exclusion.

■ **Treatment**

Supportive care. **Tetanus immune globulin.** ± penicillin.

F. **Listeriosis**

■ **Description**

Listeria monocytogenes.

■ **Symptoms**

Sepsis. *< 2mo dd !*

■ **Diagnosis**

Bacterial isolation.

■ **Treatment**

Broad antibiotics pending sensitivities. Usually sensitive to **ampicillin.**

Newborn ē sepsis ⇒ give amp ē gent

XVI. NEONATAL ETHICAL ISSUES AND INDIGENT CARE

A. **Ethics**

1. **Ethical principles**—beneficence (preservation of life), non-maleficence (minimize harm), justice (fair allocation of resources), and autonomy (involvement of patient and family).

2. **Patient-dependent issues**—patient/family interest (cultural, religious, educational), community interest (moral, financial), legal constraints.

3. **Physician role**—medical caregiver. Source of information. Source of support.

4. **Medical ethic committee.**

B. **Indigent-Care Issues**

Poor access/availability of health care: higher infant **mortality/morbidity** associated with poor prenatal care. **Poor nutrition. Debilitating infections** (AIDS, TB, sexually transmitted disease) and infestations (scabies, lice). **Delay in medical care. Prevalence of substance abuse/mental illness. Absence of family/community support.**

BIBLIOGRAPHY

Behrman RE, Kliegman RM, Nelson WE, et al. *Nelson Textbook of Pediatrics.* 14th ed. Philadelphia, Pa: WB Saunders Co; 1992.

Berlin CM. Effects of drugs on the fetus. *Pediatr Rev.* 1991;12(9):282–287.

Briggs GG, Freeman RK, Yafe SJ. *Drugs in Pregnancy and Lactation.* 2nd ed. Baltimore, Md: Williams & Wilkins; 1986.

Cloherty JP, Stark AR. *Manual of Neonatal Care.* 2nd ed. Boston, Mass: Little, Brown and Co; 1985.

Creasy RK, Resnik R. *Maternal-Fetal Medicine: Principle and Practice.* 2nd ed. Philadelphia, Pa: WB Saunders Co; 1989.

Dworkin P. *Pediatrics: National Medicine Series for Independent Study.* New York: John Wiley and Sons; 1987.

Jones KL. *Smith's Recognizable Patterns of Human Malformation.* 4th ed. Philadelphia, Pa: WB Saunders Co; 1988.

Oski FA, DeAngelis D, Feigin RD, et al. *Principles and Practice of Pediatrics.* Philadelphia, Pa: JB Lippincott; 1990.

Young EW. *Alpha & Omega: Ethics at the Frontiers of Life and Death.* New York: Addison-Wesley Publishing Co, Inc; 1989.

CHAPTER 15

Psychiatry

ALEX I. DEVER, MD

I. CHILDHOOD AND ADOLESCENT DISORDERS

A. Mental Retardation

■ **Description (Axis II)**

Occurs in 3% of live births. Overall prevalence rate 1%. Male:female ratio 15:1. Intelligence quotient (IQ) of 70 or below with impaired adaptive skills.

■ **Pathology**

Heredity, embryonic, perinatal, acquired, and environmental (ie, deprivation).

■ **Treatment**

Treat concomitant mental disorders (30 to 70%). Psychotherapy, socialization training, remediation, and tutoring. Family counseling.

B. Pervasive Developmental Disorder

■ **Description (Axis II)**

Autism. Impairments in reciprocal social interaction, verbal and non-verbal communication, restricted repertoire of interests.

■ **Pathology**

Organic. No specific site of organic damage identified.

■ **Treatment**

Haloperidol (Haldol) for hyperactivity. Lithium for aggressiveness.

C. Specific Developmental Disorders (Axis II)

1. Academic Skills Disorders

1. Developmental arithmetic disorder.
2. Developmental expressive writing disorder.
3. Developmental reading disorder.

2. Language and Speech Disorders

1. Developmental articulation disorder.
2. Developmental expressive language disorder.
3. Developmental receptive language disorder.
4. Developmental coordination disorder.

3. Motor Skills Disorder

Developmental coordination disorder.

■ **Treatment**

Educational intervention.

D. Disruptive Behavior Disorders

1. Attention Deficit Hyperactivity Disorder (ADHD)

■ **Description**

Reflects subtle neurologic impairments. More common in males. School failure. Prevalence 3%. Genetic predisposition.

■ **Diagnosis**

Distractibility, fidgety, impulsive, poor attention to tasks, talks excessively, intrudes, loses things, physically dangerous activities.

■ **Treatment**

Stimulants (ie, methylphenidate hydrochloride **[Ritalin]**); tricyclic antidepressants; individual/family therapy; special education.

2. Conduct Disorder

■ **Description**

Basic rights of others and age-appropriate societal norms violated. Physical aggression. Three types:

torture animals

ADHD - Conduct d/o - alcoholism are associated

Group type.
Solitary aggressive type.
Undifferentiated type.

■ **Treatment**

Lithium or haloperidol (Haldol) to control aggression. Individual/family therapy.

3. Oppositional Defiant Disorder

■ **Description**

Negativistic, hostile, defiant behavior.

■ **Treatment**

Individual/family therapy.

E. Anxiety Disorders

1. Separation Anxiety Disorder

■ **Description**

Excessive anxiety concerning separation from those to whom the child is attached (ie, refusal to sleep alone, go to school).

■ **Treatment**

Individual/family therapy.

2. Overanxious Disorder

■ **Description**

Excessive worry.

■ **Treatment**

Individual/family therapy; anxiolytics.

3. Avoidant Disorder

■ **Description**

Shrinking from contact with unfamiliar people, desiring contact with familiar people.

■ **Treatment**

Anxiolytics, individual/family therapy.

F. Eating Disorders

1. Anorexia

■ **Description**

Refusal to maintain minimal normal body weight, intense fear of gaining weight, distorted body image, *amenorrhea*, predominantly females, **potentially fatal.**

■ **Treatment**

family therapy Cognitive behavioral therapy; antidepressants if depressed.

2. Bulimia Nervosa

■ **Description**

Binge eating, lack of control over eating, self-induced vomiting, laxatives/diuretics, strict dieting/vigorous exercise, overconcern with body shape. Dental erosion complication of vomiting.

■ **Treatment**

Balance electrolytes/metabolic alkalosis; antidepressants helpful, psychotherapy.

3. Pica

■ **Description**

Ingestion of non-nutritive substances (ie, plaster) Lead poisoning.

4. Rumination Disorder (Infancy and Childhood)

■ **Description**

Repeated regurgitation resulting in weight loss.

■ **Treatment**

Parental guidance, behavioral techniques.

G. **Gender Identity Disorders**

1. *Gender Identity Disorder*

   ■ **Description**

   Distress about his/her assigned sex, desire to be or insisting one is of opposite sex.

   ■ **Treatment**

   Improve role models.

2. **Transsexualism**

   ■ **Description**

   Discomfort about one's assigned sex, preoccupation with acquiring sex characteristics of opposite sex. Develops after onset of puberty. **Suicide risk.**

   ■ **Treatment**

   None.

H. **Tic Disorders**

1. *Tourette's Disorder (TD)*

   ■ **Description**

   Multiple motor and one or more vocal tics. Anatomic location/complexity/severity vary over time. Persists at least 1 year.

   ■ **Pathology**

   Single autosomal dominant disorder.

   ■ **Treatment**

   Haloperidol **(Haldol)**.

2. **Chronic Motor or Vocal Tic Disorder**

   Similar to TD, either motor or vocal tic; at least 1 year.

3. **Transient Tic Disorder**

   Tics occur 2 weeks to 1 year.

I. **Elimination Disorders**

1. *Functional Encopresis*

   Voluntary or involuntary repeated passage of feces into inappropriate places; psychotherapy behavioral techniques.

2. *Functional Enuresis*

   Repeated voiding of urine into bed or clothes; involuntary or intentional. Imipramine; behavioral techniques (ie, **bell and buzzer apparatus**).

J. **Miscellaneous Childhood Issues**

1. *Stuttering*

   Abnormal brain lateralization, genetic predisposition. Specialized speech therapy.

2. *Child Abuse*

   Low birth weight, handicapped, troubled are high risk. From 2,000 to 4,000 deaths/year.

3. *Suicide*

   Increasing incidence in adolescents. Associated with depression, substance/alcohol abuse, aggressive behavior. **Must question directly** if suspicious.

Night terrors c̄ bedwetting (enuresis) during stage III/IV sleep

II. PSYCHOACTIVE SUBSTANCE USE DISORDERS

A. Overview

1. Epidemiology

Occurs in all segments of society. Adolescents most vulnerable. Males at greater risk.

2. Social Impact

Impaired work and school performance, accidents, absenteeism, violent crime, theft.

3. Comorbidity

Often coexists with depressive or anxiety disorders and personality disorders.

4. Definitions

a. *Intoxication*—maladaptive behavior associated with recent ingestion.

b. *Withdrawal*—substance-specific syndrome following cessation of regular use.

c. *Abuse*—maladaptive pattern of use for more than 1 month in hazardous situation or despite knowledge of associated problems.

d. *Dependence*—implies psychological dependence, drug-seeking behavior, physical dependence, and tolerance. Reduced social, occupational, recreational activities.

B. Alcohol Dependence and Related Disorders

■ Description

[handwritten: GABA]

Three forms of dependence: continuous use of large quantity; heavy use limited quantity; heavy use limited to weekends; binges, interspersed with long periods of sobriety.

Epidemiology—lifetime prevalence, 13%. Prevalence greater in men (3 of 4). Etiology—genetic and cultural determinants.

■ Symptoms

Intoxication—disinhibition, emotional lability, incoordination, slurred speech, ataxia, coma, **blackouts** (anterograde amnesia).

Withdrawal—**tremulousness**, agitation, **autonomic hyperactivity**, nausea and vomiting, disorientation, fever, psychosis **(delirium tremens)**, seizures.

■ Treatment

Withdrawal—(detoxification) vital signs, hydration, electrolytes, thiamine, magnesium sulfate, vitamin B$_{12}$, folate; **benzodiazepine taper.** *[handwritten: (usually librium)]*

[handwritten left margin: Chlordiazepoxide (librium)]

Overall treatment—detoxification; Alcoholics Anonymous; disulfiram, supportive psychotherapy.

1. Related Disorders

a. *Alcohol idiosyncratic intoxication (pathologic intoxication)*—marked aggression after ingesting small quantity of alcohol. Brain-injured patients predisposed.

b. *Alcohol hallucinosis.*

■ Description

Vivid persistent hallucinations shortly after cessation **without delirium.**

■ Treatment

Antipsychotic medication may help.

a. *Dementia associated with alcoholism*—follows prolonged and heavy ingestion.

b. *Alcoholic encephalopathy (Wernicke's encephalopathy).*

■ **Description**

Thiamine deficiency. *Wernicke's Encephalopathy*

■ **Symptoms**

Nystagmus, ophthalmoplegia, ataxia, confabulation, disorientation, polyneuritis.

■ **Treatment**

Thiamine replacement.

C. Opioid Dependence/Abuse

■ **Description**

Opium, morphine, diacetylmorphine (heroin), methadone, codeine.

Epidemiology—lifetime risk 0.7% in United States.

■ **Symptoms**

Intoxication—central nervous system (CNS) depression, nausea and vomiting, constipation, **pupillary constriction**, seizures. *(except meperidine)*

Withdrawal—not life threatening. Tearing, anxiety, **pupillary dilation**, piloerection, diarrhea, nausea, vomiting, tachycardia, fever.

Overdose—pinpoint pupils, respiratory depression, CNS depression.

Treatment—support vital functions, intravenous **(IV) naloxone.**

■ **Treatment**

Detoxification—**methadone; clonidine** for nausea, vomiting, diarrhea; **methadone maintenance,** therapeutic communities.

D. Amphetamines

■ **Description**

Dopamine

Oral ingestion, extremely addicting, **anorectic;** episodic or chronic regular use; causes release of **dopamine.**

Epidemiology—two percent of adult population use amphetamines at some time.

■ **Symptoms**

Intoxication—psychomotor agitation, impaired judgment, pupillary dilation, increased blood pressure (BP), tachycardia, euphoria, prolonged wakefulness and attention.

Withdrawal—dysphoric mood, fatigue, insomnia/hypersomnia, psychomotor agitation., *polyphagia*

Amphetamine/sympathomimetic delirium—lasts 1 to 6 hours (usually self-limiting).

Amphetamine/sympathomimetic delusional disorder—rapidly developing; **persecutory delusions** most common.

E. Cocaine

Dopamine

■ **Description**

Highly addictive. Snorted, smoked, or injected. Purified to free-base form to be smoked (crack). **Sensitization:** greater euphoric effects from subsequent doses.

Epidemiology—epidemic.

■ **Symptoms**

Intoxication—euphoria, psychomotor agitation, impaired judgment, tachycardia, pupillary dilation, increased BP, nausea and vomiting, visual or tactile hallucinations, paranoid ideation. **Sudden death (cardiac).**

Withdrawal—dysphoric mood, fatigue, insomnia/hypersomnia, psychomotor agitation. Peak in several days.

Cocaine delirium—tactile and olfactory hallucinations may be present. Lasts 1 to 6 hours. May lead to seizures and death.

Cocaine delusional disorder—**persecutory delusions** prominent.

F. Caffeine

■ **Symptoms**

Intoxication—restlessness, insomnia, diuresis, muscle twitching, cardiac arrhythmia, inexhaustibility. Excess of 250 mg.

Withdrawal—**headache** lasting 4 to 5 days.

G. Nicotine

■ **Description**

Dependence develops rapidly. Smoking is associated with chronic obstructive pulmonary disease (COPD), coronary heart disease, cancers, peripheral vascular disease.

■ **Symptoms**

Withdrawal—craving, irritability, anxiety, tachycardia, increased appetite; may last several weeks.

■ **Treatment**

Hypnosis, nicotine sprays, and gums.

H. Inhalants

■ **Description**

Glues, solvents, volatile cleaners, gasoline, **aromatic hydrocarbons.** Primarily adolescents in lower socioeconomic group.

■ **Symptoms**

Intoxication—belligerence, apathy, impaired judgment, impaired functioning, ataxia, confusion, nystagmus. *Withdrawal*—unknown.

■ **Treatment**

Supportive medical care acutely.

I. Phencyclidine (PCP)

■ **Description**

An atypical hallucinogen. Smoked, insufflated (snorted); **IV; angel dust.**

■ **Symptoms**

Intoxication—belligerence, impulsiveness, psychomotor agitation. **Vertical and horizontal nystagmus,** increased BP, ataxia, dysarthria, hyperacusis, muscle rigidity, seizures. **Violent acts. Analgesis. Psychosis. Delirium. Depression.**

■ **Treatment**

Isolate in non-stimulating environment. Benzodiazepines for agitation.

J. Hallucinogens

■ **Description**

Lysergic acid diethylamide (LSD), dimethyltriptamine (DMT), psilocybin, mescaline.

1. *Hallucinogen Hallucinosis*

Marked anxiety or depression, ideas of reference, **delusions,** paranoid ideation; perceptual changes, derealization, depersonalization, illusions, **hallucinations,** pupillary dilation, diaphoresis, tachycardia, tremors.

2. *Posthallucinogen Perception Disorder*

A distressing re-experiencing of the same perceptual symptoms experienced while intoxicated. **Flashback:** treat with benzodiazepine acutely or antipsychotic if persistent.

K. Cannabis

■ **Description**

Marijuana, hashish, purified tetrahydro-cannabinol (THC); usually smoked, also eaten.

■ **Symptoms**

Intoxication—euphoria, anxiety, paranoid ideation, slowed time, impaired judgment, social withdrawal; **conjunctival injection**, increased appetite, tachycardia, dry mouth, **persecutory delusions**, depersonalization, hallucinations (rarely).

Chronic use—**apathetic amotivational syndrome.**

III. AFFECTIVE DISORDERS

A. Definitions

1. Mania

Elevated, expansive, or irritable mood with grandiosity, decreased need for sleep, talkativeness, racing thoughts, increased activity, impulsivity, which causes **marked impairment.**

2. Hypomania

Same symptoms without marked impairment (ie, symptoms of lesser severity).

3. Major Depression

Depressed mood or **loss of interest** with loss of libido, weight change, insomnia/hypersomnia, anhedonia, psychomotor agitation/retardation, low energy, low self-esteem, trouble concentrating, thoughts of death or suicide for at least 2 weeks.

B. Unipolar Major Depression

■ **Description**

No history of mania/hypomania. Symptoms severe and persist at least 2 weeks. **Diurnal variation** is common with symptoms worse in early AM.

Epidemiology: average age of onset 20s to 40s, more common in women. Genetic predisposition.

■ **Treatment**

Antidepressant medications; electroconvulsive (ECT); psychotherapies may be effective (ie, cognitive/interpersonal). Antipsychotics plus ECT or tricyclic antidepressant (TCA) if psychotic symptoms are present.

C. Bipolar Disorder

■ **Description**

One or more manic episodes accompanied by one or more major depressive episodes. High suicide risk.

1. Types

a. *Type I*—history of full-blown **mania** and **major depression.**

b. *Type II*—history of **hypomania and major depression.**

c. *Rapid cycling*—alternating manic and depressive episodes with at least two or more complete cycles without remission within 1 year.

Epidemiology: prevalence 1% of population. Equal male:female ratio. Genetic predisposition.

■ **Treatment**

Mood stabilizers: lithium; carbamazepine (especially for rapid cyclers), valproic acid.

Mania—mood stabilizer ± antipsychotic/benzodiazepine; ECT.

Major depression—antidepressant medication (ie, TCA, Bupropion) ± mood stabilizer; ECT.

  Antidepressant plus antipsychotic or ECT if psychotic symptoms are present.

D. Cyclothymia

■ Description

Chronic disturbance of at least 2 years' duration. Numerous hypomanic episodes and numerous depressive episodes (not of severity/duration to qualify for mania or major depression). May respond to lithium.

E. Dysthymia

■ Description

Chronic disturbance of at least 2 years' duration. Depressed mood not of severity of major depression. **More common in females.** Antidepressant medication may help; psychotherapy.

IV. DISSOCIATIVE DISORDERS

■ Description

Alteration in normally integrative functions of identity, memory, or consciousness.

A. Multiple Personality Disorder

■ Description

Distinct personalities within the same person. Each personality may have its own set of memories, physiologic characteristics, sex, age, race. **Severe sexual and psychological abuse in childhood.** Seizure disorder, 25%. More common in females.

■ Treatment

Intensive psychotherapy.

B. Psychogenic Fugue

Unexpected travel away from home with assumption of new identity and amnesia for previous identity. Disorientation may occur. Lasts hours to months. Follows severe stress. Unaware of loss of identity. Recovery spontaneous and rapid.

C. Psychogenic Amnesia

■ Description

Sudden inability to recall important personal information. Follows severe stress. Aware of loss.

■ Treatment

Hypnosis, psychotherapy, amobarbital (Amytal) interview.

D. Depersonalization Disorder

■ Description

Persistent or recurrent feeling of detachment from one's body or self. Reality testing intact. Onset sudden. Course chronic.

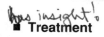 *has insight!*

■ Treatment

Uncertain.

V. PERSONALITY DISORDERS

■ Description

Persistent inflexible maladaptive **traits** of personality or subjective distress. Manifest by adolescence. Overall prevalence 6 to 9%.

■ **Treatment**

Multiple and mixed modalities, various psychotherapies, pharmacotherapies.

A. Odd/Eccentric Cluster

1. Paranoid Personality Disorder

Tendency to interpret actions of others as demeaning or threatening. More common in men. May respond to antipsychotics.

2. Schizoid Personality Disorder

Indifference to social relationships, restricted range of emotional experience. More common in men.

3. Schizotypal Personality Disorder

Peculiarities of ideation, appearance, behavior. Deficit in interpersonal relatedness. Excessive social anxiety. May respond to antipsychotics.

B. Dramatic Cluster

1. Antisocial Personality Disorder

Do not recognize the rights of others. History of conduct disorder essential. Substance abuse, precocious sexual activity, violent. Genetics plays a role. More common in men.

2. Borderline Personality Disorder

Instability of self-image, identity, relationships, and mood. Chronic feelings of emptiness. Intense personal attachments are central. Impulsivity. Inappropriate anger. More common in women. Psychotherapy, antidepressants, low-dose antipsychotics may help.

3. Histrionic Personality Disorder

Excessive emotionality and attention seeking. More common in women.

4. Narcissistic Personality Disorder

Grandiose, hypersensitive to the evaluation of others, lacking in empathy.

C. Anxious Cluster

1. Obsessive–Compulsive Personality Disorder

Perfectionism and inflexibility. Preoccupation with rules. Driven. More common in men. Familial transmission.

2. Dependent Personality Disorder

Dependent and submissive behavior. Difficulty with decision making. More common in women. Chronic physical illness predisposing factor.

3. Avoidant Personality Disorder

Social discomfort, fear of negative evaluation, timidity. Few close friends.

4. Passive–Aggressive Personality Disorder

Passive resistance to social and occupational demands expressed **indirectly.** Procrastination, intentional inefficiency.

VI. SCHIZOPHRENIA

■ **Description**

Presence of **psychotic symptoms:** delusions, hallucinations, loosening of associations, catatonic behavior. Flat affect. **Decreased social functioning.** Duration of at least 6 months.

■ Symptoms

Disturbance in content and form of thought, perceptions, affect, sense of self, volition, psychomotor behavior, relationship to external world.

> *Positive symptoms*—hallucinations, bizarre behavior, increased speech.
>
> *Negative symptoms*—flat affect, poverty of speech, low motivation, social withdrawal.

Epidemiology—lifetime prevalence 1%. More common in urban areas. Prevalence higher in blacks and Hispanics. More severe in industrialized areas. Equally common in both sexes. Onset age 15 to 35.

Etiology—no single etiologic factor. Biologic vulnerability triggered by stress. **Polygenic theory** most consistent. Monozygotic twins reared apart equal concordance rate to that of twins reared together (50%). **Dopamine** hypothesis: symptoms result of **hyperdopaminergic** activity (antipsychotic medications decrease function of D-2 dopamine receptors).

■ Pathology

Mesocortical and mesolimbic dopaminergic tracts implicated; however, no consistent structural defects. Minor (soft) neurologic signs 50 to 100% of patients. Paroxysmal saccadic eye movements 50 to 80% of patients. Course: chronic deterioration superimposed by acute exacerbations. Postpsychotic depression may occur. Increased risk medical illness, sudden death. Better prognosis if acute onset, good premorbid social history, positive symptoms, presence of mood symptoms. Families with high **expressed emotion (EE)** yield higher relapse rates.

■ Treatment

Antipsychotic medication; psychosocial treatments.

VII. SLEEP DISORDERS

A. Dyssomnias: Insomnia Disorders

■ Description

Difficulty initiating or maintaining sleep, or non-restorative sleep (adequate amount but not restful). Most common in elderly.

■ Pathology   *→ all REM in early night*

Anxiety, depression, substance use, medications.

■ Treatment

Identify and treat underlying cause. Good sleep hygiene. Short-acting sedative.

B. Disorders of Excessive Somnolence (DOES)

1. Narcolepsy

■ Description

Daytime somnolence, cataplexy (loss of muscle tone), hypnagogic hallucinations, sleep paralysis.

■ Pathology

Strong association with human leukocyte antigen (HLA)-DR2. Onset before age 15. Chronic without remission.

■ Treatment

Daytime naps. **Stimulants.** *(amphetamine)*

2. Sleep Apnea

Obstructive, central, mixed.

3. Kleine–Levin Syndrome

Young males sleep excessively for weeks. Voracious appetite, hypersexuality, hostility. Treat with stimulants.

4. Idiopathic CNS Hypersomnia

No specific treatment.

5. Sleep Drunkenness

Inability to become alert for sustained period. No specific treatment.

6. Nocturnal Myoclonus

Most prevalent after age 55. Clonazepam helps.

7. Restless Leg Syndrome

Clonazepam.

C. Sleep–Wake Schedule Disorders

■ Description

Mismatch between environmental demands and circadian rhythm (ie, jet lag). Bright light therapy when persistent.

D. Parasomnias

■ Description

Abnormal events that occur during sleep. The event is the focus, not daytime sleepiness.

1. *Dream anxiety disorder*—nightmares. Repeated awakenings, detailed recall.
2. *Sleep terror disorder (pavor nocturnus)*—panicky scream. Morning amnesia. Confusion. Treatment rarely needed.
3. *Somnambulism*—**sleep-walking.** Morning amnesia. Febrile illness as child predisposes. **Accidental injury.** In adults, rule out CNS pathology.

REM is the stage right before awakening

Seratonin improves sleep quality

dopamine blocks sleep

VIII. ANXIETY DISORDERS

A. Panic Disorder

■ Description

Recurrent **discrete** periods of intense anxiety (lasting minutes to hours) that are initially unexpected. **Agoraphobia** (fear of being in a place from which escape is difficult) is common, especially in females. Age of onset late 20s. Rule out hypoglycemia, pheochromocytoma, hyperthyroidism. Mitral valve prolapse an associated condition.

■ Symptoms

Dyspnea, paresthesias, chest pain, dizziness, palpitations, sweating, nausea, fear, **crescendo anxiety.**

■ Pathology

Locus ceruleus (NE neurons) hyperactive. Chronic with remissions.

■ Treatment

Tricyclic antidepressants (TCAs), monoamine oxidase inhibitors (MAOIs), benzodiazepines, psychotherapies (ie, cognitive) are all effective.　Paxil (paroxet)

(Zanax) alprazolam for acute anxiety

B. Obsessive–Compulsive Disorder

■ Description

Recurrent intrusive ideas, impulses, thoughts, or patterns of behavior (compulsions). Ego-alien. Course chronic. Equal among sexes.

■ Treatment

Seratonergic medications (ie, clomipramine, fluoxetine). Behavioral therapies. *(Prozac)*

paroxetine, sertriline, flutoxamine
(Paxil)   (Zoloft)   (Luvox)

C. Simple Phobia

■ Description

Persistent fear of object or situation other than fear of panic or social situation, resulting in avoidance. Exposure yields anxiety.

■ Treatment

Behavioral therapies (ie, **systematic desensitization**), flooding, implosion.

D. Posttraumatic Stress Disorder

Acute Stress Disorder is PTSD in 1st mo. after traumatic event

■ Description

Psychologically distressing events—outside range of common experiences—results in re-experiencing the event, avoidance of associated stimuli, numbing of responsiveness, increased arousal. Duration of disturbance at least 1 month. Depression and anxiety common.

■ Treatment

Psychotherapies. Antidepressants may be helpful.

E. Generalized Anxiety Disorder

■ Description

Unrealistic or excessive anxiety and worry about two or more life circumstances for at least 6 months. Signs of motor tension, autonomic hyperactivity, vigilance, scanning.

■ Treatment

Psychotherapy. Antidepressants, benzodiazepines, buspirone may help.

F. Social Phobia

■ Description

Fear of scrutiny of others. Onset late childhood. Chronic.

■ Treatment

May respond to β-blockers, MAOIs, TCAs, benzodiazepines. Behavioral and other psychotherapies.

IX. ADJUSTMENT DISORDERS

■ Description

Maladaptive reaction that occurs within 3 months of a stressor wherein symptoms are **in excess** of an expectable reaction, or impairment in occupational/social functioning results. The reaction must persist 6 months. Types:

1. *Adjustment disorder with anxious mood.*

■ Predominant Symptoms

Nervousness, worry, jitteriness.

2. *Adjustment disorder with depressed mood.*

■ Predominant Symptoms

Depressed mood, tearfulness, feelings of hopelessness.

3. *Adjustment disorder with disturbance of conduct.*

■ Predominant Symptoms

Conduct resulting in violation of rights of others or violation of age-appropriate social norms (ie, vandalism, fighting, reckless driving).

4. *Adjustment disorder with mood disturbance of emotions and conduct.*

   ■ **Predominant Symptons**

   Depression and/or anxiety and conduct.

5. *Adjustment disorder with mixed emotional features.*

6. *Adjustment disorder with physical complaints.*

   ■ **Predominant Symptoms**

   Physical (ie, fatigue, headache, backache).

7. *Adjustment disorder with withdrawal.*

   ■ **Predominant Symptoms**

   Social withdrawal without depression/anxiety.

8. *Adjustment disorder with work or school.*

   Inhibition/inability to study or write reports.

   ■ **Pathology**

   Greater vulnerability with history of serious medical illness, disability, parental loss during infancy.

   ■ **Treatment**

   Psychotherapy; antianxiety, antidepressant medication sometimes helpful.

X. ORGANIC MENTAL SYNDROMES

A. Delirium

   ■ **Description**

   Reduced attention, disorganized thinking with incoherent speech, reduced level of consciousness, sensory misperceptions (ie, illusions, disorientation, reversed sleep–wake cycle, disturbed psychomotor activity). **Onset rapid, course fluctuates, duration brief.** Most common in

children and **elderly.** Occurs in 30% of intensive care unit (ICU) patients. **Brain damage** predisposes.

   ■ **Pathology**

   Multiple, including psychoactive substance, metabolic abnormalities, cardiac failure. Common pathway for any brain insult.

   ■ **Treatment**

   Reverse the cause; low-dose antipsychotic medication.

B. Dementia

   ■ **Description**

   Impaired short- and long-term memory, with impaired abstract thinking/judgment, and impaired higher cortical functioning. Personality change. Elderly.

   ■ **Pathology**

   Alzheimer type most common. Multi-infarct dementia, acquired immunodeficiency syndrome (AIDS), CNS infection, brain trauma, toxic-metabolic (ie, pernicious anemia), 10% reversible. Otherwise slow and progressive.

   ■ **Treatment**

   Supportive; low-dose antipsychotic for agitation.

   block acetycholinesterase Tacrine & Donepazil

C. Amnestic Syndrome

   Impaired short- and long-term memory due to organic factors but does not meet other criteria for dementia.

D. Organic Delusional Syndrome

   Prominent delusions due to specific organic factor.

E. Organic Hallucinosis

Prominent recurrent hallucinations due to organic factor.

F. Acquired Immunodeficiency Syndrome

■ **Description**

Human immunodeficiency virus (HIV) infection may result in organic mood or personality disorder, depression, acute psychosis, mania, high suicide risk. AIDS encephalopathy (AIDS dementia complex); HIV-1 the direct cause. May occur before diagnosis of AIDS is made. Poor prognosis.

■ **Treatment**

Treat symptomatically; individual/group psychotherapy important. Pre- and post-HIV test counseling.

G. Other Organic Syndromes

1. Organic Mood Syndrome

Medications, reserpine.

2. Organic Anxiety Syndrome

Etiology usually endocrine (ie, thyroid, hypoglycemia) or psychoactive substance.

3. Organic Personality Syndrome

Etiology usually structural brain damage (ie, neoplasms, trauma).

XI. SOMATOFORM DISORDERS

■ **Description**

Physical symptoms suggesting physical disorder without organic findings or known physiologic mechanisms. Psychologic factors account for symptoms, which are **unintentional.**

A. Body Dysmorphic Disorder (Dysmorphophobia)

Preoccupation with imagined defect in appearance in normal-appearing person **not of delusional intensity.** Psychotherapy, serotonergic drugs (ie, clomipramine) may be helpful.

Do not DO SURGERY!

B. Conversion Disorder

■ **Description**

Involuntary alteration of physical functioning secondary to psychological conflict. Motoric (paralysis), sensory (blindness), consciousness (pseudoseizures) are typical disturbances. More common in females, low socioeconomic groups. Amobarbital (Amytal) interview; psychotherapy, hypnosis may help.

C. Hypochondriasis

Preoccupation with fear of having a serious disease though none exists, despite medical reassurance. **Not of delusional intensity.** Duration at least 6 months. Up to 10% of all medical patients.

■ **Treatment**

Antianxiety and antidepressant medication may be helpful. Psychotherapy.

D. Somatization Disorder (Briquet's Syndrome)

■ **Description**

Recurrent and multiple somatic complaints of several years' duration, not due to physical disorder, for which medical attention has been sought. Onset before 30. Chronic, fluctuating course. Rare in males. Genetic predisposition.

■ **Treatment**

Long-term psychotherapy, antidepressant medication if depressed.

E. **Somatoform Pain Disorder**

■ **Description**

Preoccupation with pain in absence of adequate physical findings or organic explanation. "Invalid role" frequent. More common in females.

■ **Treatment**

Behavioral modification/biofeedback; antidepressant medication.

XII. FACTITIOUS DISORDERS, MALINGERING

A. **Factitious Disorder with Physical Symptoms**

Intentional production of symptoms; total fabrication or self-infliction. **Munchausen syndrome.**

Sign out when confronted

B. **Factitious Disorder with Psychological Symptoms**

Intentional feigning of psychological symptoms. Goal to assume "patient role." Usually with severe personality disorder.

C. **Malingering**

■ **Description**

Voluntary production of physical or psychological symptoms to accomplish specific goal for **secondary gain** (ie, insurance payment).

■ **Diagnosis**

Vague, poorly localized complaints presented in detail. Chronic.

XIII. OTHER PSYCHOTIC DISORDERS

A. **Delusional (Paranoid) Disorder**

■ **Description**

Persistent, non-bizarre delusion (ie, well systematized). *Types* include:

Erotomanic—one is loved by another (ie, movie star).

Grandiose—one possesses great unrecognized talent.

Jealous—conviction that spouse/lover is unfaithful.

Persecutory—one is conspired against. Most common type.

Somatic—one has a physical abnormality (ie, odor).

■ **Pathology**

Unrelated to schizophrenia. Psychosocial. Factors include immigration, deafness, cruel parenting.

■ **Treatment**

Supportive psychotherapy. Antipsychotic medication may help.

B. **Schizophreniform Disorder**

■ **Description**

Identical with schizophrenia, except duration less than 6 months.

■ **Treatment**

Antipsychotic medication.

C. **Brief Reactive Psychosis**

■ **Description**

Sudden onset of psychotic symptoms, less than 1 month duration, following obvious stress with full recovery.

■ **Treatment**

Antipsychotic medication.

D. Schizoaffective Disorder

■ **Description**

Concurrent features of schizophrenia and affective disorder. Delusions or hallucinations for at least 2 weeks. Better prognosis than schizophrenia.

■ **Treatment**

Antipsychotic medication, antidepressants, lithium.

E. Induced Psychotic Disorder (Folie à Deux)

■ **Description**

Delusional system develops in a second person in association with another who is delusional. Suicide and homicide pacts.

■ **Pathology**

Primarily psychologic; chronic.

■ **Treatment**

Separate the two people. Antipsychotic medication is helpful.

XIV. SEXUAL DISORDERS

A. Paraphilias

■ **Description**

Recurrent and intense sexual arousal in response to objects or situations not normative, of at least 6 months' duration. Patient has acted on or is distressed by the urges. Types include

Exhibitionism—exposure of one's genitals to strangers, rare in females.

Fetishism—use of non-living objects (ie, undergarments); rare in females.

Frotteurism—rubbing non-consenting person.

Pedophilia—prepubescent child; most common paraphilia.

Sexual masochism—acts of being beaten, humiliated, bound, made to suffer.

Sexual sadism—psychological or physical suffering of victim; rare in females.

Transvestic fetishism—cross-dressing.

Voyeurism—observing unsuspecting persons.

B. Sexual Dysfunctions

■ **Description**

Inhibition in appetitive or psychophysiologic changes of complete response cycle (Appetitive → Excitement → Orgasm → Resolution).

1. Sexual Desire Disorders

a. *Hypoactive sexual desire disorder.*

b. *Sexual aversion disorder.*

2. Female Sexual Arousal Disorders

Inadequate lubrication: swelling response or lack of subjective excitement. Endocrine pathology must be considered.

3. Male Erectile Disorder

Inadequate erection to complete sexual activity or lack of subjective excitement. From 20 to 50% of organic etiology, usually medical illness or medication.

4. Inhibited Female Orgasm

Overall prevalence 30%.

5. Inhibited Male Orgasm

May follow gastrourologic surgery, neurologic disease, medications, interpersonal difficulties.

6. *Premature Ejaculation*

   Affects 30% of male population. Responds to behavioral techniques (squeeze technique).

7. *Dyspareunia*

   Genital pain before, during, or after intercourse. Most common in women. Pelvic pathology common (ie, cervicitis).

8. *Vaginismus*

   Involuntary spasm of musculature of vagina interferes with coitus. Sexual trauma common cause.

XV. IMPULSE-CONTROL DISORDERS

■ **Description**

Failure to resist an impulse to perform an act that is harmful to the person or others, with increasing tension before committing the act, and experience of pleasure at the time of the act. The act is **ego-syntonic.** Subsequent guilt may or may not follow. Course usually chronic.

A. Intermittent Explosive Disorder

■ **Description**

Loss of control of aggressive impulses grossly out of proportion to precipitant, resulting in serious assault or destruction of property. Males more susceptible. First-degree relatives often affected.

■ **Treatment**

Combined psychotherapy and medication. Lithium, antipsychotics, carbamazepine (Tegretol) (especially if abnormal electroencephalogram [EEG]), TCAs may help. **Benzodiazepines may cause disinhibition.**

B. Kleptomania

■ **Description**

Repeated stealing/shoplifting. More common in females.

■ **Treatment**

Insight-oriented psychotherapy.

C. Pathologic Gambling

Maladaptive gambling behavior more common in males. Treatment includes psychotherapy; **Gamblers Anonymous (GA).**

D. Pyromania

Deliberate fire setting. Onset usually childhood. More common in males. Behavioral therapy.

E. Trichotillomania

Impulse to pull one's own hair. Alopecia may result. Psychotherapy. Fluoxetine, clomipramine may be useful.

XVI. BIOLOGIC THERAPIES

A. Antipsychotic Medications

■ **Description**

Neuroleptics. Treat psychosis **regardless of etiology.** Examples: haloperidol (Haldol), trifluoraperazine (Stelazine), thioridazine (Mellaril).

Indications—acute schizophrenia and other acute psychotic disorders (ie, amphetamines); chronic schizophrenia, psychosis in context of major depression or mania, Tourette's syndrome (Haldol), acute agitation of non-psychotic nature.

Mechaninism of action—postsynaptic blockade of dopamine receptors.

Pharmacokinetics—marked interindividual differences in blood levels.

Side effects—extrapyramidal (greater for high-potency drugs [ie, Haldol]); anticholinergic/hypotension/sedation, greater for low-potency drugs (ie, chlorpromazine hydrochloride [Thorazine]). Tardive dyskinesia.

B. Lithium

Lithium carbonate.

Indications—mood stabilization in bipolar disorder, acute mania, schizoaffective disorder, intermittent explosive disorder, mental retardation with aggressiveness of self-mutilation.

Mechanism of action—uncertain. Affects norepinephrine and serotinergic systems.

Pharmacokinetics—rapid absorption, peak plasma level approximately 3 hours. Not protein bound. Half-life approximately 24 hours. Monitor blood levels: therapeutic range 0.7 to 1.2 mEq/L. Narrow margin of safety.

Side effects—tremor, GI distress, weight gain, peripheral edema, hypothyroidism, goiter.

Toxicity—confusion/disorientation, ataxia, polyuria and polydipsia (diabetes insipidus-like syndrome), possible nephrotoxicity.

C. Antidepressants

1. Tricyclic/Heterocyclic Compounds

■ Description

Examples: amitriptyline, imipramine, trazodone, doxepin, nortriptyline.

dangerous

Indications—**major depression,** dysthymia, panic disorder, enuresis.

Mechanism of action—reuptake inhibition of norepinephrine or serotonin (leading hypothesis).

Pharmacokinetics—half-life approximately 24 hours (varies). Marked interindividual differences in blood levels. Nortriptyline and protriptyline have therapeutic window.

Side effects—autonomic (ie, tremor, sweating); anticholinergic; cardiac (ie, tachycardia), atrioventricular (AV) block/bundle branch block (BBB). **Quinidine-like effect decreases frequency of premature ventricular contractions PVCs; sedation, orthostasis, weight gain, impotence, seizures.**

2. Monoamine Oxidase Inhibitors

■ Description

Phenelzine (Nardil), isocarboxazid (Marplan), tranylcypromine (Parnate). Requires tyramine-free diet (ie, no cheese, liver, red wine, smoked/preserved meats).

Indications—major depression; atypical depression (hypersomnia, hyperphagia, hypersensitivity, **reactivity**); dysthymia, panic disorder.

Mechanism of action—increase CNS norepinephrine (NE) and serotonin (5-hydroxytryptamine, 5-HT) due to inhibition of the oxidation of biogenic amines.

Pharmacokinetics—rapidly absorbed. Inhibition of platelet MAO in blood sample (80 to 90%) is a measure of effective dose.

Side effects—anticholinergic, orthostasis, insomnia, sedation, weight gain, sexual dysfunction (ie, impotence, anorgasmia).

Toxicity—hepatoxicity, hyperpyretic/hypertensive crisis (ie, when mixed with meperidine hydrochloride [Demerol], stimulants, TCAs).

Tyramine reaction: ingestion of tyramine may result in hypertensive/hyperpyretic crisis due to inhibition of MAO in gut and subsequent entrance of large quantity of pressor amine. Severe sudden headache, sweating, fever. Treat with nifedipine (Procardia) orally or phentolamine IV.

3. Fluoxetine (Prozac)

■ Description

<u>Selective</u> serotonin reuptake inhibitor.

Indications—same as TCAs, plus obsessive–compulsive disorder.
Pharmacokinetics—active metabolite with half-life approximately 7 days.
Side effects—jitteriness, headache, nausea, sexual dysfunction, insomnia, **cardiac safe.** No anticholinergic effects. No orthostasis.

4. Bupropion (Wellbutrin)

■ Description

Weak reuptake blocking effects on serotonin and norepinephrine. Affects **reuptake of dopamine.**

Indications—major depression. Rapid-cycling bipolar disorder.
Side effects—restlessness, anxiety, insomnia. Higher risk of seizure, especially in bulemics, prior history of seizures; **no sexual dysfunction. Cardiac safe.**

D. Antianxiety Medications

1. Benzodiazepines

■ Description

Widely prescribed. Abrupt discontinuation may result in symptom recurrence, rebound, or withdrawal. Examples: diazepam (Valium), alprazolam (Xanax), midazolam (Versed), triazolam (Halcion). Potency and half-life differentiate individual use (ie, hypnotic, anxiolytic).

Indications—generalized anxiety disorder, panic disorder, alcohol withdrawal, adjustment disorders, sedation, seizure disorders.
Mechanism of action—up-regulate γ-amino-butyric acid (GABA) systems.
Pharmacokinetics—well absorbed. Lorazepam effective intramuscularly IM). Metabolized by liver, excreted by kidney.
Side effects—sedation, impaired anterograde memory, impaired motor coordination, CNS/respiratory depression.
Withdrawal—anxiety, insomnia, tremor, headache, tachycardia, diaphoresis, **seizures.** Predisposing factors include high potency/short-half-life compounds (ie, Xanax); longer duration of use, higher dose, abrupt withdrawal, history of panic disorder, somatization, substance abuse, dependent personality.

2. Buspirone (Buspar) —*nonaddictive, nonsedating*

■ Description

Pharmacologically unrelated to benzodiazepines; cautious use with MAOIs. Onset of action days to weeks.

Indications—generalized anxiety disorder.
Side effects—dizziness, nausea, headache, nervousness, lightheadedness, excitement. No withdrawal symptoms. No sedation/CNS depression. No psychomotor impairment. No abuse/dependence.

3. Electroconvulsive Therapy (ECT)

■ Description

Effective, relatively safe for indicated disorders. Involves administration of electrical impulse (usually **brief pulse**) to brain to generate generalized electrical seizure by unilateral (non-dominant hemisphere) or bilateral placement of electrodes. Since onset of action rapid, preferred in acute situations (ie, inanition/intense suicidality).

Indications—major depression, especially with psychotic features (may be treatment of choice) and in elderly (more sensitive to side effects of antidepressants); mania, catatonia, neuroleptic malignant syndrome.

High-risk situations—no absolute contraindications. Due to increased blood pressure (BP) during procedure, increased intracranial pressure (brain tumor), recent myocardial infarction (MI), recent stroke, leaking aneurysms represent significant risk. Other risk factors include osteoarthritis, cardiac arrhythmias.

Side effects—transient retrograde and anterograde memory impairment, transient confusion, headache, muscle aches.

XVII. SUICIDE, VIOLENCE, LEGAL ISSUES

A. Suicide

1. Risk Factors

Demographic: bimodal distribution. Adolescence/early adulthood and elderly. Males, minorities, widowers, certain nationalities (eastern European, Scandinavian, Japanese).

2. Individual Risk Factors

Recent attempt/gesture, expressed intent, thoroughness of plan, alcohol/substance abuse, major depression, schizophrenia, psychosis (especially command hallucinations to suicide), hopelessness, recent loss (ie, spouse/job), family history of suicide.

■ Treatment

Identify and treat underlying condition. Never hold plan in confidence. Consider hospitalization.

B. Violence

1. Risk Factors

Verbal/physical threats, progressive agitation, alcohol/drug intoxication, paranoid features, mania, violent history, males, lower socioeconomic status.

2. Management

Restraints, antipsychotics/benzodiazepines IM may be used in conjunction (ie, haloperidol [Haldol]/lorazepam [Ativan]). Hospitalization.

C. Legal Issues

1. Informed Consent

Requires patient be informed about treatment, alternative treatments, potential risks and benefits; patient must understand and freely and knowingly give consent. Exception: emergencies (ie, patient in imminent physical danger).

2. Confidentiality

Hippocratic oath and law bind physician to secrecy. Exceptions: contagious disease, child abuse, suicide, gun and knife wounds, duty to warn (Tarasoff case) requires psychotherapist to warn potential victims of patient's expressed intent to harm.

3. Involuntary Commitment

Laws vary according to state. Typically requires risk or action of self-harm or danger to others.

4. Right to Refuse Treatment

Highly controversial. Issues involve status of patient, type of treatment

BIBLIOGRAPHY

American Psychiatric Association. *Diagnostic and Statistical Manual of Mental Disorders.* 3rd ed. Rev. Washington, DC: American Psychiatric Association; 1987.

Baldessarini RJ. *Chemotherapy in Psychiatry.* Cambridge, Mass: Harvard University Press; 1985.

Kaplan HI, Sadock BJ. *Comprehensive Textbook of Psychiatry.* 5th ed. Baltimore, Md: Williams & Wilkins; 1989.

Kaplan HI, Sadock BJ. *Pocket Handbook of Clinical Psychiatry.* Baltimore, Md: Williams & Wilkins; 1990.

CHAPTER 16

Pulmonary Medicine

JOEL S. GOLDBERG, DO
HECTOR STELLA, MD

I. HEALTH AND HEALTH MAINTENANCE

A. Respiratory Tract Infection

■ **Description**

Epidemiology—pneumonia more common in alcoholics, elderly, prior pulmonary disease patients, chronic disease (cancer, diabetes, immunocompromise, etc). Pneumonia is either community acquired, or nosocomial (hospital acquired). **Bronchitis** may be bacterial or viral, and in adults is often from smoking (chronic bronchitis). Source of infection may be **aspiration, inhalation,** or **hematologic/contiguous spread. Sinusitis has to be included within R.T.I. Can be chronic as well as acute and can be seen in outpatient as well as inpatient population.**

Impact—vast number of people affected, time lost from work, cost of prescription and over-the-counter cough/cold preparations, and mortality.

Prevention—vaccination where indicated (children: diphtheria, pertussis; susceptible adults: influenza, pneumococcal), and education (including hygiene, smoking cessation, etc).

Prevention of complications in HIV/AIDS patients—zidovudine (AZT) may reduce infection incidence (watch for bone marrow suppression), **aerosolized pentamidine (Pentam) or trimethoprim/sulfamethoxazole to prevent** *Pneumocystis carinii,* isoniazid for reactive purified protein derivative (PPD) patients, hygiene, patient education.

B. Chronic Bronchitis, Emphysema, Larynx and Lung Carcinoma

■ **Description**

Epidemiology—in **chronic bronchitis, emphysema, lung and larynx carcinoma,** smoking is the major cause. **Most common lung tumor type: adenocarcinoma. Most head/neck cancer** is squamous cell, and **alcohol is an additional risk factor.**

Impact—vast morbidity/mortality and cost. Lung cancer: **most common male cancer worldwide.**

Prevention—patient education, including smoking cessation and reduction in alcohol and environmental risks (nickel, arsenic, asbestos, radiation, etc).

C. Tuberculosis

■ **Description**

Epidemiology—**most often due to** *Mycobacterium tuberculosis.* **Marked impact in underdeveloped areas,** and **airborne transmission by prolonged close exposure.**

Prevention—**chemotherapy** (treat infection to prevent active disease, give isoniazid), and education (hygiene). Isoniazid for 1 year; give 10 mg/kg/day for children, up to 300 mg/day for adults.

D. Occupational and Environmental Pulmonary Disease and Asthma

■ **Description**

Epidemiology—exposure to occupational and environmental toxins results in a wide range of pulmonary disorders (acute, firefighters smoke inhalation, or over many years, asbestosis-induced mesothelioma). Risk factors for asthma may include air pollution, childhood bronchitis, and occupational exposure (common offenders include medications, chemicals, plant and animal products).

Prevention—**avoid exposure to offending agent,** including toxin/dust control, adequate ventilation, and mask/respirator protection, can also consider premedication depending on clinical scenario.

E. Postoperative Pulmonary Complications

- ■ **Description**

  Epidemiology—complications include **atelectasis (most common), respiratory failure,** pneumonia/aspiration, and **hypoxemia.**

  Risk factors—chronic obstructive pulmonary disease (COPD), **obesity, smoking,** arteriosclerotic cardiovascular disease (ASCVD), upper abdominal surgery, age > 70.

  Preoperative assessment—history and physical, pulmonary function testing.

  Prevention—chest physical therapy (PT), blow bottles, deep breathing, medication.

F. Newborn Respiratory Distress Syndrome

- ■ **Description**

  Epidemiology—**lack of surfactant** resulting in atelectasis.

  Other risk factors—maternal diabetes, cesarean section (c-section) delivery, male sex.

  Prevention—**avoid prematurity; betamethasone** given 48 to 72 hours before delivery in fetuses < 32 weeks, check lecithin/sphingomyelin (L/S) ratio (over 2:1 is OK).

G. Pulmonary Aspiration

- ■ **Description**

  Prevent aspiration in high-risk patients (elderly, neurologic disorders, intubation/tracheostomy/sedated patients). **Prevent with H$_2$-antagonists,** elevate head of bed, safe feeding tube flow rates, antacids(?), cricoid pressure during intubation, preoperative and postoperative fasting.

II. MECHANISMS OF DISEASE, DIAGNOSIS, AND TREATMENT

A. Nose, Sinus, Pharynx, Larynx, and Trachea

1. Common Cold

- ■ **Description**

  Viral rhinitis.

- ■ **Symptoms**

  Rhinitis, sneezing, headache, and cough.

- ■ **Diagnosis**

  History and physical exam.

- ■ **Pathology**

  Rhinovirus commonly, many others possible (adenovirus, respiratory syncytial virus [RSV], influenza, etc).

- ■ **Treatment**

  Symptomatic.

2. Pharyngitis

- ■ **Description**

  Pharyngeal surface inflammation.

- ■ **Symptoms**

  Fever, dry/sore throat, headache, and cough.

- ■ **Diagnosis**

  History and physical exam, throat culture.

- **Pathology**

Bacterial/viral etiology, with multiple organisms as possible agents.

- **Treatment**

Bacterial: antibiotics, otherwise supportive.

3. Tonsillitis

- **Description**

Tonsillar inflammation/infection.

- **Symptoms**

Sore throat, halitosis, high fever.

- **Diagnosis**

History and physical, throat culture.

- **Pathology**

Group A, β-hemolytic strep is **common;** other bacterial/viral agents possible.

- **Treatment**

Antibiotics as per culture report, symptomatic measures.

4. Peritonsillar Abscess

- **Description**

Quinsy.

- **Symptoms**

Dysphagia, fever, pain, trismus (hard to open mouth).

- **Diagnosis**

History and physical exam (uvula displaced by peritonsillar mass/swelling), culture of aspirate.

- **Pathology**

Extension of tonsillitis; **group A,** β-hemolytic strep common.

- **Treatment**

Surgical drainage and antibiotics.

5. Thrush

- **Description**

Moniliasis.

- **Symptoms**

White patch in mouth; **removable.**

- **Diagnosis**

History and physical exam (bleeding surface after scraping plaque off), fungal culture, KOH prep.

- **Pathology**

Excess *Candida* (*C. albicans* usually).

- **Treatment**

Antifungal (nystatin, fluconazole, etc).

6. Sinusitis

- **Description**

Localized sinus pus accumulation.

- **Symptoms**

Facial pain/pressure, fever, headache, referred pain (teeth).

- **Diagnosis**

History and physical exam (sinus tender to percussion, purulent rhinitis, decreased transillumination), x-ray and CT scan, culture from sinus.

■ **Pathology**

Strep and *Hemophilus influenzae* common; **maxillary most common.**

■ **Treatment**

Antibiotics, decongestants, drainage/irrigation.

Additional Information. **Only maxillary and ethmoid sinuses are present in children. Ethmoid sinusitis more frequent in children. Cavernous sinus thrombosis: sinusitis complication (facial edema, meningitis, ophthalmoplegia).**

7. Allergic Rhinitis

■ **Description**

Nasal inflammation.

■ **Symptoms**

Sneezing, itchy/watery eyes, nose blocked and/or runny.

■ **Diagnosis**

History and physical (blue boggy turbinates), allergy testing, nasal smear for eosinophils.

■ **Pathology**

Antibody immunoglobulin E (IgE) and allergen reaction (cytophilic).

■ **Treatment**

Antihistamines and/or decongestants, nasal sprays (cromolyn sodium, corticosteroid sprays), allergy shots.

Additional Information. **Vasomotor rhinitis:** rhinitis and nasal vascular congestion, non-allergic, etiology unknown, but positive association with anxiety patients.

8. Nasal Polyps

■ **Description**

Swollen mucosa/submucosa polypoid tissue.

■ **Symptoms**

Nasal obstructive symptoms.

■ **Diagnosis**

History and physical examination (polyp: smooth, blue, wet appearance).

■ **Pathology**

Positive association with allergic rhinitis, cystic fibrosis, and asthma with aspirin intolerance (asthma triad).

■ **Treatment**

Medical or surgical.

Additional Information. **Childhood nasal polyps: rule out cystic fibrosis.**

9. Croup

9–1. Acute Laryngotracheobronchitis

■ **Description**

Most frequent croup presentation.

■ **Symptoms**

Cold symptoms at onset, then **barking cough, slight fever, inspiratory/expiratory stridor.**

■ **Diagnosis**

History and physical examination, chest/lateral neck x-ray.

■ Pathology

Viral, children 6 months to age 3, **subglottic.**

■ Treatment

Humidification of air, racemic epinephrine, oxygen, steroids, supportive care.

9–2. Epiglottitis

■ Description

Dangerous airway-compromising infection.

■ Symptoms

High fever, respiratory obstruction, dyspnea, drooling, dysphagia, barking cough, **inspiratory** stridor.

■ Diagnosis

History and physical, **cherry-red epiglottis, lateral neck x-ray,** blood culture.

■ Pathology

Children age 2 to 7, **usually *Hemophilus influenzae* type b, supraglottic.**

■ Treatment

Antibiotics (cefuroxime [Zinacef]), or others.

Additional Information

> *Epiglottitis*—examine epiglottis only with cardiorespiratory support team available, as examination may provoke laryngospasm/complete airway loss/cardiac arrest!

Spasmodic croup—children 1 to 3, night onset, lasts few hours, usually viral, **no fever.**

10. Pertussis

■ Description

Respiratory tract infection.

■ Symptoms

Catarrhal stage (coryza, 1 to 2 weeks), **paroxysmal stage** (coughing and inspiratory whoop, 2 to 4 weeks), **convalescent stage** weeks later.

   Vomiting after coughing is common.

■ Diagnosis

History and physical exam, nasopharyngeal culture, leukocytosis.

■ Pathology

Bordetella pertussis; infants under 2 years.

■ Treatment

Erythromycin will help in catarrhal stage; otherwise, **supportive care.**

11. Nasopharyngeal Carcinoma

■ Description

Cancer of nose, pharynx, and associated structures.

■ Symptoms

Nasal obstruction, bleeding, or **discharge,** cranial nerve paralysis. May also be asymptomatic.

■ Diagnosis

History and physical examination (**posterior cervical adenopathy**), roentographic studies, nasopharyngoscopic exam.

■ Pathology

Squamous cell is most common head/neck cancer type. Etiology includes **smoking, alcohol, Epstein–Barr virus (EBV), toxin exposure.**

■ Treatment

Radiation, with possible **surgery** and **chemotherapy.**

12. Carcinoma of the Larnyx

■ Description

Laryngeal cancer.

■ Symptoms

Hoarseness, pain, dysphagia.

■ Diagnosis

History and physical examination, laryngoscopy.

■ Pathology

Squamous cell most often.

■ Treatment

Surgical resection and radiation. May use radiation alone if tumor small.

13. Chronic Laryngitis

■ Description

Chronic laryngeal inflammation.

■ Symptoms

Persisting hoarseness; recurrent acute laryngitis episodes.

■ Diagnosis

History and physical examination, laryngoscopy.

■ Pathology

Chronic irritation (smoking, overuse of voice, reflux).

■ Treatment

Voice rest, speech therapy, steroids.

14. Larynx and Pharynx Trauma

■ Description

Direct injury to larynx/pharynx.

■ Symptoms

Stridor, hoarseness, subcutaneous emphysema.

■ Diagnosis

History and physical, x-ray, laryngoscopy.

■ Pathology

Injuries include thyroid cartilage fracture, contusions, arytenoid dislocation.

■ Treatment

Observation if stable, tracheotomy if airway obstruction. **Do not intubate.**

15. Tracheoesophageal Fistula

■ Description

Communication between trachea and esophagus.

■ Symptoms

Coughing/choking with liquids, wheezing, chest (mediastinal) infections.

■ **Diagnosis**

History and physical examination, x-ray studies (air in mediastinum can be seen).

■ **Pathology**

Congenital or acquired (cancer, trauma, infection).

■ **Treatment**

Surgery.

B.   **Pulmonary Infections**

1. *Acute Bronchitis*

   ■ **Description**

   Large airway inflammation/infection.

   ■ **Symptoms**

   Fever, purulent productive cough.

   ■ **Diagnosis**

   History and physical exam, chest x-ray (not diagnostic), sputum culture.

   ■ **Pathology**

   Usually viral. May be bacterial.

   ■ **Treatment**

   Antibiotics (if culture positive), otherwise supportive (hydration, expectorants, bronchodilators).

2. *Bronchiolitis*

   ■ **Description**

   Lower respiratory tract infection, with **small airway inflammation/obstruction.**

■ **Symptoms**

Tachypnea, wheezing, fever, and **cough.**

■ **Diagnosis**

History and physical exam, chest x-ray (**overinflation**).

■ **Pathology**

Viral (RSV common); affecting infants younger than 2 (not exclusive of pediatric patients), also seen (rarely) in adults.

■ **Treatment**

Oxygen, fluids, ribavirin for RSV.

3. *Pneumonia*

   3–1. *Influenza*

   ■ **Description**

   Acute pulmonary infection, with rapid onset.

   ■ **Symptoms**

   Asymptomatic or **headache, fever/chills, myalgia.**

   ■ **Diagnosis**

   History and physical exam.

   ■ **Pathology**

   RNA virus, with **3-day incubation.**

   Treatment

   Rest, fluids, acetaminophen (Tylenol). May try **amantadine (Symmetrel) for influenza A.**

3–2. Mycoplasma

■ **Description**

Pneumonia in **young individuals,** of **slow onset.**

■ **Symptoms**

Malaise, may have **dry or purulent productive cough, fever,** sore throat.

■ **Diagnosis**

History and physical exam, chest x-ray, mycoplasma titer, cold agglutinin titer.

■ **Pathology**

Fall outbreaks due to *Mycoplasma pneumoniae.*

■ **Treatment**

Erythromycin or tetracycline.

Additional Information. **Extrapulmonary manifestations** include CNS **disease, erythema multiforme, pericarditis.**

3–3. Legionnaires' Disease

■ **Description**

Most common type of *Legionella* infection.

■ **Symptoms**

Fever/chills, myalgia, cough, nausea/vomiting.

Diagnosis

History and physical exam, leukocytosis, proteinuria, serologic testing (DNA probe), and **culture on charcoal yeast extract agar and urinary antigen.**

■ **Pathology**

Legionella pneumophilia **via soil/water source, not person-to-person.**

■ **Treatment**

Erythromycin IV.

Additional Information. **More common in male smokers, alcoholics,** and those with **chronic disease.**

Look for mental confusion, bradycardia, nausea/vomiting/ diarrhea.

3–4. Pneumococcal

■ **Description**

Most common community-acquired pneumonia.

■ **Symptoms**

Sudden onset of high fever/ chills, cough (rusty sputum), **pleurisy.**

■ **Diagnosis**

History and physical exam, chest x-ray **(consolidating lobar pneumonia),** sputum culture and Gram stain, blood culture. May remember time of exact onset of chills.

■ **Pathology**

Streptococcus pneumoniae. Risk factors include alcoholism, asplenia, and immunocompromised patients **(pneumococci are nor-**

mal flora). Complications include pleural effusion (ranging from transudates to empyemas), meningitis, and DEATH.

■ **Treatment**

Penicillin G, or erythromycin.

3–5. Streptococcal

■ **Description**

Rare.

■ **Symptoms**

Chills, fever, cough, and very ill.

■ **Diagnosis**

History and physical, chest x-ray, sputum/blood culture.

■ **Pathology**

Complication of viral illness (measles, chickenpox). May develop empyema.

■ **Treatment**

Procaine penicillin G.

3–6. Staphylococcal

■ **Description**

Staphylococcus aureus pneumonia.

■ **Symptoms**

High fever, chills, purulent productive cough.

■ **Diagnosis**

History and physical exam, chest x-ray, sputum/blood culture, Gram stain. **X-ray: effusion/ abscess/pneumatocele.**

■ **Pathology**

High mortality. Drug user or endocarditis may be source.

■ **Treatment**

β-Lactamase-resistant penicillin.

3–7. Pseudomonas

■ **Description**

Most frequent etiology of nosocomial pneumonia.

■ **Symptoms**

Fever/chills, cough.

■ **Diagnosis**

History and physical exam, chest x-ray, sputum culture, and Gram stain.

■ **Pathology**

High mortality; common in immunocompromised and mechanically ventilated patients.

■ **Treatment**

Antibiotics (aminoglycoside plus β-lactam agent).

3–8. Pneumocystis carinii

■ **Description**

Opportunistic infection; fungal(?)/parasite.

■ **Symptoms**

Dyspnea/hypoxemia, non-productive **cough, fever,** weight loss, tachypnea.

■ **Diagnosis**

History and physical exam, culture, HIV test, bronchoscopic or rare open-lung biopsy, **elevated lactate dehydrogenase (LDH) enzyme.**

■ **Pathology**

Most common opportunistic HIV infection.

■ **Treatment**

Trimethoprim/sulfamethoxazole, or pentamidine (prophylaxis on HIV population very important).

Additional Information. **Other HIV-related pulmonary infections:** bacterial (tuberculosis [TB], listeria, etc), **fungal (histoplasma, cryptococcus,** etc), and **viral (cytomegalovirus [CMV]).**

4. Tuberculosis

■ **Description**

Mycobacterial infection; pulmonary, genitourinary (GU), gastrointestinal (GI), bone and meningitis may present.

■ **Symptoms**

Asymptomatic, or **weight loss, night sweats, cough,** malaise, and hemoptysis.

■ **Diagnosis**

History and physical exam, chest x-ray, sputum **culture** and smear for **acid-fast bacilli,** skin test, tissue/body fluid exam for *Mycoplasma tuberculosis.*

■ **Pathology**

Mycoplasma tuberculosis; with immunodeficiency **(HIV), and prolonged close contact as risk factors. Airborne infection mechanism.**

■ **Treatment**

Start 4 drugs (Isoniazid 300 mg daily plus rifampin 600 mg daily, PCA and Ethambutol) until culture sensitivities arrive, then narrow treatment according to sensitivities to complete 6 months of treatment. In HIV FOLLOW STRICT CULTURE SENSITIVITIES. Always monitor liver enzymes and tailor drug therapy to individual case. Other treatment modalities include D.O.T. (Direct Observe Therapy) for the poor compliance patient.

Additional Information

Renal TB—sterile pyuria.

Isoniazid (INH)—side effects include neuropathy from pyridoxine loss, and hepatitis.

Positive TB skin test in person with history of BCG vaccine—still indicates TB infection.

5. Histoplasmosis

■ **Description**

Fungal infection.

■ **Symptoms**

Asymptomatic, or **non-productive cough, myalgia,** fever, chest pain, mild flulike presentation.

■ **Diagnosis**

History and physical exam, chest x-ray, serologic testing, in some cases might need lung biopsy.

■ Pathology

Histoplasma capsulatum infection (soil mold); bird/bat droppings in soil grow spores, which are inhaled.

■ Treatment

In mild case no treatment indicated. If more ill, then ketoconazole 400 mg/day, or amphotericin B.

Additional Information. **Progressive disseminated histoplasmosis: associated with AIDS, do blood/bone marrow culture and treat with amphotericin B.**

6. *Coccidioidomycosis*

■ Description

Mold inhalation/infection.

■ Symptoms

Asymptomatic or flulike presentation, arthralgia, erythema nodosum/ multiforme rash.

■ Diagnosis

History and physical exam, serologic testing.

■ Pathology

Coccidioides immitis; common southwest United States mold.

■ Treatment

If mild, no treatment. If severe give amphotericin B.

Additional Information. **Diabetics and blacks tend toward progressive infection.**

7. *Cryptococcosis*

■ Description

Fungal infection. **Fungal meningitis:** *Cryptococcus neoformans* **is most frequent etiology.**

■ Symptoms

Fever, cough, and dissemination in immunocompromised patients.

■ Diagnosis

Fungal culture, chest x-ray.

■ Pathology

Cryptococcus neoformans infection; in **soil and pigeon droppings. Risk factors include AIDS and corticosteroid use.**

■ Treatment

Amphotericin B plus flucytosine.

8. *Lung Abscess*

■ Description

Pus accumulation in the lung.

■ Symptoms

Purulent/putrid sputum, cough, chest pain, fever.

■ Diagnosis

History and physical, **chest x-ray (cavities and air/fluid level),** bronchoscopy/culture, lung biopsy.

■ Pathology

Anaerobic bacteria most often (bacteroides, peptostreptococcus). **Risk**

factors: **poor dentition and aspiration** (CNS disease, overdose, alcoholism, etc).

■ **Treatment**

Antibiotics (**penicillin G, 2 million units IV every 4 hours,** or cephalosporin and aminoglycoside); surgical drainage rarely.

C. **Obstructive Airway Disease**

1. **Chronic Bronchitis**

   ■ **Description**

   Large airway disorder.

   ■ **Symptoms**

   Chronic productive purulent cough, dyspnea, "blue bloater" (central cyanosis and overweight).

   ■ **Diagnosis**

   History and physical exam, chest x-ray, pulmonary function testing **(normal total lung capacity),** arterial blood gas **(hypoxemia),** productive **cough for 3 months,** yearly for at least 2 years.

   ■ **Pathology**

   Results from **smoking, allergy,** or other cause.

   ■ **Treatment**

   Stop smoking, **ipratropium bromide (Atrovent),** bronchodilator meds.

2. **Bronchiectasis**

   ■ **Description**

   Bronchial infection/inflammation, resulting in **bronchi dilation.**

■ **Symptoms**

Productive purulent cough, weight loss, hemoptysis, clubbing.

■ **Diagnosis**

History and physical exam, chest x-ray/computed tomography (CT) scan, bronchography not currently recommended. Bronchoscopy is OK.

■ **Pathology**

Etiology in **cystic fibrosis, infection** and **obstruction.**

■ **Treatment**

Antibiotics, chest PT, bronchodilators, surgery.

3. **Allergic Bronchopulmonary Aspergillosis**

   ■ **Description**

   Variant of asthma.

   ■ **Symptoms**

   Wheezing, central bronchiectasis, productive cough.

   ■ **Diagnosis**

   History and physical exam, **elevated IgE and eosinophils,** chest x-ray (infiltrates), **serologic and skin testing,** and **culture.**

   ■ **Pathology**

   Reaction to *Aspergillus fumigatus*.

   ■ **Treatment**

   Prednisone and Amphotericin B (for *Aspergillus* infection).

4. Asthma

■ Description
Episodic dyspnea/wheezing.

■ Symptoms
Dyspnea, wheezing, or coughing.

■ Diagnosis
History and physical exam, pulmonary function testing (including methacholine bronchoprovocation test and pre- and postbronchodilator studies), chest x-ray.

■ Pathology
Airway hyperreactivity (many different pathways present, leading to airway hyperreactivity; also consider an inflammatory process).

■ Treatment
Inhaled corticosteroids, inhaled cromolyn sodium (not in acute state), sympathomimetics, theophylline, ipratropium bromide, IV steroids use for status or severe exacerbations.

5. Emphysema

■ Description
Chronic obstructive pulmonary disease.

■ Symptoms
Dyspnea, wheezing, cough.

■ Diagnosis
History and physical exam, may present as "pink puffer" (thin, noncyanotic), chest x-ray (flat diaphragm and abnormal retrosternal space), pulmonary function testing **(decreased forced expiratory volume in 1 second [FEV$_1$] and increased total lung capacity [TLC]).**

■ Pathology
Lung damage and enlarged air space beyond terminal bronchiole. Etiology: protease-antiprotease theory.

■ Treatment
Ipratropium bromide, bronchodilators, corticosteroids, oxygen, and **quit smoking!**

6. α$_1$-Antitrypsin Deficiency

■ Description
Inherited glycoprotein lack.

■ Symptoms
Emphysema at early age (or in nonsmoker!), dyspnea, cough.

■ Diagnosis
History and physical exam, **serum protein electrophoresis (no α-globulin peak), chest x-ray (basal bullae, not only found at the bases),** pulmonary function testing.

■ Pathology
Excess elastase (without α$_1$-antitrypsin to inactivate it), results in lung damage.

■ Treatment
See emphysema. Also **α$_1$-proteinase inhibitor** may be tried.

7. Cystic Fibrosis

■ Description
Exocrine gland disorder.

■ Symptoms

Steatorrhea, cough, sputum production.

■ Diagnosis

History and physical exam, **sweat chloride test** (over 60 mEq/L), chest x-ray.

■ Pathology

Autosomal recessive disorder.

■ Treatment

Antibiotics, chest PT.

Additional Information. If azoospermia noted, or *Pseudomonas aeruginosa* in sputum, **think cystic fibrosis in outpatients.**

D. Atelectasis and Aspiration

1. *Atelectasis*

■ Description

Lung collapse (segment, lobe, or lung).

■ Symptoms

Fever, leukocytosis.

■ Diagnosis

History and physical exam, chest x-ray, bronchoscopy.

■ Pathology

Bronchi obstruction (frequently mucus/secretions plug). **Most frequent postop pulmonary problem.** Risk factors include COPD/smoking, obesity, age over 70, and upper abdominal/thoracic surgery.

■ Treatment

Chest PT, incentive spirometry, O.O.B. (out of bed), deep breathing exercises, continuous positive airway pressure (CPAP) and bronchoscopy.

2. *Aspiration*

■ Description

Aspiration of material (secretion, emesis/gastric content, foreign body, etc), into pulmonary tree.

■ Symptoms

Chronic cough, **pneumonia, pulmonary edema, leukocytosis.**

■ Diagnosis

History and physical exam, x-ray studies, bronchoscopy (for foreign body).

■ Pathology

Abnormal gastroesophageal sphincter tone or abnormal glottic function, decrease level of consciousness/alertness, (sedation, coma, postop, etc).

■ Treatment

Prevention (H_2-antagonists), aspiration precautions. Treat infection, supportive care (oxygen).

Additional Information. **Mendelson syndrome: gastric aspiration, often postop, may cause adult respiratory distress syndrome (ARDS). Most risky time for aspiration during surgery is during anesthetic induction.**

E.   **Pneumothorax and Hemothorax**

1. *Pneumothorax*

■ **Description**

Air in pleural space.

■ **Symptoms**

Dyspnea, chest pain.

■ **Diagnosis**

History and physical exam, chest x-ray, hypoxemia.

■ **Pathology**

Traumatic or spontaneous (primary or secondary). **Catamenial pneumothorax: pneumothorax with menstruation.**

■ **Treatment**

Small—observe if stable.

Over 15%—**chest tube/Heimleck valve (percutaneous pneumothorax valve), important to correlate with clinical demands.**

Most common chest tube insertion complication—hemothorax.

2. *Hemothorax*

■ **Description**

Blood in pleural space.

■ **Symptoms**

Dyspnea; if massive, shock.

■ **Diagnosis**

History and physical, **decubitus film (can detect decrease in hematocrit if severe enough), true blood will clot unlike other bloody effusions.**

■ **Pathology**

Etiology—usually **trauma, also seen as a postprocedural complication.**

■ **Treatment**

Very small—observe.

All others—**chest tube** (32 to 40 French with 20 cm water suction), **possible thoracotomy** (for continued bleeding over 200 mL/hour).

F.   **Pneumoconiosis**

1. *Asbestosis*

■ **Description**

Asbestos (a silicate)-induced interstitial lung disorder.

■ **Symptoms**

Asymptomatic, or exertional dyspnea, cough.

■ **Diagnosis**

History and physical exam, chest x-ray (pleural thickening/plaques, effusion, and opacities), pulmonary function testing (restrictive disease), lung biopsy.

■ **Pathology**

Histologic hallmark—ferruginous bodies. Asbestosis may lead to **mesothelioma and GI cancer. Additional risk if patient smokes.**

■ **Treatment**

None (stop smoking).

Additional Information. Prevention: in areas of known possible asbestos exposure (removal sites, industrial pipe maintenance, etc), body suits and respirator masks (EPA approved) required as other government-regulated measurements are to be followed).

2. Silicosis

■ Description

Silica-induced fibrosing lung disease; with **no increased lung cancer risk.**

■ Symptoms

Asymptomatic or **exertional dyspnea and cough.**

■ Diagnosis

History and physical, chest x-ray **(upper lobe nodules** and **eggshell hilar node calcification).**

■ Pathology

Found with sandblasters/miners; TB and bacteria may coexist with silicosis. Silicosis may be **acute, chronic, or accelerated** in type.

■ Treatment
None.

3. Sarcoidosis

■ Description

Granulomatous disorder.

■ Symptoms

Asymptomatic, or **fever, dyspnea, skin/eye/CNS/cardiac symptoms** (erythema nodosum, iritis, arrhythmia, nerve palsy).

■ Diagnosis

History and physical exam, chest x-ray **(bilateral enlarged hilar adenopathy),** biopsy **(non-caseating epithelioid granuloma, with no AFB**

organisms) only true diagnostic feature (other features are helpful but not diagnostic), elevated angiotensin-converting enzyme, possibly elevated calcium, skin test anergy. Pulmonary function test.

■ Pathology

Etiology unknown; more common in blacks.

■ Treatment

Corticosteroids. Cutaneous sarcoid: chloroquine (Plaquenil).

G. Respiratory Failure

1. Newborn Respiratory Distress

■ Description

Hyaline membrane disease.

■ Symptoms

Respiratory distress (cyanosis, grunting, tachypnea).

■ Diagnosis

History and physical exam, chest x-ray **(air bronchograms** and fine reticular pattern).

■ Pathology

Deficient surfactant, and high lung surface tension.

■ Treatment

Oxygen, continuous distending airway pressure (CDAP), or CPAP, and mechanical ventilation.

Additional Information. **Transient tachypnea of the newborn: tachypnea without distress/cyanosis,** usually c-section baby.

2. Adult Respiratory Distress Syndrome (ARDS)

■ **Description**

Acute lung damage syndrome, from **increased pulmonary (alveolar) permeability.**

■ **Symptoms**

Dyspnea, tachypnea, tachycardia.

■ **Diagnosis**

History and physical exam, **hypoxemia with increase $P_{O_2}:F_{I_{O_2}}$ (ratio),** chest x-ray **(non-cardiogenic pulmonary edema, bilateral diffuse infiltrates), stiff lungs** (reduced lung compliance).

■ **Pathology**

Etiology includes **infection, aspiration, shock, drugs,** and multiple other conditions.

■ **Treatment**

Supportive, positive end-expiratory pressure (PEEP), and treat cause.

3. Acute and Chronic Respiratory Failure

■ **Description**

Inadequate oxygenation (P_{O_2} reduced or P_{CO_2} elevated); of acute or chronic nature.

■ **Symptoms**

Dyspnea, hypoxemia (headache, confusion, tachycardia, shock).

■ **Diagnosis**

History and physical exam, pulmonary function testing, **arterial blood gas (hypoxemia/hypercapnia).**

■ **Pathology**

Etiology includes ARDS, pulmonary edema, drugs, and neuromuscular conditions. **Reduced P_{O_2} etiology: impaired diffusion, ventilation-perfusion mismatch, hypoventilation, right-left shunt,** and **reduced inspired P_{O_2}.**

■ **Treatment**

Oxygen, control airway, ventilator (assisted ventilation [A/C] and intermittent mandatory ventilation [IMV]).

4. Respiratory Failure with COPD

■ **Description**

Pulmonary deterioration in COPD, progressing to respiratory failure.

■ **Symptoms**

Exacerbation of COPD symptoms, and hypoxemia (arrhythmia, somnolence, cough, dyspnea).

■ **Diagnosis**

History and physical exam, arterial blood gas, chest x-ray.

■ **Pathology**

Etiology may be infection in COPD patient, resulting in increased airway resistance, and increasing Pa_{CO_2}.

■ **Treatment**

Oxygen, mechanical ventilation, medications.

H. Pulmonary Vascular Disorders

1. Pulmonary Embolism

■ **Description**

Pulmonary thrombus, via the right side of the heart, from the venous system.

■ **Symptoms**

Chest pain, cough, hemoptysis, tachycardia/tachypnea **or non-specific symptoms** (apprehension).

■ **Diagnosis**

History (sudden onset!) and physical exam (fever, rales, or normal), arterial **blood gas (increase A-a gradient, lung scan** (ventilation/perfusion [V/Q]), chest x-ray, ECG with sinus tachycardia and/or $(S_1, Q_3, V_{1-3}$ **T-wave inversion),** pulmonary angiography (gold standard), search for deep-vein thrombosis (DVT) in lower extremities.

■ **Pathology**

Mostly from deep leg vein thrombi and pelvic venous system (less frequent etiology).

■ **Treatment**

Anticoagulation (heparin, then coumadin), thrombolytic medication (use with massive pulmonary embolism [PE] and hypotension), embolectomy (use in non-responding shock case). In pregnancy where coumadin is contraindicated, need to use heparin S/Q until term is reached (keeping therapeutic PTT).

If cannot use anticoagulation, vena caval Greenfield filter. Prevention important for high-risk groups (orthopedic surgery, pelvic/abdominal surgery associated with malignancy, surgery with history of DVT or PE).

Anticoagulation: heparin 5,000 to 10,000 U (80 U/kg) **bolus IV, then 1000 U/hour (18 U/kg/hour IV), (partial thromboplastin time [PTT] 1.5 to 2 times control), duration 5 to 10 days. After 96 hours, start coumadin (to bring prothrombin time [PT] to 1.5 times control).** Continue coumadin 3 months.

Monitor platelet count: **heparin-induced thrombocytopenia.**

2. Pulmonary Hypertension

■ **Description**

Abnormal pulmonary artery pressure.

■ **Symptoms**

Chest pain, dyspnea, lethargy, hemoptysis.

■ **Diagnosis**

History and physical exam **(shortened second heart sound split and louder P_2, weak peripheral pulse/cold hands),** ECG (right heart-strain pattern), chest x-ray, polycythemia. Increase pulmonary wedge pressure (PCWP) and increase pulmonary artery pressures (PAP). **Pulmonary function tests are of no value.**

■ **Pathology**

Major etiology is **hypoxia,** but may also be from obstruction, shunts, or unknown etiology (primary pulmonary hypertension).

■ **Treatment**

Oxygen, vasodilators, anticoagulation(?).

3. Cor Pulmonale

- **Description**

Right ventricular hypertrophy (RVH) secondary to pulmonary disease.

- **Symptoms**

Dyspnea, weight gain, wheezing.

- **Diagnosis**

History and physical exam (cyanosis, edema, ascites, clubbing), ECG (RVH), chest x-ray. **Large pulmonary artery (main and left/right descending), and RVH;** echocardiogram.

- **Pathology**

Overworked right ventricle.

- **Treatment**

Oxygen, bronchodilators, diuretics.

4. Pulmonary Edema

- **Description**

Congestive heart failure.

- **Symptoms**

Dyspnea, diaphoresis, anxiety, wheezing, tachycardia, cyanosis.

- **Diagnosis**

History and physical exam (rales/crackles and/or wheezing, peripheral edema, increased JVD, orthopneic and PND symptoms, most times related to cardiac complaints but not exclusively cardiac in origin, with or without pink/frothy sputum), arterial blood gas, chest x-ray (Kerley B lines, bilateral diffuse infiltrates [puffiness], cardiomegaly, effusion), echocardiogram

(in some cases might be helpful evaluating left ventricular function). Diagnosis done with history, physical exam, and chest x-ray in most of the cases.

- **Pathology**

Excess pulmonary capillary pressure (left ventricle overload, acute myocardial infarction [MI]).

- **Treatment**

Oxygen, medication (furosemide [Lasix], morphine sulphate, venodilators, dopamine [if hypotensive]. Swan–Ganz catheter helpful.

5. Vasculitis

5–1. Goodpasture Syndrome

- **Description**

Pulmonary hemorrhage.

- **Symptoms**

Hemoptysis, glomerulonephritis, anemia, chills/fever/chest pain.

- **Diagnosis**

History and physical exam, and **anti-glomerular basement membrane (GBM) antibodies,** renal biopsy.

- **Pathology**

Antiglomerular basement membrane antibody.

- **Treatment**

Prednisone and cyclophosphamide, plasmapheresis.

5–2. Wegener's Granulomatosis

■ Description

Necrotizing upper and lower pulmonary granulomatous vasculitis.

■ Symptoms

Cough, dyspnea, lethargy, conjunctivitis, glomerulonephritis, fever, purulent sinusitis.

■ Diagnosis

History and physical exam, biopsy/tissue histology (lung biopsy).

■ Pathology

Small artery/vein vasculitis, with granulomas.

■ Treatment

Corticosteroids and cyclophosphamide.

Attention. There are other vasculitis but these are the most frequent asked in test questions. Be aware of the others.

I. Pleural Disorders

1. Pleurisy

■ Description

Pleural inflammation.

■ Symptoms

Inspiratory pain (usually unilateral, and of rapid onset), dyspnea.

■ Diagnosis

History and physical exam, chest x-ray.

■ Pathology

Etiology unknown.

■ Treatment

Indomethacin, intercostal nerve block.

Additional Information. Pleurodynia—epidemic infection in young people, coxsackie B virus, supportive treatment.

2. Pleural Effusion

■ Description

Pleural fluid collection.

■ Symptoms

May be asymptomatic or present as per primary etiology, also dyspnea, pleuritic chest pain.

■ Diagnosis

History and physical exam, chest x-ray (lateral decubitus film), pleural fluid exam.

■ Pathology

Increased capillary permeability or hydrostatic pressure, or decreased lymph drainage or oncotic pressure.

■ Treatment

Treat primary etiology.

Additional Information

1. Transudate—pleural fluid protein divided by serum protein under 0.5 and pleural lactate dehydrogenase (LDH) divided by serum LDH under 0.6. Noted in congestive heart failure (CHF), and renal/liver disease.

2. Exudate—protein and LDH numbers above the transudate values. Empyema or complicated

parapneumonic effusions (LDH > 1000 or pH of fluid < 7.20 and/or decrease glucose concentration). Noted in **infections, malignancy, and trauma.**

J. Pulmonary Neoplasm—Primary and Metastatic Tumors

■ Description

Lung cancer.

■ Symptoms

May be **asymptomatic** or **hemoptysis, cough, dyspnea,** weight loss, fever/chills.

■ Diagnosis

History and physical exam, chest x-ray/CT, bronchoscopy/cytology, biopsy.

■ Pathology

Etiology of lung cancer includes **smoking,** and **environmental/occupational toxin exposure.** Types include **adenocarcinoma (mostly peripheral** and **most frequent type), small cell (oat cell), squamous cell (usually proximal), large cell (undifferentiated),** mesothelioma, sarcoma, melanoma, and others.

■ Treatment

Staging (thoracotomy/bronchoscopy/mediastinoscopy), followed by **surgical excision. Radiation and/or chemotherapy depending on tumor type and stage.**

Additional Information. **Metastatic cancer to the lung may come from colon, breast, melanoma, cervix,** and others.

> *Radiation*—**good for small cell; but not for large cell.**
> *Chemotherapy*—**best therapy for small cell; poor for other types.**

Other lung cancer symptoms—**superior vena caval syndrome, hypercalcemia, Cushing's,** and **carcinoid syndromes.**

Pancoast syndrome—**shoulder pain; Horner syndrome, apex tumor.**

III. PRINCIPLES OF MANAGEMENT

A. Intubation, Tracheostomy, and Assisted Ventilation

■ Description

1. *Intubation*—endotracheal tube: via oral or nasal route, with position confirmed by x-ray and auscultation (where available, also can use PH detector for airway as an aid to confirmed position). Nasal tube is more difficult to suction through than oral tube (and has increased infection risk after 5 days). Endotracheal intubation may be maintained without time limit (in prolonged intubations or recurrent intubations watch for tracheostenosis, also watch for increased balloon pressures and tracheal trauma).

2. *Tracheostomy*—tracheostomy tube: easier to suction through than oral tube. More comfortable to patients for prolonged/extended periods of time. Air must be humidified. As all tubes, bypass normal nose/upper airway humidification. Same precautions as above.

3. *Assisted ventilation*—decision to intubate is clinical in nature (ABG also useful). Clinical signs to look for: paradoxical respirations, increased JVD, pulsus paradoxicus, and increased lethargy are a few of the most popular signs that should be used.

   a. *Initial settings:* FIO_2, 100%; tidal volume, 10 mL/kg; A/C or IMV, 10 to 14 breaths/minute (always need to correlate with clinical scenario).

b. *Most common modes of mechanical ventilation use*—intermittent mandatory ventilation (IMV): delivers set respiratory rate per minute with set tidal volume with each of those breaths. Patient can generate in-between machine breaths, his/her own breaths, and own tidal volume, allowing for patient's own muscles to be exercised.

c. *Assisted ventilation (A/C)*—patient receives set rate per minute with set volumes with each breath. Any extra breaths generated by the patient, in addition to the ones already set, will be assisted (the machine will complete/supplement each breath [volume]) for patient.

Additional Information. **Positive end-expiratory pressure (PEEP). Added to A/C or IMV to produce constant positive ventilation pressure;** most useful for pulmonary edema, ARDS, or other conditions where oxygenation is poor, with settings of 3 to 20 cm water.

Complications of PEEP—**reduced cardiac output** and **pneumothorax.**
Ventilator problem—**disconnect patient from machine, and ventilate by bag. Hard to ventilate: suction patient,** and **rule out pneumothorax, tube position problem, or obstruction. Treat as indicated.**

B. **Massive Hemoptysis**

■ **Description**

Blood flow of 200 to 600 mL into the pulmonary system within 24 hours.

■ **Symptoms**

As described, hemoptysis, hypoxia, dyspnea, lethargy, wheezing.

■ **Diagnosis**

History and physical exam, chest x-ray and lab, bronchoscopy.

■ **Pathology**

Bronchiectasis, TB, vasculitis, fungal cavitations, abscess, and coagulopathies most commonly.

■ **Treatment**

Oxygen, fluids, bronchoscopy, A-gram embolization, correct coagulopathy, and surgery.

BIBLIOGRAPHY

Adams GL. *Fundamentals of Otolaryngology.* 6th ed. Philadelphia, Pa: WB Saunders Co; 1989.

Bass JB, et al. Treatment and Tuberculosis Infection in Adults and Children. *Am Rev Resp Dis:* May 1994; 1359–74.

Baum GL. *Textbook of Pulmonary Diseases.* Vols. 1, 2. 4th ed. Boston, Mass: Little, Brown and Co; 1989.

Civetta JM. *Critical Care.* Philadelphia, Pa: JB Lippincott Co; 1992.

Dosman JA. *The Medical Clinics of North America, Obstructive Lung Disease.* Vol. 74. Philadelphia, Pa: WB Saunders Co; May 1990.

Fraser and Pare. *Diagnosis of Disease of the Chest: Vols. I, II, and III.* Philadelphia, Pa: WB Saunders Co; 1995.

Freundlich IM. *A Radiologic Approach to Diseases of the Chest.* Baltimore, Md: Williams & Wilkins; 1992.

George RB. *Chest Medicine, Essentials of Pulmonary and Critical Care Medicine.* 2nd ed. Baltimore, Md: Williams & Wilkins; 1990.

Guenter CA. *Pulmonary Medicine.* 2nd ed. Philadelphia, Pa: JB Lippincott Co; 1982.

Light RW. *Pleural Diseases.* 2nd ed. Philadelphia, Pa: Lea & Febiger; 1990.

Middleton E. *Allergy Principles and Practices.* Vols. I and II. 3rd ed. Mosby; 1988.

Murray JF. *Textbook of Respiratory Medicine.* Philadelphia, Pa: WB Saunders Co; 1994.

Pennington JE. *Respiratory Infections: Diagnosis and Management.* New York: Raven Press; 1988.

Pinsky MR. *Pathophysiologic Foundations of Critical Care.* Baltimore, Md: Williams & Wilkins; 1993.

Schroeder SA. *Current Medical Diagnosis and Treatment.* 30th ed. Norwalk, Conn: Appleton & Lange; 1991.

Simmons DH. *Current Pulmonology.* Vols. 1 to 3. New York: John Wiley and Sons; 1981.

CHAPTER 17

Renal System and Urology

JOEL S. GOLDBERG, DO

I. HEALTH AND HEALTH MAINTENANCE

A. Urinary Tract Infection

■ Description

Epidemiology—more frequent in females (except in neonates), and increases with age.

Impact—recurrent infections and renal damage.

Risk factors—obstructive uropathy (calculus, stricture/valves), vesico-ureteral reflux, diabetes mellitus, sexual activity, and pregnancy.

Prevention—patient education, for both prevention/hygiene, early intervention/treatment, and prophylactic antibiotics where indicated.

B. Toxic Nephropathy

■ Description

Epidemiology—common causes include **analgesics, penicillin/sulfa, phenytoin sodium (Dilantin), cimetidine (Tagamet), heavy metals, and aminoglycosides.** Noted in chronic pain patients with continued analgesic use.

Impact—papillary necrosis/renal failure.

Risk factors—compounds listed, occupational/environmental exposure to toxins, and both calcium disorders (sarcoid, multiple myeloma, etc), and antineoplastic agents.

Prevention—patient education and early intervention/diagnosis (discontinue the offending agent). Special consideration is given to the elderly in whom reduced renal function may contribute to elevated serum toxin levels and earlier toxicity.

C. Renal Failure/Disease Prevention

■ Description

Prevention of acute renal failure and of urinary tract disease secondary to formation of calculi and/or obstruction. Where **absorptive hypercalciuria** is noted, **reduced-calcium diet, ion-exchange resin (sodium cellulose), hydration,** and **orthophosphates. For renal hypercalciuria** use **thiazides. For hyperuricosuria** use **allopurinol.** For **struvite/chronic infection stones, use repeat cultures/antibiotics.** For **hypercystinuria, alkalinize the urine.** For **obstructions,** treat/remove obstruction when indicated.

D. Limiting Renal Disease Progression

■ Description

Control underlying disorder (hypertension, diabetes mellitus, etc). Dietary measures include protein/potassium/phosphorus restriction for chronic renal failure. Limit extra dietary magnesium, treat acidosis, and supply additional calcium when required.

E. Economic Impact

■ Description

Nephrotoxic agents, uncontrolled hypertension/diabetes, and infections may ultimately lead to the need for dialysis. Increasing range of indications include drug overdose, severe hyperkalemia and hypercalcemia, congestive heart failure (CHF), and pulmonary edema.

Impact includes both benefits to the patient, and risks (sepsis, hypotension, etc) along with ever-increasing costs involved. Expanding indications and prolongation of life result in increased need for continued services, and increased health care financial burden.

II. MECHANISMS OF DISEASE AND DIAGNOSIS

A. Male Reproductive System Disorders

1. Prostatitis

■ **Description**

Prostate inflammation/infection.

■ **Symptoms**

Dysuria, chills/fever, low back pain, frequency.

■ **Diagnosis**

History and physical exam, **large (boggy if chronic) tender gland.** Avoid prostate massage (bacteremia risk).

■ **Pathology**

Escherichia coli (usually aerobic gram-negative rods).

■ **Treatment**

Antibiotics (trimethoprim-sulfamethoxazole, for example).

2. Epididymitis

■ **Description**

Epididymitis inflammation/infection.

■ **Symptoms**

Tender enlarged testicle and/or epididymis, fever.

■ **Diagnosis**

History and physical exam, **scrotum may be red/tender.** Pyuria, epididymitis tender. Urethra/urine culture and Gram stain. Elevating scrotum may reduce epididymitis pain, but increase torsion pain **(Prehn's sign).**

■ **Pathology**

Organisms include *Neisseria gonorrhoea, E. coli,* and *Chlamydia.*

■ **Treatment**

Tetracycline, or antibiotic as per culture.

3. Orchitis

■ **Description**

Testicular inflammation.

■ **Symptoms**

Fever, testicular size increase, and erythema.

■ **Diagnosis**

History and physical (H and P), rule out mumps, usually no urethral symptoms/discharge.

■ **Pathology**

Complication of mumps, tuberculosis (TB), and other infections.

■ **Treatment**

Antibiotic (if bacterial), scrotal support, ice first 24 to 48 hours, then warm soaks.

4. Urethritis

■ **Description**

Urethral infection.

■ **Symptoms**

Discharge, dysuria.

■ **Diagnosis**

History and physical examination, urethral culture/Gram stain.

■ **Pathology**

Sexual transmission common. Gono-coccal (GC) and non-gonococcal ure-thritis (NGU) (*Chlamydia, Trichomonas,* herpes simplex).

■ **Treatment**

Antibiotics, doxycycline.

5. **Sexually Transmitted Diseases (STDs)**

5–1. **Gonorrhea**

■ **Description**

Gonococcal infection.

■ **Symptoms**

Dysuria, urethritis/discharge (thick yellow).

■ **Diagnosis**

H and P, culture/Gram stain (gram-negative intracellular dip-lococci).

■ **Pathology**

Neisseria gonorrhoeae.

■ **Treatment**

Antibiotics (ceftriaxone 250 mg intramuscularly [IM], plus doxy-cycline 100 mg twice daily for 1 week). *(for concurrent chlamydial infection which is assumed*

5–2. **Syphilis**

■ **Description**

Spirochetal STD.

■ **Symptoms**

Penile painless lesion: chancre (primary syphilis). → *often not noticed*

2° syphilis: maculopapular rash over hands & feet (palms & soles)

3° syphilis: neurosyphilis · tabes dorsalis

■ **Diagnosis**

RPR, VDRL
FTA-ABS

History and physical, serologic test for syphilis (STS) and fluo-rescent treponemal antibody ab-sorption (FTA-ABS) studies.

■ **Pathology**

Treponema pallidum.

■ **Treatment**

Benzathine penicillin G, 2.4 million U IM (if allergic to penicillin, give doxycycline).

5–3. **Chlamydia**

■ **Description**

Common STD.

■ **Symptoms**

Dysuria, frequency, or asympto-matic.

■ **Diagnosis**

Urethral culture/Gram stain, *Chlamydia* culture.

■ **Pathology**

Chlamydia trachomatis.

■ **Treatment**

Doxycycline 100 mg twice daily for 1 week.

5–4. **Human Immunodeficiency Virus (HIV)/Acquired Immunodeficiency Syndrome (AIDS)**

■ **Description**

Human immunodeficiency virus.

■ Symptoms

Night sweats, fever, adenopathy, weight loss, prostatic cryptococcus, and urinary tract lymphoma.

■ Diagnosis

History and physical, serologic testing (HIV and Western blot for confirmation).

■ Pathology

Cell-mediated immunity defect.

■ Treatment

Consult current literature.

6. Testicular Torsion

■ Description

Testicular rotation and loss of blood supply. **Most common cause of scrotal swelling in children.**

■ Symptoms

Testicular pain/swelling, vomiting and/or abdominal pain. May have initially only abdominal pain; check scrotum!

■ Diagnosis

History and physical, pain unchanged or worse with testicular elevation. Urine negative, and affected testicle may be elevated in position.

■ Pathology

Abnormal tunica vaginalis attachment allowing room for testicular twisting ("bell-clapper deformity").

■ Treatment

Surgery (within 4 to 6 hours, if possible).

7. Undescended Testicle

■ Description

Non-descended testicle (cryptorchidism).

■ Symptoms

None. Pick up on exam only (50% of premature males have undescended testicle).

■ Diagnosis

History and physical exam. Rule out retractile testis (hyperactive cremaster muscle pull).

■ Pathology

Abnormal descent (normally testicle pulled down by gubernaculum).

■ Treatment

Surgery by age 1 **(orchiopexy)**. Hormones have been tried (human chorionic gonadotropin [hCG]).

8. Neoplasm of the Testis—Seminoma

■ Description

Testicular tumor. (equivalent of dysgerminoma in ♀)

■ Symptoms

Painless mass. May have fullness/pain at times, or metastatic disease symptoms.

■ Diagnosis

History and physical examination, ultrasound, and transillumination. **Pos-**

sible elevated β-hCG. α-Fetoprotein (AFP), usually normal, removal and biopsy.

■ Pathology

Cause unknown, more frequent if undescended testicle history. Usually ages 40 to 50.

■ Treatment

Seminoma most common, treat with orchiectomy and radiotherapy (plus chemo if bulky/distant metastatic).

9. Prostate Neoplasm—Benign Prostatic Hyperplasia

■ Description

Glandular hyperplasia.

■ Symptoms

Obstruction (hesitancy, dribbling, reduced stream force), and urgency, nocturia, frequency, renal failure.

■ Diagnosis

History and physical examination. Intravenous pyelogram (IVP) (bilateral hydronephrosis), ultrasound, retrograde urography, cystoscopy.

■ Pathology

Hyperplasia, increasing incidence with age, etiology unknown, resulting in increased intravesical pressure, increased residual urine.

■ Treatment

Transurethral prostatectomy (TURP), alpha-blockers (prazosin, phenoxybenzamine), finasteride (Proscar).

10. Prostate Cancer

■ Description

Most common cancer in elderly males.

■ Symptoms

Long bone fracture/x-ray lesion, **obstructive uropathy,** frequency, urgency, hematuria, weight loss, or asymptomatic.

■ Diagnosis

History and physical, serum prostate-specific antigen (PSA) study, **ultrasound, and biopsy.**

■ Pathology

Adenocarcinoma usually, with spread to bone (vertebrae), lung (less often), liver. Stage A (histologic cancer, found in transurethral prostatectomy [TURP]), B (palpated cancer in gland), C (outside capsule without metastasis), and D (metastatic). **Etiology unknown,** but genetics/hormones/environment play a role.

■ Treatment

Check current literature, treat by stage: currently A/B, radical prostatectomy or radiation; C, radiation; D, hormone treatment (orchiectomy, luteinizing hormone-releasing hormone [LH-RH] agonists, etc). **Most cancer in peripheral zone** of prostate.

11. Penile Disorders—Hypospadias

■ Description

Most frequent urologic anomaly, with meatus below penis tip.

■ **Symptoms**

None. May be associated with chordee (**ventral penile curve**).

■ **Diagnosis**

Physical examination.

■ **Pathology**

Urethral ridges do not fuse, possibly hereditary.

■ **Treatment**

Surgical if meatus too proximal. Look for associated anomalies.

Additional Information. **Most common etiology of ambiguous genitalia, adrenal hyperplasia** (check for Y chromosome).

12. *Hydrocele and Varicocele*

■ **Description**

Hydrocele—fluid around testis (in tunica vaginalis layers).
Varicocele—pampiniform plexus vein dilation.

■ **Symptoms**

Non-tender scrotal mass.

■ **Diagnosis**

Transillumination, H and P, ultrasound. Varicocele may be absent when supine, increase if straining/standing (Valsalva).

■ **Pathology**

Hydrocele—**patent processus vaginalis.**
Varicocele—inefficient pampiniform valves.

■ **Treatment**

Observation, surgical if not resolving on own, or if resulting in infertility (varicocele), or symptoms (pressure).

13. *Urethral Stricture*

■ **Description**

Fibrotic urethral narrowing.

■ **Symptoms**

May be **asymptomatic**, prostatitis, obstruction (abnormal stream angle/spraying, or narrow stream), cystitis.

■ **Diagnosis**

Cystourethrogram, H and P, flow studies, culture, cystoscopy.

■ **Pathology**

May have history of **gonorrhea**, trauma, or other infections.

■ **Treatment**

Dilation.

B. **Bladder/Collecting System Disorders**

1. *Cystitis, Dysuria, Hematuria, and Pyuria*

■ **Description**

Cystitis is bladder infection.

■ **Symptoms**

Cystitis presents as dysuria, frequency, nocturia, urgency.

■ **Diagnosis**

History and physical exam, urine analysis, and culture.

■ **Pathology**

Cystitis usually from *E. coli.*

■ **Treatment**

Antibiotics.

Additional Information

Dysuria may be symptom of cystitis, or urethral syndrome in females.

Pyuria is **leukocytes in urine,** but **not necessarily infection (pyuria and negative culture: rule out TB).**

Hematuria may be sign of infection, cancer, in runners, renal disease. Always abnormal in males; cystoscope to rule out tumor.

Casts suggest **renal disease** (leukocyte, pyelonephritis; red blood cell [RBC] casts, glomerulitis).

2. *Carcinoma of the Bladder*

■ **Description**

Bladder cancer, **most are transitional cell.**

■ **Symptoms**

Hematuria, with/without other symptoms (dysuria, frequency, etc).

■ **Diagnosis**

History and physical, urinary cytology, **cystoscopy,** biopsy.

■ **Pathology**

Increased incidence in **smokers** and with **carcinogen/toxin exposure.**

■ **Treatment**

Surgical with/without intravesical chemo, transurethral resection of bladder tumor (TURBT). Radiation in addition in advanced disease. Consult current literature.

3. *Urolithiasis*

■ **Description**

Ureter calculus.

■ **Symptoms**

Severe pain, nausea/vomiting, flank pain, hematuria. **Caliceal,** may be asymptomatic; **proximal ureter,** severe intermittent flank pain, colic; **distal ureter**/ureterovesicle junction, radiating pain, bladder irritation, groin pain.

■ **Diagnosis**

History and physical examination, IVP, urine analysis. **Uric acid stones not visible on plain x-ray.**

■ **Pathology**

Etiology in infection or metabolic abnormality.

■ **Treatment**

Medical (absorptive hypercalciuria, fluids, low-calcium diet, orthophosphates; renal hypercalciuria, thiazides; cystine stones, hydration and alkalinization of the urine) and/or surgical. Most stones under 4 mm in distal ureter will pass (increase fluids/strain urine).

4. *Ureteral Reflux*

■ **Description**

Reflux of urine into ureter with voiding.

■ **Symptoms**

Infection/pyelonephritis, kidney damage/uremia.

- **Diagnosis**

History and physical, urine analysis and culture, IVP, **voiding cystoure-thrography.**

- **Pathology**

Weak trigone tone, short intramural ureter.

- **Treatment**

Medical (watch and wait, antibiotics), surgical (urinary diversion, uretero-vesicle junction repair [ureteroneocy-totomy])

5. Neurogenic Bladder

- **Description**

Neurologic etiology of bladder control loss.

- **Symptoms**

Voiding dysfunction.

- **Diagnosis**

History and physical examination, urodynamic testing (cystometrogram [CMG], flowmeter, etc).

- **Pathology**

Sensory, motor, uninhibited, reflex, and **autonomous.**

> *Sensory*—no sensation of full bladder, diabetics, herniated disc.
> *Motor*—sensation OK, but cannot initiate contraction, disc, polio, tumor.
> *Uninhibited*—no control, brain/CNS lesion or disease.
> *Reflex-spinal cord injury, autonomous*—no connection from bladder to brain, spinal trauma.

- **Treatment**

Medical (medication, bethanechol; suprapubic/abdominal pressure, Credé, catheter), and surgical (sphincterotomy).

6. Urinary Incontinence

- **Description**

Involuntary voiding.

- **Symptoms**

Loss of urine with activity, coughing, or without reason.

- **Diagnosis**

History and physical examination, urine analysis and culture, urodynamic studies, cystoscopy, IVP.

- **Pathology**

Vast etiology (stress incontinence, infection, obstruction, medications, neurogenic bladder, detrusor instability, etc).

- **Treatment**

Depends on etiology, medical/surgical. Includes intermittent catheterization, antibiotics, α-adrenergics for stress incontinence, anticholinergics for detrusor instability.

7. Enuresis

- **Description**

Involuntary voiding, typically **night** bedwetting.

- **Symptoms**

Unable to retain urine, day or night.

■ Diagnosis

History and physical, excretory urogram, urine analysis, and culture.

■ Pathology

Psychological, organic disease, or delayed CNS/neuromuscular development (most common etiology).

■ Treatment

Wait, 1-desamino-8-D arginine vasopressin (DDAVP), imipramine.

8. Obstruction

■ Description

Urinary tract obstruction. Leads to hydronephrosis.

■ Symptoms

Dribbling, infection, alteration in stream size, urgency. May have flank pain, hematuria, and fever (upper tract).

■ Diagnosis

History and physical exam, IVP, cystoscopy.

■ Pathology

Stricture, urethral valve (lower), prostate (mid), kidney/ureter lesion (upper tract).

■ Treatment

Surgical.

9. Hydronephrosis

■ Description

Kidney/ureter damage from ureter obstruction.

■ Symptoms

May be asymptomatic, also flank/back pain, infections. In infant may have multiple non-specific symptoms.

■ Diagnosis

History and physical exam, ultrasound, IVP, retrograde study, cystoscopy.

■ Pathology

Obstruction or reflux, in child often uteropelvic junction obstruction; in adult may be benign prostatic hypertrophy (BPH), calculus, tumor, aortic aneurysm.

■ Treatment

Surgical.

C.   Disorders of the Kidneys

1. Pyelonephritis (Acute and Chronic)

■ Description

Ascending infection/inflammation into the kidney.

■ Symptoms

Chills/fever, vomiting, flank pain, anorexia.

■ Diagnosis

History and physical exam, urine analysis (white blood cell [WBC] casts, pyuria) and culture, blood culture, complete blood count (CBC). Chronic pyelonephritis: renal damage with persisting infection.

■ Pathology

Usually *E. coli*. Also *Pseudomonas*.

■ **Treatment**

Antibiotics (IV cephalosporin and aminoglycoside). If recurrent/chronic infection, rule out organic disease and coexisting medical conditions.

2. Glomerulonephritis

■ **Description**

Kidney inflammation with glomeruli as area of disorder.

■ **Symptoms**

Hematuria, proteinuria, reduced glomerular filtration rate (GFR) resulting in **hypertension, edema.**

■ **Diagnosis**

History and physical exam, urine analysis and culture, serologic studies to attempt to define cause.

■ **Pathology**

Inflammation/immune deposits resulting in glomerular injury.

■ **Treatment**

None. Treat primary disease and complications. Chronic glomerulonephritis: end stage of any glomerular disorder, small kidneys, renal failure.

3. Minimal Change Disease

■ **Description**

Idiopathic glomerular disease.

■ **Symptoms**

Proteinuria, hematuria, edema.

■ **Diagnosis**

History and physical exam, urine analysis, **biopsy.**

■ **Pathology**

Etiology unknown.

■ **Treatment**

Steroids.

4. Immunoglobulin A (IgA) Nephropathy

■ **Description**

Berger's disease (a variety of Henoch–Schönlein purpura).

■ **Symptoms**

Gross hematuria after viral infection, fever, proteinuria, dysuria.

■ **Diagnosis**

History and physical exam, possible elevated serum IgA, **biopsy.**

■ **Pathology**

Immune deposits of IgA on glomeruli.

■ **Treatment**

None.

5. Diabetic Nephropathy

■ **Description**

Glomerulus microvascular damage.

■ **Symptoms**

Azotemia, proteinuria.

■ **Diagnosis**

History and physical exam, renal biopsy.

■ **Pathology** (diabetic nephropathy)

Microvascular glomerular damage and Kimmelstiel–Wilson lesions (nodular deposits in glomeruli).

■ **Treatment**

Dialysis, transplant.

6. Nephrotic Syndrome

■ **Description**

Syndrome secondary to glomerular disease.

■ **Symptoms**

Significant proteinuria (over 3.5 g/day), hypoalbuminemia, edema, hyperlipidemia, lipiduria. (no HTN or hematuria)

■ **Diagnosis**

History and physical exam, urine analysis, serum immune complex/complement studies, biopsy.

■ **Pathology**

A result of medication, infection, allergic reactions, systemic disease, and other states, where capillary wall permeability increased to protein. Most common etiology: idiopathic!

When idiopathic, often minimal Δ disease ≡ no LM changes!

■ **Treatment**

Treat etiology where possible. Mild diuretic, reduce dietary sodium, prednisone.

7. Proteinuria

■ **Description**

Elevated urinary protein.

■ **Symptoms**

Asymptomatic.

■ **Diagnosis**

Urine analysis or dipstick, followed by 24-hour urine protein collection.

■ **Pathology**

Includes reduced protein reabsorption (Fanconi syndrome), elevated glomerular protein permeability (nephrotic syndrome), elevated plasma protein level (overflow, Bence Jones).

■ **Treatment**

Define and treat primary cause.

8. Interstitial Nephropathy

■ **Description**

Interstitial inflammation.

■ **Symptoms**

Polyuria, nocturia, acute renal failure, fever, rash, joint pain.

■ **Diagnosis**

History and physical examination, eosinophilia, renal biopsy.

■ **Pathology**

Wide variety of infections, toxins (heavy metals), calcium disorders, drugs, and systemic disorders as etiologic agents.

(Cipro, zyloprim, maxi)
(allopurinol)

■ **Treatment**

Remove offending agent, treat primary disease.

Additional Information

Interstitial nephritis—no marked proteinuria, rarely elevated BP, high uric acid.

Glomerulonephritis—marked proteinuria, elevated BP, minimal uric acid elevation.

9. Renal Failure

9–1. Acute

■ Description

Acute renal function reduction, and buildup of nitrogenous byproducts (azotemia). Anuria: no urine flow.

■ Symptoms

May have reduced output, azotemia. Facial edema, fluid retention.

■ Diagnosis

History and physical, urine analysis, **reduced urine volume/elevated serum creatinine,** kidneys, ureters, bladder (KUB), blood and urine studies (osmolality, electrolytes, etc), other x-ray studies. **Oliguric renal failure: 24-hour urine under 400 mL;** if more urine output, termed **high-output (non-oliguric) acute renal failure.** *(≥ 400 ml / 24 hours)*

■ Pathology

Prerenal (hypovolemia), **renal** (interstitial nephritis), or **postrenal** (obstruction).

■ Treatment

Treat/correct etiology where possible. Medical management including **fluid/electrolyte** and **protein/calorie** adjustment. Dialysis.

Additional Information

Prerenal azotemia—urine osmolality over 500, **urinary Na under 20,** try fluid challenge. *(highly concentrated urine b/c kidney thinks theres no blood!)*

Renal failure—urine osmolality under 400, **urinary Na over 40.** *Kidney can not concentrate* *Peritoneal dialysis*—use short term, watch for peritonitis.

9–2. Chronic

■ Description

Long-term renal function reduction.

■ Symptoms

May have reduced urine output, **lethargy, hypertension, myopathy, pruritus,** pericarditis, **anemia.**

■ Diagnosis

See Renal Failure.

■ Pathology

Etiology in numerous disorders.

■ Treatment   *(low protein)*

Treat complications, proper diet, balance electrolytes, and treat anemia and osteodystrophy.

Additional Information. Most common skeletal lesion in chronic renal failure (CRF): **osteitis fibrosa.** **Lack of erythropoietin results in CRF anemia. Serum phosphate is elevated with reduced GFR** (eg, chronic renal failure).

Total serum calcium is reduced in CRF.

10. Renal Osteodystrophy

■ Description

Skeletal abnormality secondary to chronic renal failure (CRF).

(Renal Osteodystrophy)

■ Symptoms

Children—growth retardation, rickets.

Adults—may be asymptomatic, or bone pain, proximal muscle weakness.

■ Diagnosis

History and physical exam, x-ray findings.

■ Pathology

Subperiosteal bone resorption. Results in osteitis fibrosa and osteomalacia.

■ Treatment

Control serum calcium/phosphorus (phosphate binders), parathyroidectomy. Drug of choice for hypocalcemia/secondary hyperparathyroidism is vitamin D.

D.O.C ⇒ vit D
failing kidney can not convert 10-VitD to 10,25OH-VitD!

11. Papillary Necrosis

■ Description

Kidney papilla necrosis. May be a complication of pyelonephritis. *(or independent problem)*

■ Symptoms

Hematuria, fever, flank pain, renal failure.

■ Diagnosis

History and physical exam, IVP, urine analysis, and culture.

■ Pathology

Ischemic, usually associated infection. Chronic disease, toxins, obstructions.

■ Treatment

Treat primary etiology (infection, etc).

12. Hypertensive Renal Disease

12–1. Pre-eclampsia

■ Description

Pregnancy-related hypertensive disease, with proteinuria.

■ Symptoms

Edema, proteinuria, and hypertension after 24th week. May also have oliguria, disseminated intravascular coagulation (DIC), and hyperreflexia, headache.

blurry vision

■ Diagnosis

Symptoms plus history and physical exam, urine analysis; BP 140/90 or higher for 4 to 6 hours, or 30 mm Hg increase (systolic) or 15 mm Hg (diastolic) compared to early pregnancy readings. May have nephrotic syndrome.

■ Pathology

Etiology unknown. Glomerular capillary endotheliosis is the pathologic renal alteration.

■ Treatment

Bed rest, sedation, antihypertensives (hydralazine), delivery. For severe pre-eclampsia, give magnesium sulfate (loading dose 4 to 6 g, then 1 to 2 g/hour).

prevent seizures = Eclampsia

12–2. Eclampsia

■ Description

Pre-eclampsia and seizures.

■ Symptoms

Edema, proteinuria, hypertension, and seizures.

- **Diagnosis**

History and physical exam. **No test, measure BP/urinary protein.** *plus pt must have seizure!*

- **Pathology**

See Pre-eclampsia.

- **Treatment**

Control BP, prevent seizures (magnesium sulfate).

Additional Information. **Monitor magnesium sulfate by deep tendon reflexes, urinary output, respirations,** serum magnesium level.

13. Renovascular Hypertension

- **Description**

Renal artery stenotic lesion. *Causes ↑ bp*

- **Symptoms**

Hypertension, may be **rapid onset at any age, difficult to control, childhood** or **older adult onset.**

- **Diagnosis**

History and physical exam (epigastric bruit), IVP, renal/digital subtraction angiography (DSA), renal vein renin ratio over 1.5.

- **Pathology**

young ♀ c̄ HTN ← (Fibromuscular hyperplasia) or **atheroma.**
↳ *old ♂ c̄ sudden ↑ in HTN*

- **Treatment**

Surgical (including angioplasty) or medication (captopril).

14. Nephrosclerosis

- **Description**

Renal sclerosis.

- **Symptoms**

Hypertensive renal disease. Renal failure, proteinuria, hematuria, small kidneys, or no symptoms.

- **Diagnosis**

History and physical exam, urine analysis.

- **Pathology**

Renal vascular lesions.

- **Treatment**

Treat blood pressure.

15. Lupus Nephritis

- **Description**

Lupus may present as interstitial nephritis or glomerulonephritis.

- **Symptoms**

Hematuria, proteinuria, hypertension, edema, red cell/hyaline casts. *⊕ other st of Lupus ⊕ AN*

- **Diagnosis**

History and physical exam, urine analysis, lupus symptoms (rash, fever, weight loss, joint symptoms, etc), serologic testing (antinuclear antibodies [ANA], anti-DS–DNA, etc), renal biopsy.

- **Pathology**

Interstitial fibrosis and inflammation. Includes several histologic types (minimal, mesangial, focal, diffuse, and **membranous**).

■ Treatment

Prednisone, cyclophosphamide, azathioprine.

16. Inherited Disorders—Polycystic Kidney Disease

■ Description

Hereditary cystic kidney disorder.

■ Symptoms

Hematuria, flank pain, hypertension, pyelonephritis, uremia.

■ Diagnosis

History and physical (enlarged kidney), **IVP, ultrasound. Child: bilateral flank mass.**

■ Pathology

assoc c̄ berry aneurysm in brain ←

Adult polycystic kidney disease— autosomal dominant, cysts. → *presents as renal failure in adulthood*
Infantile polycystic disease— autosomal recessive, collecting duct dilation → *early renal failure, can be dx @ u/s*
assoc c̄ liver cysts

■ Treatment

Blood pressure control, antibiotics, dialysis, renal transplant.

Additional Information. **Cysts also in liver** and **pancreas. Positive association of polycystic kidney disease and intracranial aneurysms.**

17. Neoplasms—Wilms' Tumor

■ Description

Rare but **treatable childhood tumor (nephroblastoma).**

■ Symptoms

Asymptomatic abdominal mass, hematuria, fever, abdominal pain.

■ Diagnosis

History and physical exam, IVP, **ultrasound/CT, biopsy.**

■ Pathology

Peak incidence age 3. ✶

■ Treatment

Stage 1 (kidney)—radical nephrectomy, chemotherapy (actinomycin/vincristine).
Stage 2 (extrarenal, but surgically excised)—similar.
Stage 3 and 4—same as 1 or 2 plus radiotherapy.

Additional Information

*Nephroblastoma—*usually **unilateral,** usually **not metastatic,** no marker.
*Neuroblastoma—*cross midline, **metastatic, possible positive marker** vanillylmandelic acid (**VMA**).

18. Adenocarcinoma

■ Description

Most common primary renal cancer; called **hypernephroma.**

■ Symptoms

Hematuria, flank pain, mass, hypertension, anemia, multiple other systemic symptoms possible.

■ Diagnosis

History and physical, KUB, IVP, CT/ magnetic resonance imaging (MRI), ultrasound.

- **Pathology**

Cause unknown. **Analgesics and smoking raise risk of developing hypernephroma,** as do toxins, polycystic kidney disease, and other conditions.

- **Treatment**

If local disease, **radical nephrectomy;** addition of radiation/hormones if metastatic.

D. Electrolyte and Acid–Base Disorders

1. Hyponatremia

- **Description**

Sodium under 130.

[handwritten: Serum Osm = $2Na + \frac{BUN}{28} + \frac{Gluc}{18}$]

- **Symptoms**

Confusion, vomiting, coma, nausea, lethargy.

[handwritten annotations across top: low Na — low Osm → most common; normal Osm → pseudohyponatremia; high Osm → DKA, hyperglycemic coma, mannitol, D50]
[handwritten: low volume dehydration; normal vol SIADH; high vol CHF nephrosis cirrhosis; (hyperlipidemia, hyperproteinemia)]

- **Diagnosis**

History and physical examination (decreased deep tendon reflex, seizures), electrolytes.

- **Pathology**   *[handwritten: (aldosterone deficiency?)]*

~~Excess salt loss~~ (diuretic use), water retention (renal/cardiac failure, syndrome of inappropriate antidiuretic hormone [SIADH]).

- **Treatment**

Salt loss—give saline.
Water excess—restrict water.

Additional Information. **With pigmentation increase, low BP, low sodium; think Addison's disease.** Hyponatremia also seen in TURP syndrome: intraoperative irrigation absorbed by prostate sinuses; stop procedure, give diuretic.

2. Hypernatremia

- **Description**

Elevated sodium, over 145.

- **Symptoms**

Thirst, hypotension, oliguria, hyperpnea, coma.

- **Diagnosis**

History and physical exam, electrolytes.

- **Pathology**   *[handwritten: (Diabetes insipidus)]*

Excess water loss, impaired thirst, and solute loss (diabetic ketoacidosis).

- **Treatment**

Replace water.

Additional Information. **Replace water with half-normal saline or 5% D and W (with caution).** **Too rapid, brain swelling.**

3. Hypokalemia

- **Description**

Potassium (K) under 3.5 mEq/L.

- **Symptoms**

Arrhythmia, muscle weakness/ cramps, rhabdomyolysis.

[handwritten: Slow correction of all Na+ disturbances to prevent brain injury]

- **Diagnosis**

History and physical exam, serum electrolytes, electrocardiogram (ECG) (smaller/wider T wave, U wave, AV block).

- **Pathology**

Etiology **in gastrointestinal (GI) and urinary loss, decreased intake** (uncommon), **shift into cells** (delirium tremens, hypothermia, increased insulin as in hyperglycemia therapy).

■ Treatment

Potassium replacement via potassium chloride, control loss. **Rapid replacement not advised, stay under 20 mEq/hour IV.**

Additional Information. **Periodic paralysis: low, normal, or high potassium, muscle weakness.**

4. Hyperkalemia

■ Description

Potassium over 5 mEq/L.

■ Symptoms

Diarrhea, weakness.

■ Diagnosis

History and physical, serum electrolytes, ECG (wide QRS, peaked T).

May degenerate to sine-wave ECG

■ Pathology

Reduced renal excretion, excess intake, adrenocortical insufficiency.

■ Treatment

Ca++ gluconate acutely to counter ↑K+ ECG Δ's; then give NaHCO3, glucose + insulin, Kayexalate

Stop potassium, exchange resin (sodium polystyrene sulfonate [Kayexalate]), insulin/50% glucose, dialysis. *If really bad, do dialysis 1st!*

5. Volume Depletion

■ Description

Water deficiency. → *Salt deficiency!*

■ Symptoms

Thirst, dehydration (sunken eyes, reduced skin turgor, etc), coma.

■ Diagnosis

History and physical, **increased serum sodium, blood urea nitrogen (BUN), and osmolality.**

■ Pathology

Excessive water loss, reduced intake, or "third spacing."

■ Treatment

Fluids. **If high sodium/glucose, use hypotonic fluids. If low sodium, use ISO or hypertonic fluids.**

6. Volume Excess

■ Description

Water excess.

■ Symptoms

Weakness, nausea, seizure, coma.

■ Diagnosis

History and physical, electrolytes (low sodium, BUN).

■ Pathology

SIADH, renal failure, CHF.

■ Treatment

Restrict water.

7. Water Intoxication

■ Description

Too much water!

■ Symptoms

Low sodium, stupor, seizures.

■ **Diagnosis**

History and physical examination, electrolytes, urine analysis, serum osmolality.

■ **Pathology**

Psychiatric etiology typical.

■ **Treatment**

Stop fluids.

8. *Alkalosis*

8–1. *Metabolic*

■ **Description**

Elevated pH and carbon dioxide.) ?
not necessarily

■ **Symptoms**

May have symptoms of hypokalemia, lethargy, tetany.

■ **Diagnosis**   *(sometimes)*

History and physical, **elevated anion gap,** blood gas **(elevated pH and serum bicarbonate).**

■ **Pathology**

Reduced acid or gain of bicarbonate.

■ **Treatment**

Correct electrolyte abnormality, and primary cause.

8–2. *Respiratory*

■ **Description**

Elevated pH with low carbon dioxide.

■ **Symptoms**

Syncope, tetany, anxiety, perioral paresthesias.

■ **Diagnosis**

History and physical, blood gas.

■ **Pathology**

Hyperventilation.

■ **Treatment**

Control hyperventilation, rebreathing in paper bag.

9. *Acidosis*

9–1. *Metabolic*

■ **Description**

Reduced blood pH and bicarbonate.

■ **Symptoms**

Thirst, lethargy, coma, dehydration, and primary disease symptoms.

■ **Diagnosis**

History and physical exam, arterial blood gas. Evaluation of individual disorders (ketoacidosis: ketonemia, hyperglycemia; toxins: blood level, etc).

■ **Pathology**

Elevated anion gap—diabetic ketoacidosis, lactic acidosis, starvation, methanol/salicylate/ethylene glycol ingestion. *Normal anion gap*—diarrhea, renal tubular acidosis. Anion gap = **sodium − (bicarb + chloride).**

Treatment

Correct primary etiology (salicylate: alkalinize plasma, methanol/ethylene glycol: give ethanol, etc) and fluid/electrolyte status.

Lactic acidosis: acidosis, associated with shock and metabolic disorders, considerable mortality.

9–2. Respiratory

■ **Description**

Reduced pH and elevated P_{CO_2}.

■ **Symptoms**

Lethargy, disorientation, coma, headache, anxiety.

■ **Diagnosis**

History and physical, arterial blood gas (hypercapnia).

■ **Pathology**

Inadequate ventilation.

■ **Treatment**

Correct primary ventilatory defect.

Additional Information. **Sleep apnea: nocturnal apneic episodes, hypoxemia, hypercapnia. May be central, obstructive, or mixed. Symptoms include lethargy, confusion, arrhythmia. Treat with surgical obstruction removal, weight loss, respiratory stimulant.**

[handwritten: assoc c̄ obesity = Pickwickian syndrome]

10. Hypomagnesemia

■ **Description**

Low magnesium.

■ **Symptoms**

Tetany, lethargy, delirium, CNS irritability, muscle cramps.

■ **Diagnosis**

History and physical exam, serum magnesium, ECG (long QT).

■ **Pathology**

Etiology includes **alcoholism, malnutrition, diabetic ketoacidosis, diuretics.**

■ **Treatment**

Replace magnesium (IV or IM).

11. Hypercalcemia

■ **Description**

Calcium over 2.9.

■ **Symptoms**

Renal failure, **nausea/vomiting,** confusion, ECG (short QT, long PR).

■ **Diagnosis**

History and physical exam, serum calcium.

■ **Pathology**

Etiology includes **sarcoid, cancer, milk-alkali, hyperthyroid/parathyroid.**

■ **Treatment**

Treat etiology, **saline, furosemide (Lasix),** disodium etidronate.

12. Hypocalcemia

■ **Description**

Low calcium (under 2.2).

■ **Symptoms**

Tetany, Chvostek's sign, Trousseau's sign, perioral paresthesia, muscle cramps.

■ **Diagnosis**

History and physical, serum calcium.

■ **Pathology**

Etiology includes renal failure, vitamin D deficiency, hypoparathyroidism, malabsorption.

■ **Treatment**

Control etiology, give calcium and vitamin D.

E. **Kidney and Urinary System Trauma**

■ **Description**

Renal injury, minor (contusion, cut, hematoma), and major (deeper cut/rupture, pedicle injury). Ureteral injury: most often surgical mishap, external cause most often gunshot.

■ **Symptoms**

Pain, shock, flank ecchymosis.
Injury to upper urinary tract—hematuria.
Injury to posterior urethra—blood at meatus, distended bladder, voiding difficulty.
Ureter ligation—presents as pain, nausea/vomiting, fever postop.

■ **Diagnosis**

History and physical examination, IVP, CT, angiography, KUB. Evaluate urethra with retrograde study. If blood at meatus: do not catheterize. Do retrograde cystography to evaluate bladder.

■ **Pathology**

Renal—blunt, by auto accident most common.
Pedicle injury—left renal vein most often injured, usually penetrating injury.
Ureter—often surgical injury, hysterectomy commonly.

■ **Treatment**

Kidney—penetrating, surgical exploration; blunt, medical, or surgical.
Bladder—contusion, catheter; rupture, surgery.
Ureter—surgical (may need stent, anastomosis, bladder reimplantation, depending on injury).
Urethra—partial rupture, suprapubic cystotomy; complete rupture, drainage, and suprapubic cystotomy.

F. **Kidney Transplant Rejection**

■ **Description**

Allograft rejection. Acute type most common.

■ **Symptoms**

Lethargy, edema, oliguria, fever. Elevated BP, diminishing renal function and proteinuria may indicate chronic graft rejection.

■ **Diagnosis**

History and physical exam, renal scan, renal biopsy.

■ **Pathology**

Immunologic host reaction, where activated helper T cells and macrophages damage donor tissue.

■ **Treatment**

Rejection types: hyperacute (immediate, no treatment, nephrectomy), acute accelerated (after several days, no treatment, nephrectomy), acute (after 1 to 3 weeks, try immunosuppressives), chronic (no treatment).

G. **Hepatorenal Syndrome**

■ **Description**

Cirrhosis and renal failure.

■ **Symptoms**

Cirrhosis (jaundice, ascites, etc), renal failure (azotemia, oliguria).

■ **Diagnosis**

History and physical examination, clinical picture (oliguria and severe liver disease), no urine sediment. Low wedge pressure may suggest pre-renal azotemia (not hepatorenal syndrome).

■ **Pathology**

Cause unknown.

■ **Treatment**

Treat etiology if possible, dialysis(?), fluids to rule out hypovolemia.

III. PRINCIPLES OF MANAGEMENT: ETHICAL AND SOCIAL CONSIDERATIONS

The use of chronic dialysis and renal transplantation is increasing. Indications for these procedures are increasing also. Chronic dialysis costs are high, and consideration must be given to both the potential complications involved, and the patient's quality of life expected. Decisions to institute dialysis or perform transplantation must involve the physician, the patient, and the patient's family.

As in all other specialties, special consideration is required for the elderly, where incidence of particular diseases (eg, prostate carcinoma), ability to seek and comply with treatment, effect of medications and potential interactions, and psychosocial and economic concerns may have a significant and unique impact.

BIBLIOGRAPHY

Brenner BM. *Acute Renal Failure.* 2nd ed. New York: Churchill Livingstone; 1987.

Brenner BM. *The Kidney.* 4th ed. Vols. 1 and 2. Philadelphia, Pa: WB Saunders Co; 1991.

Dalton JR. *Basic Clinical Urology.* Philadelphia, Pa: Harper & Row; 1983.

Gower PE. *Handbook of Nephrology.* 2nd ed. London: Blackwell Scientific Publications; 1991.

Hanno PM. *A Clinical Manual of Urology.* Norwalk, Conn: Appleton-Century-Crofts; 1987.

Heptinstall RH. *Pathology of the Kidney.* 4th ed. Vols. 1, 2, 3. Boston, Mass: Little, Brown and Co; 1992.

Kassirer JP. *Diseases of the Kidney.* 46th ed. Boston, Mass: Little, Brown and Co; 1988.

Kursh ED. *Urology, Problems in Primary Care.* Oradell, NJ: Medical Economics Books; 1987.

Mandal AK. *The Medical Clinics of North America,* Vol. 74, Number 4, *Renal Disease.* Philadelphia, Pa: WB Saunders Co; 1990.

Maxwell MH. *Clinical Disorders of Fluid and Electrolyte Metabolism.* 4th ed. New York: McGraw-Hill; 1987.

Rose BD. *Clinical Physiology of Acid-Base and Electrolyte Disorders.* 3rd ed. New York: McGraw-Hill; 1989.

Schrier RW. *Renal and Electrolyte Disorders.* 3rd ed. Boston, Mass: Little, Brown and Co; 1986.

Tanagho EA. *Smith's General Urology.* 13th ed. Norwalk, Conn: Appleton & Lange, 1992.

CHAPTER 18

Surgical Principles

RALPH P. IERARDI, MD
MORRIS D. KERSTEIN, MD

I. ESOPHAGUS

A. Achalasia

■ Description

Motility disorder in which primary peristalsis is deficient. Gastroesophageal (GE) sphincter fails to relax with swallowing. Circular muscle of distal esophagus is thickened. Auerbach's plexus absent.

■ Symptoms

Dysphagia, regurgitation of undigested food and aspiration while recumbent, minimal pain.

■ Diagnosis

Esophagram—marked dilation above constricted distal esophagus. Abnormal peristalsis.

Endoscopy—exudes an esophageal stricture whether benign or malignant.

Esophageal manometry—uncoordinated peristalsis, primary peristalsis absent, GE sphincter has above-normal resting pressure and does not relax with swallowing.

Complications of untreated achalasia: megaesophagus, increased risk of squamous cell carcinoma.

■ Treatment

Pneumatic dilatation. Longitudinal esophageal myotomy is surgical procedure of choice.

B. Hiatal Hernia and Reflux Esophagitis

1. Sliding Hiatal Hernia

■ Description

Esophagogastric junction and proximal stomach displaced into mediastinum. Ninety-five percent of hiatal hernias are sliding. Symptoms caused by accompanying esophageal reflux.

■ Symptoms

Retrosternal burning pain especially lying supine, lifting, or straining; regurgitation of bitter fluid; nocturnal cough, recurrent pneumonia from aspiration; dysphagia. Bleeding rare.

■ Diagnosis

Chest x-ray: air fluid level in mediastinum. Gastroesophageal reflux may be evident on esophagram. Esophagoscopy to rule out other lesions and document esophagitis. Distal esophagus pH monitoring most sensitive test.

■ Treatment

Antacids, H^2 blockers. Sleep with head elevated. Change eating habits. Surgical antireflux procedures—Nissen fundoplication, Hill repair, Belsey fundoplication.

2. Paraesophageal Hiatal Hernia

■ Description

Esophageal (EG) junction in normal anatomic position. Stomach herniates through hiatus usually to left of esophagus. May strangulate or volvulize leading to rapid death (20 to 30%).

■ Symptoms

Fullness after meals, postprandial pain in the chest, bowel sounds in chest, early postprandial vomiting, breathlessness while eating. Chronic blood loss in up to ⅓ of patients due to recurrent bleeding from the gastric mucosa.

■ Diagnosis

Chest x-ray: air fluid level in mediastinum. Esophagram establishes the diagnosis.

■ Treatment

Because of high rate of complications, all paraesophageal hiatal hernias should be surgically repaired with or without an accompanying antireflux procedure.

C. Esophageal Cancer

■ Description

Squamous carcinoma most common cell type: distal third 30%, middle third 50%, upper third 20%. Spreads by lymphatics, vascular invasion, and direct extension. Adenocarcinoma 5 to 10% of primary carcinomas of esophagus. Extraesophageal extension present in high percentage of patients at time of diagnosis. Highly aggressive. Five-year survival rate only 3% when lymph nodes are involved.

■ Symptoms

Progressive dysphagia, odynophagia, chest pain, weight loss.

■ Diagnosis

Esophagram—irregular mass narrowing lumen of esophagus, minimal proximal dilatation.

Esophagoscopy—biopsy for tissue diagnosis.

Bronchoscopy—for upper- and middle-third lesions to rule out tracheobronchial involvement.

Computed tomographic (CT) scan—helps with staging.

■ Treatment

Surgery; only 30% resectable. Esophagectomy, total or partial, depending on tumor location and size. Stomach used to re-establish gastrointestinal (GI) tract continuity. Resection may also provide palliation in low-risk patients. Radiation therapy preoperative may shrink tumor mass allowing resection. Combined with chemotherapy may be effective adjuvant therapy. Endoscopic laser therapy used to establish esophageal patency in unresectable obstructing tumors.

D. Esophageal Perforation

1. Instrumental Perforation Causes

Endoscopy, dilation, paraesophageal surgery, SB tube, intubation, sclerotherapy.

■ Description

Susceptible at areas of narrowing: cricopharyngeal area, midportion near aortic arch and mainstem bronchi, diaphragmatic hiatus.

■ Symptoms

Dysphagia, pain, fever, neck tenderness and crepitus (with cervical perforations), chest pain, dyspnea, shock, mediastinal air (Hamman's sign).

■ Diagnosis

X-rays: soft tissue air, mediastinal air, pleural effusion, pneumothorax, mediastinal widening. Esophagram shows site of perforation.

■ Treatment

Antibiotics. Surgical repair required in all cases except those with small, localized perforations.

■ Criteria for Non-operative Therapy

Contained mediastinal leak, free drainage back into esophagus, minimal symptoms, no sign of sepsis. Surgical repair possible within 24 hours of perforation. After 24 hours, resection combined with diverting procedures may be necessary ("spit fistula").

2. *Spontaneous Perforation*

■ Description

Postemetic perforation usually following an alcoholic binge (Boerhaave syndrome). Posterior, distal esophagus most usual site.

■ Symptoms

Sudden, severe pain in lower chest and upper abdomen; shock; rigid abdomen.

■ Differential Diagnosis

Pancreatitis, myocardial infarction, perforated peptic ulcer, dissecting aortic aneurysm.

■ Diagnosis

Same as instrumental perforation.

■ Treatment

Same as instrumental perforation.

II. STOMACH AND DUODENUM

A. Peptic Ulcer Disease

1. *Duodenal Ulcer*

■ Description

Associated with acid hypersecretion. Increased number of parietal cells. Peak incidence between the ages of 20 and 60. Typically periods of remission and exacerbation. Ninety-five percent occur in duodenal bulb, 5% are postbulbar.

■ Symptoms

Epigastric pain, pain relieved by food and/or antacids, nocturnal awakenings.

■ Diagnosis

Upper GI series 75 to 80% accurate. Ulcer crater or scarring of duodenal bulb. Endoscopy is 95% accurate and is diagnostic procedure of choice.

■ Treatment

Medical—aim to keep intraluminal pH above 5.5. Use antacids or H_2 blockers. Recurrence after ulcer healing is common. Maintenance therapy with H_2 blockade is common.

Surgical—indications for surgery are hemorrhage, perforation, obstruction, and intractability.

Surgical procedures—vagotomy and pyloroplasty, vagotomy and antrectomy, highly selective vagotomy; laproscopic vagotomy for perforated ulcer; omentopexy (Graham patch) with vagotomy if chronic symptoms exist.

2. *Gastric Ulcer*

■ Description

Appear later in life. Peak incidence in fifth decade. More common in men. Usually no acid hypersecretion. Cause factor is mucosal injury that renders mucosa susceptible to gastric acid. Majority occur on lesser curve of stomach. Malignant potential.

■ Types

1. Ulcer located at incisura angularis.
2. Ulcers located in stomach and duodenum.
3. Ulcer located in pylorus or prepyloric area.
4. Ulcer located high in stomach (juxta-cardia).

■ Symptoms

Similar to duodenal ulcer. Pain localizes to left of midline.

■ Diagnosis

Upper GI series can localize. Endoscopy important. Must biopsy ulcer 8 to 12 times to rule out malignancy.

■ Treatment

Principles are similar to those of treatment of duodenal ulcer. Because recurrence rate is higher after medical therapy, surgical therapy should be considered earlier. Procedure of choice is antrectomy with Billroth I anastomosis. No vagotomy with type I gastric ulcers.

B. Gastric Carcinoma

■ Description

Adenocarcinoma is the most common (95%); classified into ulcerating (25%), polypoid (25%), superficial spreading (15%), linnitus plastica (10%), and advanced (35%). Dietary (nitrosamines, smoked/salted or pickled foodstuffs) and environmental factors. Major factors influencing survival are level of spread through gastric wall and lymph node involvement. Age range: 50 to 70, male:female—3:2.

■ Symptoms

Early—vague, nondescript symptoms.
Late—indigestion, postprandial fullness, eructation, loss of appetite, heartburn, vomiting. Pain pattern is similar to peptic ulcer disease.

■ Diagnosis

Barium meal—polypoid mass, ulcer crater not extending outside boundary of gastric wall, non-distensible stomach.

CT scan—evaluation of metastatic spread.
Endoscopy—with biopsy, 90% accurate. Endoscopic ultrasound may be of value in determining depth of tumor and presence of enlarged lymph nodes.

■ Treatment

Radical subtotal gastrectomy for cure, distal lesions; radical total gastrectomy for proximal lesions. Half of those operated on are resectable. Chemotherapy reserved for unresectable or recurrent disease. Gastrojejunostomy for palliative bypass in unresectable disease.

III. SMALL INTESTINE

A. Intestinal Obstruction

■ Description

Can be classified into

Simple—no vascular compromise.
Strangulating—vascular obstruction.
Paralytic ileus—impairment of muscle function, closed-loop blockage at two points.

Can be caused by adhesions (70%), hernia (8%), tumor (9%), inflammatory disease (4%), volvulus, or intussusception.

■ Symptoms

Crampy abdominal pain, vomiting, obstipation, distention, failure to pass flatus.

■ Diagnosis

High-pitched bowel sounds on physical examination. Peritoneal signs signify peritonitis and strangulation. X-ray: distended small-bowel loops in stepladder pattern, air-fluid levels.

■ Treatment

Replace electrolyte losses, intravenous fluids, nothing by mouth (NPO). Nasogastric tube decompression. Consider trial of long-tube decompression. Operative therapy: exploratory laparotomy with lysis of adhesions.

■ Results

Morbidity—30% (60% with strangulated bowel).

Morbidity—20% with neoplasia, 20% with adhesion and hernia.

B.   Neoplasms

■ Description

Jejunum and ileum, 5% of all tumors of GI tract. Benign are more common. Most are asymptomatic; 10% become symptomatic.

Benign tumors—leiomyomas (18 to 20%), lipomas (15%), neurofibromas (10%), adenomas (15%), polyps (15%), hemangiomas (13%), fibromas (10%).

Malignant tumors—adenocarcinomas (30 to 50%), lymphomas (15%), leiomyosarcomas (20%), carcinoids (30 to 50%).

■ Symptoms

Bleeding and obstruction. Carcinoid syndrome (flushing, pain, diarrhea, bronchoconstriction, valvular disease) from release of vasoactive substances from metastatic carcinoid tumors.

■ Diagnosis

Often made at time of laparotomy. Small-bowel series (enteroclysis is most sensitive). Endoscopy (procedure of choice with duodenal neoplasms). Arteriography (useful with vascular neoplasms: hemangiomas). CT/MRI may complement staging. Biochemical analysis of urine samples (5-hydroxyindoleacetic acid in carcinoid tumors).

■ Treatment

Wide resection. Bypass for palliation.

C.   Radiation Injury

■ Description

Pathogenesis involves progressive obliterative vasculitis. May be diagnosed many years remote from time of radiation therapy.

■ Symptoms

Obstruction due to stricture, bleeding from ulcerated mucosa, necrosis with perforation, fistula formation, abscess formation.

■ Treatment

Avoid surgery if possible. (TPN used with severe symptomatic disease, poor nutritional status.) Minimal dissection. Resection or bypass with wide margins. May need to exteriorize if bowel viability is in question.

D.   Meckel's Diverticulum

■ Description

Congenital anomaly, persistent omphalomesenteric duct. A true diverticulum. Found in 2% of the population. Two feet from ileocecal valve; 2 inches long. May contain heterotopic tissue (pancreas, gastric mucosa, other types). Four percent symptomatic, usually in childhood.

■ Symptoms

May mimic appendicitis. Bleeding. Intestinal obstruction from intussusception.

■ **Diagnosis**

X-ray and small-bowel series unreliable. Technetium scan will localize heterotopic gastric mucosa, if present (accuracy, 90%).

■ **Treatment**

Surgical resection (with GI bleeding, excise diverticulum with sufficient margin of ileum to encompass ulceration). Incidental finding at laparotomy: leave alone.

E.   Crohn's Disease

■ **Description**

Chronic inflammatory disease of the GI tract. Unknown cause. Peak age of onset is between second and fourth decades. Transmural involvement of bowel wall, non-caseating granulomas, aphthous ulcers, malignant potential, extraintestinal manifestations are common. Obstruction and perforation with abscess and fistula formation. Skip lesions. Seventy percent come to operation for complications of the disease. Anal manifestations of the disease are common.

■ **Symptoms**

Crampy abdominal pain, diarrhea, nausea and vomiting, fear of eating, weight loss.

■ **Diagnosis**

Physical   examination—abdominal mass right lower quadrant.

Endoscopy—reddened mucosa, skip lesions. Biopsy.

Small bowel series—string sign, fistulas. Thickened bowel wall.

■ **Treatment**

Medical therapy—antibiotics, steroids, sulfasalazine, 5-ASA, immunosuppressive agents (6-mercaptopurine, azathi-

aprine), bowel rest, central hyperalimentation.

Surgical therapy—(use eventually required in 75%). For complications, excision, bypass, stricturoplasty.

Recurrence—(40% within 5 years, 60% within 10 years, 75% within 15 years). The major problem in surgical treatment.

IV.   COLON, RECTUM, ANUS

A.   Carcinoma of the Colon and Rectum

■ **Description**

Second most common malignancy. Pathogenesis unclear. Likely environmental influence. Diets high in fat, low in fiber: higher incidence. Screening: digital examination, stool for occult blood, sigmoidoscopy.

■ **Symptoms**

Right-sided lesions—dull abdominal pain, occult bleeding.

Left-sided lesions—change in bowel habits, visible blood, change in stool caliber.

Rectal lesions—tenesmus, incomplete evacuation, blood-streaked stool.

■ **Diagnosis**

Digital examination, barium enema, colonoscopy, CT scan, liver function tests, chest x-ray. Carcinoembryonic antigen level (provides a baseline level for future comparison).

■ **Treatment**

Operative excision with adequate margins. Rectal carcinoma: level of resection depends on location of tumor. Lesions less than 8 cm from anal verge may need abdominoperineal resection; greater than 8 cm, low anterior resection.

B. Diverticular Disease

1. Diverticulosis

■ Description

Males and females equal incidence. Sixty-five percent of population by age 85. Bleeding occurs in 15%. Hemorrhage arises in right colon in 70 to 90%. Seventy percent stop bleeding spontaneously; 30% have recurrent bleeding.

■ Symptoms

Blood per rectum, minimal pain.

■ Diagnosis

Endoscopy, bleeding scan, arteriography.

■ Treatment

Selective infusion of vasopressin, segmental colonic resection if bleeding site is localized, subtotal colectomy if bleeding not localized.

2. Diverticulitis

■ Description

Inflammation of diverticulae. Limited to sigmoid colon in 90%. Inflammation is usually contained by pericolic fat and mesentery.

■ Symptoms

Left lower quadrant (LLQ) pain, anorexia, nausea and vomiting, fever, abdominal mass.

■ Diagnosis

Clinical presentation, CT scan, barium enema and colonoscopy when acute inflammation lessened (usually > 1 week following acute episode).

■ Treatment

Bowel rest, antibiotics, intravenous fluids, analgesia. Surgical resection when inflammation has subsided (approximately 8 weeks following recent attack). Operations for diverticular disease:

> *One-stage procedure*—resection and 1° anastomosis.
>
> *Two-stage procedure*—Hartman operation (sigmoid resection, and decending colostomy, mucous fistula). OR sigmoid resection, primary anastomosis, and proximal diverting colostomy.
>
> *Three-stage procedure*—colostomy and drainage.

C. Ulcerative Colitis

■ Description

Mucosal inflammation, crypt abscesses, mucosa sloughs, colon becomes shortened. Two peaks in incidence: second and sixth decades. Can involve rectum alone or entire colon. Malignant potential increases with time (2 to 5% at 10 years, then 1% 1 year thereafter). Extraintestinal manifestations (arthralgias, ankylosing spondylitis, sclerosing cholangitis, and liver dysfunction, uveitis, nephrolithiasis).

■ Symptoms

Bloody diarrhea, fever, crampy abdominal pain, tenesmus, urgency, incontinence.

■ Diagnosis

Endoscopy—friable, erythematous mucosa.

Barium enema—loss of haustral markings, stricture, stovepipe colon.

■ **Treatment**

Medical—intravenous fluids, NPO, steroid enemas, correct electrolyte abnormalities, sulfasalazine.

Surgery—reserved for treatment of complications (hemorrhage, perforation, toxic megacolon, carcinoma, intractability).

Total proctocolectomy with ileostomy. Proctocolectomy with ileoanal anastomosis (ileal J-pouch).

D. **Hemorrhoids**

■ **Description**

Internal hemorrhoids above dentate line. External below dentate line. Location of internal hemorrhoids: right anterior, R posterior, L lateral. Hereditary. Straining. Portal hypertension. Pregnancy.

■ **Symptoms**

Bleeding, pruritis ani, pain.

■ **Diagnosis**

Physical examination, anoscopy.

■ **Treatment**

Medical symptomatic relief (high-fiber diet, stool softeners, bulk agents [psyllium]). Surgical excision, rubber band ligation, anal dilatation.

E. **Anal Fissure**

■ **Description**

Superficial linear ulceration. Sentinel pile (skin tag). Squamous epithelium; therefore, very painful. Straining at stool. Constipation. Condition is cyclic.

■ **Symptoms**

Exquisite pain, painful defecation, blood on toilet paper.

■ **Diagnosis**

Sentinel pile, painful digital examination, endoscopy when acute episode resolved.

■ **Treatment**

Local cleansing agents, sitz baths, topical ointments, stool softeners, lateral internal sphincterotomy.

V. **APPENDIX—APPENDICITIS**

■ **Description**

Appendix: variable location in relation to the cecum. Teniae converge on appendix. Closed-loop obstruction of lumen, vascular congestion, serosal inflammation, perforation.

■ **Symptoms**

Pain, anorexia, vomiting, diarrhea, cutaneous hyperesthesia, guarding and rebound at McBurney's point, Rovsing's sign, psoas sign, obturator sign.

■ **Diagnosis**

Physical examination. Fecalith in right lower quadrant (RLQ) is diagnostic, altered R psoas shadow. Leukocytosis (may be absent).

■ **Treatment**

Appendectomy.

VI. **GALLBLADDER**

A. **Acute Cholecystitis**

■ **Description**

Bacterial or chemical inflammation of the gallbladder. Stones in 95%. Incidence higher in females. Obstruction of the cystic duct. Bacteria in 50 to 75% (*E. coli*, *Klebsiella, Enterobacter*).

■ Symptoms

Right upper quadrant (RUQ) or epigastric pain. Pain radiates to tip of scapula. Nausea and vomiting.

■ Diagnosis

Physical examination: Murphy's sign. Mild jaundice. Ultrasound detects stones. HIDA scan 90% accurate.

■ Treatment

Antibiotics. Cholecystectomy, delayed or immediate. Cholecystostomy in poor-risk patients. **Variant forms:** empyema of gallbladder, gangrene, achalculous cholecystitis.

B. Chronic Cholecystitis

■ Description

Repeated attacks of acute cholecystitis. Stones almost always present.

■ Signs and Symptoms

Pain in RUQ and epigastric pain. May radiate to tip of scapula. Nausea and vomiting. Attacks often follow large meals.

■ Diagnosis

Physical examination. Ultrasound to identify stones. Oral cholecystography if symptoms are typical but ultrasound negative.

■ Treatment

Chemical stone dissolution: methylterbutyl ether. Extracorporeal shock wave lithotripsy (ESWL). Laparoscopic cholecystectomy or conventional open cholecystectomy. Variant forms: hydrops of gallbladder, calcified ("porcelain gallbladder"), gallbladder polyps.

C. Cholangitis

■ Description

Infection in the biliary tree. Bacteria, obstruction, increased pressure. Most commonly associated with choledocholithiasis.

■ Symptoms

Fever and chills. Jaundice. Biliary colic (Charcot's triad). Severe: hypotension and mental confusion.

■ Diagnosis

Clinical presentation. RUQ tenderness. Elevated white blood cell count, bilirubin, and alkaline phosphatase. Ultrasound of RUQ to document gallstones. CT scan to rule out periampullary malignancies or liver abscesses.

■ Treatment

Antibiotics. Triple antibiotics if severe (60% of cases with multiple organisms). Endoscopic sphincterotomy with stone extraction. Exploratory laparotomy, cholecystectomy with common bile duct exploration and T-tube drainage.

D. Gallstone Ileus

■ Description

Antecedent cholecystointestinal or choledochointestinal fistula. Gallstone obstructs at intestinal narrowing. More common in women (usually distal ilium).

■ Symptoms

Pain in RUQ. Distention. Nausea. Vomiting. Colicky abdominal pain.

■ Diagnosis

Air in biliary tree (55 to 60%). Dilated small-bowel loops. Opaque stone in the intestinal tract (15 to 20%). Non-opaque stone in intestinal tract identified by ultrasound.

■ Treatment

Exploratory laparotomy, enterotomy with removal of stone. Repair of biliary-enteric fistula to prevent recurrence. Cholecystectomy if medically stable.

E. Gallbladder Carcinoma

■ Description

Most common malignancy of biliary tract. Association with gallstones and porcelain gallbladders. Adenocarcinoma in 82%. More common in females. One to 2% of those undergoing cholecystectomy. Tends to be diagnosed in advanced stage.

■ Symptoms

Non-specific. Pain. Weight loss. Jaundice. Anorexia. RUQ mass.

■ Diagnosis

Advanced disease: CT scan. Curable, localized disease found at time of cholecystectomy.

■ Treatment

If tumor localized to mucosa and submucosa, cholecystectomy. Serosal or lymph node involvement: cholecystectomy with node resection and hepatic wedge resection. **Results:** overall 5-year survival, 2 to 5%.

VII. LIVER

A. Hepatocellular Carcinoma

■ Description

More common in Africa and Asia. Cirrhosis and hepatitis B predisposes. Eighty percent of primary liver tumors. Present in advanced stage.

■ Symptoms

Pain, distention, weight loss, fatigue, anorexia, fever, jaundice ascites.

■ Diagnosis

Tumor marker: alpha-fetoprotein elevated. CT scan with or without percutaneous biopsy. Arteriography. **Intraoperative ultrasound.**

■ Treatment

Only 25% are resectable (5-year survival: 18 to 36%). Can remove up to 80% of liver. Transplantation. Palliation: intra-arterial chemotherapy, hepatic artery ligation.

B. Pyogenic Liver Abscess

■ Description

Follows an acute abdominal infection. Routes: portal system, ascension from the biliary tree, hepatic artery, direct extension, trauma. Untreated, 100% mortality rate; treated, 20% mortality rate. Right lobe more common. Solitary or multiple. Bacteria: *E. coli*, *Klebsiella*, enterococcus, bacteroides. May rupture into adjacent peritoneal, pericardial, or thoracic cavities.

■ Symptoms

Fever, malaise, chills, anorexia, weight loss, abdominal pain, RUQ tenderness, jaundice, hepatomegaly.

■ Diagnosis

Chest x-ray: atelectasis, pneumonia, effusion (all right-sided), CT scan, ultrasound, arteriography.

■ Treatment

Eliminate abscess and underlying cause. Percutaneous drainage if single, operative drainage if multiple or multilocated abscess.

C. Amebic Liver Abscess

■ Description

Prevalence higher in tropical zones, travelers to tropical countries. More common in males, peak incidence fourth decade. Follows infestation with *Entamoeba histolytica*. Ninety percent in right lobe. May grow to large size.

■ Symptoms

Recent diarrheal syndrome in minority. Similar to pyogenic abscess.

■ Diagnosis

Serum antibody for *Entamoeba histolytica* (indirect hemagglutinin test). Only ⅓ have positive amoebic stool cultures.

■ Treatment

Metronidazole 750 mg by mouth, three times a day for 10 days. Operative treatment reserved for rupture.

VIII. PORTAL HYPERTENSION

■ Description

Present when portal venous pressure exceeds 15 mm Hg. Collaterals between portal and systemic venous circulations. Leads to esophageal varices. Increased resistance to portal flow; prehepatic, hepatic (cirrhosis), posthepatic.

■ Symptoms

Ascites. Hepatic encephalopathy, hypersplenism, hemorrhoids, caput medusa, esophageal variceal bleed. Stigmata of cirrhosis: spider angiomata, palmar erythema, testicular atrophy, gynecomastia, hepatomegaly. Jaundice.

■ Diagnosis

Liver function tests, liver biopsy, hepatitis profile, endoscopy if bleeding.

■ Treatment

Acute variceal bleed—injection sclerotherapy, vasopressin infusion, balloon tamponade, emergency portosystemic shunt.
Shunt procedures—end-to-side portacaval shunt, side-to-side shunts, selective shunts.

IX. PANCREAS

A. Acute Pancreatitis

■ Description

Inflammation from escape of active pancreatic enzymes. Eighty percent due to alcohol and biliary disease. Trauma, hyperlipidemia, hypercalcemia, pancreas divisum. Ninety percent mild cases; 10% life-threatening.

■ Symptoms

Epigastric and back pain, fever, tachycardia, hypotension, nausea, vomiting, epigastric tenderness, flank ecchymosis (Grey–Turner's sign), periumbilical ecchymosis (Cullen's sign).

■ Diagnosis

Serum amylase and lipase, hypocalcemia, hyperbilirubinemia, leukocytosis, CT scan (dynamic angio-CT also measures amount of pancreatic necrosis). Upper gastrointestinal (UGI) series, sentinal loop on plain film abdomen, ultrasound of biliary tree.

■ **Treatment**

Bowel rest, NPO, intravenous fluids, analgesia, nasogastric tube, antibiotics. Total parenteral nutrition (TPN) for prolonged cases. Surgery: correct biliary disease; reserved for complications of pancreatitis (abscess, etc). Pancreatic debridement and open packing/closed lavage for pancreatic necrosis.

B. **Chronic Pancreatitis**

■ **Description**

Recurrent abdominal pain of pancreatic origin. Irreversible damage. Exocrine and endocrine insufficiency. Most often alcohol related.

■ **Symptoms**

Epigastric and back pain, anorexia and weight loss, insulin-dependent diabetes mellitus (IDDM), steatorrhea.

■ **Diagnosis**

Clinical findings:

Plain films—pancreatic calcifications.

CT scan—calcifications, size of pancreas.

Endoscopic retrograde cholangiopancreatography (ERCP)—identify ductal abnormalities.

■ **Treatment**

Analgesia, correct exocrine and endocrine function. Surgery: ampullary procedures; transduodenal sphincteroplasty. Ductal drainage procedures: side-to-side pancreaticojejunostomy (Puestow procedure).

C. **Pancreatic Carcinoma**

■ **Description**

Ninety percent duct cell adenocarcinoma; 65% arise in pancreatic head. Present in advanced stage.

■ **Symptoms**

Jaundice, weight loss, abdominal pain, pain in epigastrium and back, palpable gallbladder (Courvoisier's sign).

■ **Diagnosis**

Liver function tests (LFTs) reflect ductal obstruction. Elevated carcinoembryonic antigen (CEA), occult blood in stool, computed tomography (CT) scan to evaluate size of tumor and relation to surrounding structures, ERCP or percutaneous transhepatic cholangiography, arteriography (define anatomy/resectability), percutaneous biopsy.

■ **Treatment**

Resection for cure, if possible: pancreaticoduodenectomy. Bypass for palliation: choledochojejunostomy, gastrojejunostomy.

D. **Endocrine Tumors of the Pancreas**

1. *Insulinoma*

Most common. Beta cell origin. Eighty percent solitary benign; 10% malignant. Whipple's triad. Fasting hypoglycemia (insulin: glucose ratio > .3). Preoperative localization: arteriography. Resection is curative. Debulk for palliation. Medical therapy: diazoxide.

2. *Gastrinoma*

Second most common. Hypergastrinemia and peptic ulcer disease. Zollinger–Ellison syndrome. Elevated fasting gastrin. 50% malignant. Resection for cure. Preoperative localization. Explore if localization attempts fail. Somatostatin.

3. *Glucagonoma*

From alpha cells. Elevated plasmin glucagon is diagnostic. Hyperglycemia. Majority are malignant. Necrolytic migratory erythema. Present in advanced stage. Resect for cure. Debulk for relief of symptoms.

X. SPLEEN

A. Trauma

■ Description

Most commonly injured organ in blunt trauma. Associated with rib fractures left chest.

Symptoms

Non-specific abdominal pain. Left upper quadrant (LUQ) pain. Pain referred to L shoulder (Kehr's sign).

■ Diagnosis

Clinical suspicion. Gross blood on diagnostic peritoneal lavage. CT scan findings in stable patients.

■ Treatment

Splenectomy. Splenic salvage in appropriate cases. Non-operative therapy in children.

B. Immune Thrombocytopenic Purpura

■ Description

Persistently low platelet count. Anti-platelet factor (circulating immunoglobulin) directed against a platelet antigen. Majority are young women.

■ Symptoms

Spontaneous bleeding. Spleen normal size or small.

■ Diagnosis

Thrombocytopenia. Bone marrow aspirate megakaryocytes.

■ Treatment

Steroids, response in 3 to 7 days. Complete remission with steroids is rare. Elective splenectomy. Emergent splenectomy with central nervous system (CNS) bleeding.

C. Hodgkin's Disease

■ Description

Malignant lymphoma; Reed–Sternberg cells; asymptomatic lymphadenopathy: cervical, axillary, inguinal. Four pathologic subtypes: lymphocyte predominance, nodular sclerosis, mixed cellularity, lymphocyte depletion. Metastasize in predictable patterns.

■ Symptoms

Asymptomatic lymphadenopathy, night sweats, weight loss, pruritus, malaise.

■ Diagnosis

Hematologic tests, bone marrow aspirate, LFTs, CT scan abdomen and chest, chest x-ray, lymph node biopsy, lymphangiogram. Staging laparotomy: splenectomy, liver biopsy, lymph node sampling, oophoropexy.

■ Treatment

Radiation, chemotherapy. Staging laparotomy: when result may change therapy.

D. Non-Hodgkin's Lymphoma

Clinical course and natural history more diverse than Hodgkin's. Pattern of spread is variable. Two thirds have asymptomatic lymphadenopathy. Onset may be in extranodal site. May present as asymptomatic splenomegaly. Constitutional symptoms commonly present. Chemotherapy and radiation therapy.

E. Postsplenectomy Sepsis

■ Description

Risk highest for splenectomy for thalassemia and reticuloendothelial (RE) diseases like Hodgkin's, lowest for trauma and idiopathic thrombocytopenic purpura (ITP). Risk may be as high as 1% per year. Risk greatest for children younger than four years, and within 2 years of splenectomy.

■ Symptoms

Preceded by upper respiratory infection (URI). Followed by nausea, vomiting, headache, confusion, shock, coma, death within 24 hours.

■ Diagnosis

Clinical suspicion. Blood cultures positive for *Streptococcus pneumoniae* in 50%. Encapsulated organisms predominate (pneumococcin, H. *influenzae*).

■ Treatment

Broad-spectrum antibiotics. Supportive care. Prophylaxis: Pneumovax, prophylactic antibiotics.

XI. ARTERIAL DISEASE

A. Arterial Embolism

■ Description

Heart is the source in 90%. Left ventricular thrombus after infarct; left atrium in atrial fibrillation; valvular disease; paradoxical embolus right-to-left intracardiac shunt (prosthetic valve, subacute bacterial endocarditis, rheumatic heart disease). Acute onset; occurs at bifurcations.

■ Symptoms

Pulselessness, pain, pallor, paresthesias, paralysis.

■ Diagnosis

Physical examination, duplex scan, arteriography.

■ Treatment

Heparinization, balloon embolectomy.

B. Aortoiliac Occlusive Disease

■ Description

Arteriosclerosis involves arteries singly or in combination. Slow progression of occlusive disease allows for collateral formation.

■ Symptoms

Claudication, rest pain, tissue loss. Leriche syndrome: buttock claudication, impotence, diminished femoral pulses, bruit, thrill, elevation pallor, dependent rubor.

■ Diagnosis

History and physical examination. Non-invasive tests: ankle/brachial index, pulse volume recording, duplex scan, arteriography.

■ Treatment

Medical—control risk factors, control hypertension, lower cholesterol, stop smoking, trental, exercise program.
Surgical—bypass, endarterectomy, angioplasty.

C. **Abdominal Aortic Aneurysm**

■ **Description**

Typically involve infrarenal aorta, but may extend above renals. Most are fusiform. Atherosclerosis. More common in males.

■ **Symptoms**

Intact aneurysms are asymptomatic. Expanding or leaking causes back pain and abdominal pain. Pulsatile abdominal mass.

■ **Diagnosis**

Physical examination, calcific outline on plain x-ray, ultrasound, CT scan, arteriography.

■ **Treatment**

Asymptomatic less than 5 cm: observe. Greater than 5 cm: aneurysmectomy with aortobifemoral graft or tube graft.

D. **Femoropopliteal Occlusive Disease**

■ **Description**

Arteries involved singly or in combination.

■ **Symptoms**

Claudication, rest pain, tissue loss.

■ **Diagnosis**

Physical examination, non-invasive tests, arteriography.

■ **Treatment**

Control risk factors, trental, exercise programs. Surgery for disabling claudication, rest pain, or tissue loss.

E. **Cerebrovascular Disease**

■ **Description**

Lesions of the extracranial cerebral vessels. Decreased cerebral perfusion from occlusive lesions, thrombosis, or embolization.

■ **Symptoms**

Transient ischemic attacks, stroke, vertebral-basilar insufficiency (ataxia, vertigo, diplopia), diminished pulses, bruits.

■ **Diagnosis**

Duplex scan, arteriography.

■ **Treatment**

Medical therapy. Antiplatelet agents (aspirin, persantine, ticlopide). Avoid stroke. Endarterectomy.

XII. VENOUS DISEASE

A. **Deep Venous Thrombosis**

■ **Description**

Those at risk: elderly, bedridden, hip replacement and other orthopedic procedures, pelvic and abdominal procedures, trauma. Virchow's triad: stasis, intimal damage, hypercoagulability.

■ **Symptoms**

Asymptomatic in 50%, swelling, tenderness, Homan's sign (calf pain with dorsiflexion of foot). *Phlegmasia alba dolens:* milk leg. *Phlegmasia cerulea dolens:* venous gangrene.

■ **Diagnosis**

Duplex scan, venography, impedance plethysmography, fibrinogen scan.

■ **Treatment**

Bed rest, heparin, then coumadin for 3 to 6 months. Compressive hose, Greenfield filter if anticoagulation contraindicated, venous thrombectomy.

B. **Varicose Veins**

■ **Description**

Dilated, tortuous veins in the leg.

Primary—normal deep system.
Secondary—diseased deep system.

■ **Symptoms**

Dull ache, feeling of leg heaviness relieved by elevation. Dilated veins along anatomic distribution of greater and lesser saphenous veins. May be accompanied by signs of chronic deep venous disease.

■ **Diagnosis**

Clinical examination, Trendelenburg test, duplex scan, Perthes' test.

■ **Treatment**

Support hose, sclerotherapy, ligation and stripping.

C. **Thrombophlebitis**

Inflammation and thrombosis of vein, pain, swelling, warmth. Treat with hot compresses, leg elevation, analgesics, excision of vein if purulent, systemic anticoagulation if process extends to deep venous system.

D. **Pulmonary Embolus**

■ **Description**

Relatively common complication. Deep venous thrombosis in pelvis veins and iliofemoral region more likely to embolize.

■ **Symptoms**

Dyspnea, pleuritic chest pain, hemoptysis, tachycardia, tachypnea, fever, rales, shock. May be asymptomatic in 10 to 20%.

■ **Diagnosis**

Chest x-ray: decreased vascular markings (Westermark's sign). Electrocardiogram (ECG): right axis deviation. Arterial blood gas (ABG): hypoxia, hypocarbia. Ventilation-perfusion scan. Pulmonary arteriogram.

■ **Treatment**

Systemic anticoagulation, thrombolytic therapy, Greenfield filter. Surgical thrombectomy for patients with massive pulmonary edema (PE), hemodynamic instability.

XIII. HERNIA

A. **Indirect Hernia**

■ **Description**

Fifty percent of all hernias. Congenital defect. Patent processus vaginalis. Lateral to inferior epigastric vessels. Chronic intra-abdominal pressure elevation. Rule out colon disease.

■ **Symptoms**

Pain, groin mass.

■ **Diagnosis**

Physical examination.

■ **Treatment**

High ligation of sac. Close defect in transversalis fascia.

B. Direct Hernia

■ **Description**

Weakness in the inguinal floor (Hesselbach's triangle).

■ **Treatment**

Cooper's ligament repair.

XIV WOUND INFECTIONS

■ **Description**

Usually caused by break in sterile technique, carrier in operating room, ruptured viscus, large wound inoculum. Local factors: devitalized tissue, foreign body, hematoma, seroma. Systemic risk factors: age, steroids, immunosuppression, diabetes, obesity, length of operation.

■ **Symptoms**

Fever, pain, erythema, drainage, swelling.

■ **Diagnosis**

Physical examination, cultures.

■ **Treatment**

Drainage, debridement, antibiotics, prophylactic antibiotics perioperatively.

XV. THYROID

A. Hyperthyroidism

■ **Description**

Increased levels of thyroid hormone. Loss of normal feedback. Graves' disease, autoimmune. Thyroid-stimulating immunoglobulins in 90% with Graves' disease.

■ **Symptoms**

Heat intolerance, sweating, insomnia, muscle weakness, weight loss, nervousness, irritability, staring appearance, fine hair or alopecia, exophthalmos, vitiligo, onycholysis.

■ **Diagnosis**

T_4 and T_3 levels high. Thyroid-stimulating hormone (TSH) is low. Elevated radioactive iodine uptake.

■ **Treatment**

Antithyroid drugs—propylthiouracil or tapazole, radioiodine (^{131}I). Subtotal thyroidectomy.

B. Non-toxic Nodular Goiter

■ **Description**

Compensatory response to decreased production of thyroid hormone, inadequate intake of iodine, medications that impair hormone production, enzyme deficiency.

■ **Symptoms**

Compression of neck structures, cough, fullness in neck, neck mass.

■ **Diagnosis**

Increased TSH. Decreased levels of thyroid hormone.

■ **Treatment**

Thyroid hormone replacement. Surgery reserved for compressive symptoms, cosmesis, threat of malignancy.

C. Thyroid Carcinoma

■ Description

Low overall mortality. Favorable prognosis for most cell types. Papillary, 60 to 70%. Follicular, 15 to 20%. Medullary. Anaplastic very aggressive. Previous neck irradiation. Best prognosis is papillary.

■ Symptoms

Solitary neck mass most common. Lymphadenopathy.

■ Diagnosis

Thyroid function tests, thyroid scan, ultrasound, fine-needle aspiration, neck exploration.

■ Treatment

Surgery: thyroid lobectomy and isthmusectomy, subtotal thyroidectomy, total thyroidectomy. Procedure depends on cell type and size of tumor. Postoperative thyroid suppression, radioactive iodine for metastatic disease.

XVI. PARATHYROID—PRIMARY HYPERPARATHYROIDISM

■ Description

Cause unknown. Increase in serum parathyroid hormone. Single or multiple adenomas or hyperplasia.

■ Signs and Symptoms

Weakness, anorexia, nausea, constipation, renal colic, renal stones, osteoporosis, osteitis fibrosa cystica, subperiosteal resorption, pancreatitis, gallstones, depression, anxiety.

■ Diagnosis

Increased serum calcium, decreased serum phosphate. Increased serum parathyroid hormone: carboxy-terminal fragment longer half-life, biologically inactive. Chloride:phosphate ratio greater than 33. Localization: CT scan, venous catheterization, and sampling. Thallium-technetium subtraction scan.

■ Treatment

Surgery: one enlarged gland, remove; generalized hyperplasia, remove 3.5 glands or total parathyroidectomy with reimplantation.

XVII. ADRENAL

A. Primary Hyperaldosteronism

■ Description

Excess aldosterone secretion. No adrenocorticotropic hormone (ACTH) regulation. One percent of all cases of hypertension. More common in women. Adenoma in 75%, hyperplasia in 25%.

■ Symptoms

Hypertension, headache, weakness, polydipsia, edema.

■ Diagnosis

Elevated serum aldosterone levels, decreased serum renin level. Hypernatremia, hypokalemia, hypochloremia, alkalosis. Localization: CT scan, venous catheterization, and sampling.

■ Treatment

Adenoma—surgical removal, adrenalectomy.

Hyperplasia—medical therapy, spironolactone.

B. **Hypercortisolism**

■ **Description**

Cushing's disease—pituitary ACTH excess that leads to hyperplasia.

Cushing's syndrome—adrenal source of cortisol, low ACTH. Syndrome more common in women, young age. Seventy-five percent of adrenal tumors are benign, 98% unilateral.

■ **Symptoms**

Change in menstrual cycle, virilization, weight gain, lassitude, muscle weakness, psychiatric disturbance, hypertension, edema, purple striae, buffalo hump.

■ **Diagnosis**

Plasma cortisol levels, low-dose dexamethasone suppression test, urinary-free cortisol excretion, ACTH assay, high-dose dexamethasone suppression test, metapyrone test, CT scan.

■ **Treatment**

Cushing's disease—transsphenoidal hypophysectomy.

Cushing's syndrome—adrenalectomy.

C. **Pheochromocytoma**

■ **Description**

Catecholamine-producing tumors for amine precursor uptake and decarboxylation (APUD) cells. Neural crest origin. Adrenal medulla or sympathetic system. Of all patients with hypertension, 0.1%. Malignant, 10%; bilateral, 10%; in adrenal or periadrenal area, 90%.

■ **Symptoms**

Sustained or paroxysmal hypertension, perspiration, pallor, flushing, palpitation, trembling, weakness, anxiety.

■ **Diagnosis**

Urine for catecholamine metabolites: Vanillylmandelic acid (VMA), normetanephrine, metanephrine. Urinary-free epinephrine and norepinephrine. Localization: meta-iodobenzylguanidine (MIBG) scan, CT scan.

■ **Treatment**

Surgery: preparation with alpha blocking agent phenoxybenzamine, followed by beta blockade (propranolol hydrochloride [Inderal]). Adrenalectomy with careful intraoperative monitoring.

XVIII. LUNG

A. **Lung Cancer**

■ **Description**

Peak incidence 50 to 70 years. Cigarette smoking, exposure to asbestos, other toxic agents. Cell types: squamous (40 to 70%), adenocarcinoma (15%), bronchoalveolar (5%), undifferentiated (20 to 30%). Most common malignancy in males.

■ **Symptoms**

Cough, dyspnea, chest or shoulder pain, hoarseness, weight loss, clubbing, hemoptysis. May be asymptomatic.

■ **Diagnosis**

Chest x-ray, sputum cytology, CT scan, bronchoscopy, transpleural needle biopsy, mediastinoscopy, open-lung biopsy.

■ **Treatment**

Thoracotomy with wedge resection, lobectomy, or pneumonectomy. Radiation. Chemotherapy.

B. Lung Abscess

■ **Description**

Can have multiple causes: aspiration, pneumonia, septic embolus, bronchial obstruction, trauma, transdiaphragmatic extension.

■ **Symptoms**

Cough, pleuritic pain, fever. Copious, malodorous sputum.

■ **Diagnosis**

Increased white blood cell count. Sputum for Gram stain, culture, and sensitivity. Chest x-ray, CT scan, magnetic resonance imaging (MRI) scan, bronchoscopy.

■ **Treatment**

Antibiotics. Drainage: tube thoracostomy, percutaneous. Surgery: when unresponsive to medical therapy. Resection of involved segment or lobe.

C. Pneumothorax

■ **Description**

May be spontaneous, traumatic, or iatrogenic. Air or gas enters pleural space.

■ **Symptoms**

Chest pain, cough, dyspnea, decreased breath sounds, hyperresonance.

■ **Diagnosis**

Physical examination, chest x-ray.

■ **Treatment**

Small pneumothorax with minimal symptoms: can try conservative therapy.
Symptomatic or large pneumothorax: tube thoracostomy.

XIX. BREAST

A. Breast Cancer

■ **Description**

Most common cancer in women; can occur in males. Risk factors: previous cancer, heredity, early menarche, late menopause. Ductal or lobular accounts for 85%; spreads by lymphatic and hematogenous routes.

■ **Symptoms**

Painless lump, nipple discharge, erythema, asymmetry, nipple inversion, bone pain, weight loss. Edema of overlying skin (peau d'orange); hard, irregular, fixed mass in advanced cases.

■ **Diagnosis**

Liver function tests may be elevated in advanced cases, hypercalcemia with bone metastasis, chest x-ray, CT scan abdomen, mammography, breast biopsy, fine-needle aspiration.

■ **Treatment**

Mastectomy. Breast conservation: lumpectomy with axillary dissection, radiation therapy; stage I and stage II. Adjuvant chemotherapy (cylophosphamide, methotrexate, 5-FU. Antiestrogen therapy (tomoxifan).

B. Mammary Dysplasia

■ **Description**

Incidence peaks age 35 to 40. Most common breast complaint. Common cause of breast mass. Atypical hyperplasia premalignant.

■ **Symptoms**

Breast pain varying with menstrual cycle. Breast masses may appear in cyclic manner. Tender mass; thickened, nodular areas.

■ Diagnosis

Physical examination, mammography.

■ Treatment

Biopsy dominant masses to rule out carcinoma. Avoid caffeine. Danazol in severe cases. Simple mastectomy with breast reconstruction in very severe cases.

C. Fibroadenoma

■ Description

Common cause of breast mass in young women, peak age to 25. May grow to large size. Unusual to find cancer invading fibroadenoma.

■ Symptoms

Asymptomatic mass, found incidentally. Firm, freely movable.

■ Diagnosis

Physical examination, needle biopsy.

■ Treatment

Excisional biopsy.

D. Intraductal Papilloma

■ Description

Benign; may degenerate if allowed to enlarge. Grows within ducts. Nipple discharge, bloody.

■ Symptoms

Nipple discharge. May be too small to feel on physical examination.

■ Diagnosis

Physical examination. Note area of discharge on nipple and areolar palpation.

■ Treatment

Excision.

E. Breast Abscess

■ Description

Most associated with lactation.

■ Signs and Symptoms

Fever, erythema, tender mass.

■ Diagnosis

Physical examination.

■ Treatment

Antibiotics, operative drainage, biopsy wall of abscess and skin to rule out inflammatory carcinoma.

XX. SKIN AND SOFT TISSUE

A. Melanoma

■ Description

Increasing incidence, ultraviolet irradiation. Genetic predisposition: fair skin, blonde hair, blue eyes higher risk. Four types: lentigo maligna, superficial spreading, acral lentiginous, nodular. Prognosis depends on level of invasion, thickness, and ulceration.

■ Symptoms

Change in existing nevus: bleeding, ulceration, irregular border, size change.

■ Diagnosis

Biopsy: full thickness.

■ Treatment

Wide local excision, amputation, lymph node dissection, isolated limb perfusion, immunotherapy.

B. Soft Tissue Sarcomas

■ Description

Uncommon. One percent of malignant tumors. Liposarcomas, malignant fibrous histiocytomas, leiomyosarcomas, fibrosarcomas, rhabdomyosarcomas are most common. Hematogenous spread to lung.

■ Symptoms

Painless mass, enlarging. May become painful and interfere with function. Most often in lower extremities.

■ Diagnosis

Biopsy along longitudinal axis of extremity (do not cross fascial compartments). CT scan or MRI of area. Chest x-ray.

■ Treatment

Surgical resection: avoid simple enucleation. Irradiation, surgery, and chemotherapy in combination (limb sparing).

BIBLIOGRAPHY

Sabiston D. *Textbook of Surgery.* 14th ed. Harcourt, Brace, Jovanovich: Philadelphia, Pa: WB Saunders; 1986.

Schwartz ST. *Principles of Surgery.* New York: McGraw-Hill Books, Inc; 1994.

Hardy JD. *Textbook of Surgery.* Philadelphia, Pa: JB Lippincott Co; 1988.

CHAPTER 19

Symptoms, Signs, and Ill-Defined Conditions

JOEL S. GOLDBERG, DO

I. CARDIORESPIRATORY SYSTEM AND CHEST

A. Cough

■ **Description**

Protective respiratory reflex, induced by stimulation of respiratory tree receptors.

■ **Symptoms**

Cough.

■ **Diagnosis**

History and physical, chest x-ray, pulmonary function testing, asthma work-up, sputum analysis (culture and cytology), upper gastrointestinal (GI) (rule out reflux/aspiration).

■ **Pathology**

A result of allergy/asthma, infection, foreign body (pulmonary aspiration or object contacting tympanic membrane), tumor, cardiac disease, thyroid disorder, other pulmonary disease (chronic obstructive pulmonary disease [COPD]/smoking, asbestosis, bronchiectasis, etc), drugs (acetylcholine esterase [ACE] inhibitors, inhaled cromolyn), and psychogenic factors.

■ **Treatment**

As per individual condition.

Additional Information. **Cough complications: syncope, rib fractures. Asthma may present with cough only, without wheezing.**

B. Hemoptysis

■ **Description**

Bloody sputum production.

■ **Symptoms**

Production of **bloody sputum (coughing up blood).**

■ **Diagnosis**

History and physical examination, **chest x-ray, bronchoscopy,** pulmonary angiography, lab studies (prothrombin time [PT], partial thromboplastin time [PTT], platelets).

■ **Pathology**

A result of **carcinoma, bronchitis,** tuberculosis (TB), pulmonary embolism, coagulation disorder, Goodpasture's syndrome, mycetomas, **bronchiectasis,** hemosiderosis, Wegener's disease, and mitral stenosis.

■ **Treatment**

Supportive, control cough (codeine), intubation, and tamponade or thoracotomy for massive hemorrhage/tumor.

C. Epistaxis

■ **Description**

Nasal hemorrhage.

■ **Symptoms**

Nasal bleeding (slight or brisk), hypotension.

> *Anterior bleed*—often one side only.
> *Posterior bleed*—both sides, coughing/choking on blood.

■ **Diagnosis**

History and physical examination.

■ **Pathology**

Anterior (**Kiesselbach's** or **Little's plexus bleeding,** trauma, low humidity), or **posterior** sites. Additional etiologies: hypertension, nasal foreign body, tumor, vascular abnormalities/arteriosclerosis, leukemia, bleeding disorders, and infection.

■ **Treatment**

Anterior—**pressure/packing, and/or cautery.**

Posterior—**posterior pack/balloon,** artery ligation.

Additional Information. **Posterior pack blocks sphenopalatine artery (anterior bleeding from ethmoid arteries).**

Most frequent bleeding site: Kiesselbach's area.

D. Dyspnea

■ **Description**

Air hunger.

■ **Symptoms**

Subjective complaint of **uncomfortable shortness of breath, of more than expected severity for activity level.**

■ **Diagnosis**

History and physical examination, cardiac (electrocardiogram [ECG], 2-D echocardiogram, stress test), and pulmonary evaluation (chest x-ray, pulmonary function tests [PFTs]).

■ **Pathology**

Most frequently pulmonary or cardiac disease, of acute or chronic nature. Deconditioning and psychogenic factors may be present.

■ **Treatment**

Treat primary problem.

Additional Information

Orthopnea—supine dyspnea.
Platypnea—upright dyspnea.
Hyperpnea—increase minute volume.

E. Chest Pain

■ **Description**

Chest pain.

■ **Symptoms**

Chest pain. May be pleuritic (pleurisy), exacerbated by chest wall palpation (costochondritis), or exercise (angina), or episodic (spasm?) and atypical (other disorders).

■ **Diagnosis**

History and physical examination, cardiac work-up (ECG, 2-D echocardiogram, stress testing, arteriography), chest x-ray. Other studies may include lung scan, ultrasound of aorta, and GI work-up.

■ **Pathology**

Rule out **angina pectoris:** ischemic cardiac pain. Other etiologies include pleurisy, pericarditis, costochondral disease, gastrointestinal disease, neuritis, embolism, aneurysm, pulmonary hypertension, and others.

■ **Treatment**

Treat as per specific etiology.

Additional Information. **Pleurisy:** increased pain with inspiration and movement. **Intercostal neuritis:** increased pain with coughing and sneezing.

F. Palpitations

■ Description

Subjective sensation of additional/irregular or strong heart beats, or chest discomfort related to cardiac rhythm.

■ Symptoms

As described. Depending on etiology, may also experience chest pain, anxiety, and syncope.

■ Diagnosis

History and physical examination, ECG, 2-D echocardiogram, Holter monitor, lab studies (complete blood count [CBC], thyroid functions, etc).

■ Pathology

Sensation of abnormal beats (palpitations) may reflect significant cardiac pathology or be of no importance whatsoever.

■ Treatment

As per individual condition.

G. Cyanosis

■ Description

Blue color of mucous membranes and/or skin, and nail beds.

■ Symptoms

As described. May be associated with other symptoms depending on specific disorder.

■ Diagnosis

History and physical examination, cardiopulmonary evaluation (ECG/echo/chest x-ray/cath/PFTs). **Newborn with cyanosis:** oxygen (100%) will improve hypoxemia with pulmonary disorders, but have negligible effect with intracardiac shunt lesions.

■ Pathology

Reduced arterial hemoglobin from central (cardiac shunt or pulmonary pathology), or peripheral (vasoconstriction) mechanisms.

■ Treatment

As per individual condition.

Additional Information. **Anemia may obscure detection of cyanosis. Most frequent cause of cardiac-related cyanosis after age 2: tetralogy of Fallot (cyanosis and clubbing of both fingers and toes). Cyanosis without hypoxia: rule out methemoglobinemia. Tricuspid atresia: cyanotic newborn; diagnosis by ECG/echo/cath; treat by surgery; most frequent cause of death is hypoxia. Congenital cardiac lesions resulting in cyanosis: great vessel transposition, pulmonary or tricuspid atresia, and tetralogy of Fallot.**

H. Hypoxemia

■ Description

Inadequate blood oxygen.

■ Symptoms

Lethargy, mental status change, arrhythmia, headache, palpitations, impaired judgment.

■ Diagnosis

History and physical examination (cyanosis, tachycardia, etc), cardiopulmonary evaluation, arterial blood gases (ABGs), response to oxygen, A-a gradient (see the following), and **hemoglobin. Most specific physical sign of hypoxemia: cyanosis.**

■ **Pathology**

Etiologies include **ventilation-perfusion (V/Q) mismatch, right-to-left shunt, diffusion abnormality, alveolar hypoventilation,** and **reduced inspiratory oxygen content.**

■ **Treatment**

As per condition, but **oxygen** is critical.

Additional Information. **Most frequent cause of hypoxemia: mismatch of V/Q.**

Alveolar-arterial oxygen gradient— $\bar{P}(A\text{-}a)O_2$, usually under 15.

Increased A-a gradient—mismatch of V/Q or intrapulmonary shunt.

Normal A-a gradient—alveolar hypoventilation, or reduced inspired oxygen.

Unimproving hypoxemia and pulmonary edema **in septic patient—**suspect AIDS-related disease syndrome (ARDS).

I. Shock

■ **Description**

Inadequate tissue perfusion.

■ **Symptoms**

Hypotension, tachypnea, mental confusion, cyanosis, tachycardia.

■ **Diagnosis**

History and physical examination (weak pulse, reduced urinary output, fever, poor skin color, etc). Other procedures as indicated (blood cultures, hemodynamic monitoring, etc).

■ **Pathology**

Primary etiology includes **cardiogenic** and **hypovolemic** disorders. Other sources include trauma and sepsis.

■ **Treatment**

Cardiopulmonary resuscitation (CPR) (including ventilatory support, cardiac monitoring, acid/base management, and fluids/vasopressors), and treatment of primary disorder.

Additional Information

Early septic shock—reduced systemic vascular resistance (SVR) with elevated cardiac output.

Cardiogenic shock—increased SVR with decreased cardiac output.

J. Respiratory Failure

■ **Description**

Inadequate oxygen or carbon dioxide exchange.

■ **Symptoms**

Tachypnea, tachycardia, mental confusion, cyanosis, wheezing/dyspnea.

■ **Diagnosis**

History and physical examination, **most important test is ABGs;** lung scan, pulmonary function testing, and chest x-ray may all be helpful.

■ **Pathology**

$PaCO_2$ **over 50** or PaO_2 **under 60.**

■ **Treatment**

Oxygen (with or without intubation and mechanical ventilation), and treatment of primary problem (drug overdose, infection, trauma, etc).

II. SKIN

A. Edema

■ **Description**

Increased tissue fluid.

■ Symptoms

Tissue swelling.

■ Diagnosis

History and physical examination; appropriate studies to evaluate vascular, cardiac, renal, and hepatic systems.

■ Pathology

Interstitial fluid excess. Etiology includes venous insufficiency, nephrotic syndrome, medications (calcium channel blockers), malabsorption, cirrhosis, and congestive heart failure.

■ Treatment

Treat primary condition; reduction of salt and fluids, diuretics (cardiac causes).

Additional Information. **Elevated total body sodium results in pitting edema. Periorbital edema: rule out renal disease.**

B. Jaundice

■ Description

Yellow skin and **mucous membranes** (icterus), secondary to elevated bilirubin levels.

■ Symptoms

Yellow skin/mucosa, may have **dark urine, pruritus,** light-colored stools, and symptoms of individual etiologic disorder.

■ Diagnosis

History and physical examination (examine conjunctiva), liver function tests, computed tomography (CT)/ultrasound, liver scan/biopsy, HIDA scan, endoscopic retrograde cholangiopancreatography (ERCP).

■ Pathology

Unconjugated—etiology includes excess bilirubin production (hemolytic disorders), or **faulty liver conjugation or uptake** (genetic disorders).

Conjugated—**reduced liver production** (hepatic disease of various types, including inflammation, infection, and obstruction).

■ Treatment

Treat primary condition.

Additional Information

Dubin–Johnson syndrome—**genetic, conjugated jaundice disease, elevated urine coproporphyrin type 1 rather than type 3.**

Gilbert syndrome—genetic, most frequent unconjugated disorder, glucuronyl transferase deficiency.

Neonatal jaundice—most frequent type is physiologic (no treatment needed); **high prolonged bilirubinemia may cause kernicterus (brain damage),** aggressive therapy required as per current literature/tables.

Carotenemia—"jaundice," normal bilirubin, excess carrot ingestion.

Obstructive jaundice—serum glutamic-oxaloacetic transaminase (SGOT) under 300, and **alkaline phosphatase** three times normal.

Drugs causing jaundice—griseofulvin, erythromycin estolate, oxacillin, and **chloramphenicol.**

C. Clubbing

■ Description

Nail deformity.

■ Symptoms

Loss of nail plate-to-finger angle (convex nails), with fingernail thickness greater than distal interphalangeal (DIP) joint thickness.

■ Diagnosis

Physical examination.

■ Pathology

Common to many cardiopulmonary disorders (bronchiectasis, pulmonary hypertension, atrial septal defect, lung cancer, cystic fibrosis, cyanotic congenital heart disease, etc), possibly secondary to hypoxemia. May also be familial.

■ Treatment

Treat primary condition.

D. Pruritus

■ Description

Itching.

■ Symptoms

Sensation of itching, via skin nerve-ending stimulation.

■ Diagnosis

History and physical examination, routine lab studies, and evaluation for any underlying disease as indicated.

■ Pathology

May relate to local factors (dry skin, allergy), medications, or systemic pathology (uremia, malignancy, endocrine/thyroid disease).

■ Treatment

Symptomatic treatment, corticosteroids topical/oral, antihistamines.

III. DIGESTIVE SYSTEM AND ABDOMEN

A. Abdominal Pain

■ Description

Abdominal pain.

■ Symptoms

Abdominal pain (may include signs of peritonitis, referred pain, abdominal rigidity, etc).

■ Diagnosis

History (important factors include speed of onset, duration, radiation, type and severity of pain), and physical examination, laboratory testing (CBC, sequential multiple analyzer-12 [SMA-12], amylase, etc), **flat plate/kidneys, ureters, and bladder (KUB)/decubitus films, urine analysis (UA),** and other studies as indicated (CT, ultrasound, intravenous pyelogram [IVP]), paracentesis/colpocentesis.

■ Pathology

Wide etiology including both acute and chronic events, and both abdominal and referred pain (cardiac).

■ Treatment

As per individual condition.

Additional Information. **Peritonitis patients remain still. Viscus perforation causes severe pain.**

> *Referred pain*—hepatic to right shoulder; uterine to back.
>
> *Obstruction*—bowel sounds high-pitched, distention, pain.
>
> *Cervical motion tenderness*—rule out pelvic inflammatory disease (PID).

Vomiting blood—lesion above ligament of Treitz.

Grey Turner's sign—flank ecchymosis.

Cullen's sign—periumbilical ecchymosis.

B. Infantile Colic

■ **Description**

Prolonged infant crying/abdominal pain.

■ **Symptoms**

Crying episodes, with clenched fists and legs pulled up.

■ **Diagnosis**

History and physical examination.

■ **Pathology**

Uncertain, but most often resolves by 12 weeks of age.

■ **Treatment**

Reduce infant stress, increase parent relaxation, hot water bottle for infant, simethicone drops (Mylicon), and burping.

C. Hepatomegaly

■ **Description**

Enlarged liver.

■ **Symptoms**

May be none or abdominal mass.

■ **Diagnosis**

History and physical examination, ultrasound, CT.

■ **Pathology**

Numerous possible etiologies (hemolytic anemia, hepatocellular disease and neoplasm, volume overload, etc).

■ **Treatment**

Treat primary condition.

D. Splenomegaly

■ **Description**

Enlarged spleen.

■ **Symptoms**

May be none, or abdominal mass, pain.

■ **Diagnosis**

History and physical examination, ultrasound, CT, and radioisotope scan.

■ **Pathology**

Numerous possible etiologies (hemolytic anemia, portal hypertension and hepatocellular disease, mononucleosis, sarcoid, leukemia/lymphoma, storage disorders, idiopathic).

■ **Treatment**

Treat primary condition.

Additional Information

Felty syndrome—splenomegaly, rheumatoid arthritis, and **granulocytopenia.**

Gaucher's disease—excess cerebroside, splenomegaly.

E. Ascites

■ **Description**

Excess peritoneal fluid.

■ **Symptoms**

Enlarging tender abdomen, and nausea.
May also have edema, weight gain, and
dyspnea.

■ **Diagnosis**

History and physical examination, **paracentesis,** ultrasound.

■ **Pathology**

> *Exudate*—protein greater than 3 g/100
> mL (**TB, cancer,** and others).
> *Transudate*—cirrhosis, and congestive
> heart failure (CHF).

■ **Treatment**

As per individual condition. For **cirrhosis: restrict salt, diuretics, Le Veen
shunt.**

Additional Information

> *Most frequent cause of ascites*—cirrho-
> sis.
> *Treatment for ascites fluid removal*—
> paracentesis.
> *Meig syndrome*—ovarian tumor, tran-
> sudative ascites.
> *Spontaneous bacterial peritonitis*—
> ascites complication with fever, ele-
> vated number ascitic polymorphonu-
> clear cells (over 250/μL), **pain.**

F. **Dysphagia**

■ **Description**

Difficulty swallowing.

■ **Symptoms**

Difficulty swallowing, weight loss, regurgitation.

■ **Diagnosis**

History and physical examination, swallowing function study, **endoscopy.**

■ **Pathology**

Esophageal constriction may be due to
**tumor, achalasia, stricture, esophageal
ring** (Schatzki's ring may cause intermittent dysphagia), or **neuromuscular disorders.**

■ **Treatment**

As per individual condition.

Additional Information

> *Odynophagia*—painful swallowing.
> *Chalasia*—lower esophageal sphincter
> (LES) **does not close.**
> *Achalasia*—pressure of LES elevated,
> with poor esophageal peristalsis.
> *Barrett's esophagitus*—**esophageal col-
> umnar epithelium** (instead of squa-
> mous epithelium), **secondary to reflux,**
> with **stricture and adenocarcinoma** as
> potential **complications.**
> *Globus hystericus*—**psychogenic, con-
> tinuous "lump in throat" feeling, may
> improve after swallowing.**
> *Plummer–Vinson syndrome*—**esopha-
> geal web** and **iron deficiency anemia.**

G. **Nausea and Vomiting**

■ **Description**

Nausea and vomiting.

■ **Symptoms**

Nausea, possibly followed by tachycardia, hypersalivation, and vomiting.

■ **Diagnosis**

History and physical examination, x-ray
studies (obstruction series), lab studies,
endoscopy.

■ **Pathology**

Etiology includes multiple disorders, including pancreatic and biliary tract disease, pregnancy, gastroenteritis, myocar-

dial infarction, migraine, ileus and obstruction, and others.

■ Treatment

Treat primary condition. Antiemetics include scopolamine, meclizine, and corticosteroids.

Additional Information. **Vomitus with fecal odor: distal obstruction.**

Obstruction treatment: correct obstruction after **fluids** and **nasogastric (NG) suction.**

H. Diarrhea

■ Description

Acute or chronic diarrheal illness **(increased stool weight per 24 hours).**

■ Symptoms

Diarrhea, mild or severe, dehydration.

■ Diagnosis

History and physical examination, stool exam (culture, ova and parasites, leukocytes), sigmoidoscopy, lab studies (SMA-12, pancreatic enzymes, human immunodeficiency virus [HIV], electrolytes, etc).

■ Pathology

Physiology includes **secretory, osmotic, impaired motility,** and **absorptive disorders.** Etiology includes **infection, medications,** and **inflammatory bowel disease.**

■ Treatment

Rehydration, treat primary condition (amebiasis/giardiasis: metronidazole; pseudomembranous colitis: vancomycin, etc), antidiarrheals.

Additional Information. **Positive association of chronic diarrhea and AIDS.**

Methylene blue stool stain—look for leukocytes (suggests invasive bowel infection).

Effect of fasting on diarrhea types— secretory, no effect; osmotic, diarrhea stops.

I. Fecal Incontinence

■ Description

Fecal incontinence. In children termed encopresis.

■ Symptoms

Inability to maintain stool continence.

■ Diagnosis

History and physical examination.

■ Pathology

Anal sphincter disorder (idiopathic, postsurgical, trauma, Crohn's, etc). May also relate to impaction, diabetes, and neuromuscular disease.

■ Treatment

Anal sphincter exercises (consult physician), biofeedback, and medication.

J. Anorexia Nervosa

■ Description

Self-inflicted weight loss disorder.

■ Symptoms

Weight loss, depression, amenorrhea, distorted self-image.

■ Diagnosis

History and physical examination, lab studies (SMA-12, CBC), rule out GI disease: GI studies (upper GI, endoscopy, barium enema [BE], etc).

■ **Pathology**

Typically in adolescent females, with unknown etiology (though family and social situations/pressures play a role).

■ **Pathology**

Psychiatric/psychological care, medication (cyproheptadine, chlorpromazine).

Additional Information

Anorexia—lack of hunger.

Anorexia nervosa complications—metabolic abnormality, arrhythmia, gastric rupture.

Bulemia—binge eating and self-induced vomiting.

K. Failure to Thrive in Infancy

■ **Description**

Lack of weight gain, or growth.

■ **Symptoms**

Insufficient weight gain or growth, lethargy, emotional/behavioral disorders.

■ **Diagnosis**

History and physical examination, laboratory and other studies as indicated.

■ **Pathology**

Etiology most often includes psychological disorders and deprivation/abuse.

■ **Treatment**

Treat any coexisting medical disorder; family counseling, social service intervention, and possible child foster placement.

IV. NERVOUS SYSTEM AND SPECIAL SENSES

A. Headache

■ **Description**

Head pain.

■ **Symptoms**

Migraine—throbbing, unilateral, nausea/vomiting.

Cluster—periorbital, severe pain, unilateral autonomic signs.

Tension—bilateral, neck muscles tight, tight band feeling.

Acute CNS—acute-onset severe headache, neurologic signs.

■ **Diagnosis**

History and physical examination, lab testing (glucose, CBC), x-ray head/sinuses, electroencephalogram (EEG), CT/magnetic resonance imaging (MRI) studies, lumbar puncture (LP).

■ **Pathology**

May include **migraine, cluster, tension, CNS disease, exertional,** and others (carbon monoxide, nitrites, temporal arteritis, temporomandibular joint [TMJ], etc), as a result of inflammation or alteration of pain-sensitive CNS structures.

■ **Treatment**

As per individual condition.

B. Delirium

■ **Description**

Alteration of consciousness.

■ **Symptoms**

Confusion, memory difficulty, disorientation, agitation, perception disturbance.

■ **Diagnosis**

History and physical examination, lab studies (infection, endocrine and metabolic/toxin studies), CT, EEG.

■ **Pathology**

Etiology includes **infection, medication, metabolic disease, cardiac disease, sleep deprivation,** and CNS **disease.** Most frequent in elderly hospital patients, and resulting from complex and multiple factors.

■ **Treatment**

Treat primary condition, provide orientation for the patient, nursing support, avoid restraints, allow sleep (intensive care unit [ICU] psychosis), and medication if necessary (low-dose haloperidol [Haldol]).

Additional Information. **Acute onset of symptoms: think delirium, not dementia.**

C. **Coma**

■ **Description**

State of **unconsciousness,** and unresponsiveness, resulting from metabolic, CNS pathology, and other causes.

■ **Symptoms**

Unresponsiveness.

■ **Diagnosis**

History and physical examination, EEG, CT, laboratory studies (SMA-12, CBC, drug screen, PT, PTT, ABGs, thyroid functions), **lumbar puncture.**

■ **Pathology**

Only two causes: extensive bilateral cerebral disorder or brain-stem disorder.

■ **Treatment**

Cardiopulmonary resuscitation, **dextrose** (50 mL of 50% given IV), **naloxone, thiamine** (100 mg IV), correct metabolic abnormalities, and treatment as per individual condition.

Additional Information

Pupils reactive and small—narcotics, metabolic, and pontine pathology.

Pupils fixed and dilated—anoxia, and scopolamine overdose (OD).

Pupils face hemiparesis side—pontine lesion.

Pupils face strong side—unilateral cerebral hemisphere lesion.

Other antidotes—benzodiazepines (give flumazenil).

D. **Convulsions**

■ **Description**

Seizure, and/or uncontrolled contraction of muscles.

■ **Symptoms**

As described for following seizure disorders:

Grand mal—tonic/clonic, incontinence, postictal lethargy.

Petit mal—staring/absence spells, patient possibly unaware.

Partial—simple (consciousness not lost), or complex (possible unconsciousness). Both may have sensory and/or motor signs.

■ **Diagnosis**

History and physical examination, EEG, CT/MRI, laboratory studies, including blood cultures and toxicology screening.

■ **Pathology**

Convulsions—wide etiology (epilepsy, poisoning, infection, heat stroke, etc).

Seizures—generalized or partial (focal). Wide variety of CNS causes (trauma, metabolic, drugs/drug withdrawal, congenital disease, etc).

■ **Treatment**

Neurologic work-up, medication (see Chapter 11, Neurology).

E. **Insomnia**

■ **Description**

Sleep disorder.

■ **Symptoms**

Inability to sleep, or disrupted sleep (waking up early or during the night).

■ **Diagnosis**

History and physical examination, psychological evaluation, routine laboratory studies, sleep studies, EEG.

■ **Pathology**

Psychological and/or medical etiology. May result from medication, depression, and/or alcohol use.

■ **Treatment**

Treat coexisting medical disorders, psychological evaluation, progressive relaxation/biofeedback, non-medicinal measures (warm milk, exercise, avoidance of reading/eating in bed and caffeine, etc), medication.

Additional Information. **Average sleep time:** consists of 25% REM (rapid eye movement, dreaming) stages, and **the rest is non-REM.** Duration of REM sleep: five nightly episodes of **10 to 30 minutes** each.

F. **Syncope**

■ **Description**

Fainting.

■ **Symptoms**

Sudden loss of consciousness.

Vasovagal—may have diaphoresis, ringing in the ears, and blurry vision prior to faint.
Orthostatic—postural-related symptoms.
Cardiac—possibly exercise induced.

■ **Diagnosis**

History and physical examination, Holter monitor, ECG, EEG, and laboratory studies (rule out hypoglycemia and seizure disorders).

■ **Pathology**

Reduced cerebral blood perfusion, via reduced cardiac output/venous return, or other disorders.

■ **Treatment**

Treat primary disorder.

Additional Information. **Valsalva induced: micturition and cough syncope.**

G. **Ataxia**

■ **Description**

Disorder of muscle coordination.

■ **Symptoms**

Balance loss, may have limb, gait, or dysarthric ataxia.

■ **Diagnosis**

History and physical examination, CT/MRI.

■ **Pathology**

Cerebellar or brain-stem pathology. Multiple disorders (drugs/alcohol, B_{12} deficiency, hypothyroidism, viral infection, etc.).

■ **Treatment**

Treat primary condition.

Additional Information

> *Midcerebellar disease*—wide stance, short steps.
> *Lateral cerebellar disease*—wide stance, swaying.
> *Hemiparesis*—weak arm, reduced arm motion, weak leg.
> *Parkinsonian gait*—short steps, diminished arm swing, stooped.
> *Senile gait*—slow, may appear similar to parkinsonian gait.
> *Dyskinetic gait*—involuntary jerking or dancelike movements.
> *Cerebral atrophy gait*—may have short steps, similar to parkinsonism.

H. Weakness

■ **Description**

Muscle and/or neurologic disease resulting in reduced muscle strength.

■ **Symptoms**

Weakness (may include reduced deep tendon reflexes, and fasciculations).

■ **Diagnosis**

History and physical examination, laboratory studies, CT/MRI, lumbar puncture, electromyogram (EMG)/nerve conduction velocity (NCV), pulmonary function studies.

■ **Pathology**

Neurologic (most often myasthenia gravis, polio), infectious, endocrine, psychological, and other conditions (botulism, medication, etc).

■ **Treatment**

As per individual condition

Additional Information.

> *Proximal weakness*—often a myopathy, Guillain–Barré, nerve root lesion, and spinal muscular atrophy.
> *Distal weakness*—often a neuropathy.
> *Cranial/facial weakness*—myotonic dystrophy, and neuromuscular junction disease.
> *Painful weakness*—polymyositis and myotonic dystrophy.
> *Weakness*—also consider multiple sclerosis (MS) and chronic fatigue syndrome.

I. Dysphasia

■ **Description**

Speech disorder (aphasia).

■ **Symptoms**

Receptive (posterior)—difficulty with comprehension, speech remains fluent.
Expressive (anterior)—difficulty with expression, speech fluency disturbed.

■ **Diagnosis**

History and physical/neurologic examination.

■ **Pathology**

Brain pathology (cerebrovascular accident [CVA], trauma, infection), typically of **dominant temporal lobe.**

■ **Treatment**

Treat primary condition, speech therapy when stable.

Additional Information

> *Broca dysphasia*—non-fluent with good comprehension.
>
> *Wernicke dysphasia*—fluent with poor comprehension.
>
> *Global dysphasia*—non-fluent, poor comprehension.
>
> **Cortical locations include speech (left motor cortex), and reading/writing (left angular gyrus).**

J. Dyslexia

■ Description

Reading disorder.

■ Symptoms

Reading disorder without associated intellectual or visual disability.

■ Diagnosis

History and physical examination, reading tests.

■ Pathology

Cortical developmental disorder.

■ Treatment

Tutoring.

K. Vertigo

■ Description

Vestibular disorder.

■ Symptoms

Inappropriate perception of motion, often of abrupt onset (peripheral disease) with associated nausea and vomiting. May have nystagmus (peripheral disease, horizontal; central pathology vertigo, vertical nystagmus).

■ Diagnosis

History and physical examination, CT/MRI, electronystagmography (ENG), brainstem auditory-evoked responses (BAER), and audiologic testing.

■ Pathology

Vestibular disorder.

■ Treatment

Medication, attempt to fatigue response, and surgery.

Additional Information

> *Ménière's disease*—endolymphatic hydrops, tinnitus, hearing loss and episodic vertigo, give **diuretic** and reduce salt intake to treat.
>
> *Acoustic neuroma*—tinnitus, hearing loss, and chronic vertigo.
>
> *Vestibular neuronitis*—nausea/vomiting, and vertigo with **normal hearing,** possibly viral etiology, treat with antihistamines and fluids.

L. Diplopia

■ Description

Double vision.

■ Symptoms

Double vision; may demonstrate head tilt/compensation (head turns toward weak lateral rectus muscle with sixth nerve lesion).

■ Diagnosis

History and physical examination, laboratory studies, CT/MRI.

■ Pathology

Loss of eye muscle strength (neurologic disease, infection, tumor and trauma).

■ **Treatment**

Treat individual condition.

Additional Information

> *Oculomotor (third nerve) weakness*—rule out aneurysm and tumor with unreactive pupil. Muscle weakness with normally reactive pupil is less ominous (may be ischemic in elderly).
>
> *Trochlear (fourth nerve) weakness*—usually trauma induced; cannot look down on inward deviation (superior oblique).
>
> *Abducens (sixth nerve)*—cannot look outward, most often tumor.

V. URINARY SYSTEM

A. Dysuria

■ **Description**

Pain with urination.

■ **Symptoms**

Pain with urination, possibly associated with other urinary tract signs and symptoms (frequency, urgency).

■ **Diagnosis**

History and physical examination, urine analysis and culture, cystoscopy, x-rays.

■ **Pathology**

Urinary tract inflammation; suggestive of infection, though other etiologies possible (stone, foreign body, tumor, etc).

■ **Treatment**

Treat primary disorder and antibiotics as per culture.

B. Pyuria

■ **Description**

White blood cells in the urine.

■ **Symptoms**

Asymptomatic, or symptoms of infection (urgency, frequency, nocturia, etc).

■ **Diagnosis**

Midstream urine analysis, and culture, KUB (rule out stone, and foreign body).

■ **Pathology**

Urinary system inflammation (suggestive of infection), with **polymorphonuclear leukocytes in the urine.**

■ **Treatment**

Antibiotics as per culture, and/or treatment of other coexisting disorders.

Additional Information

> *Sterile pyuria*—**rule out renal TB.**
> *Casts*—**renal inflammation.**

C. Glycosuria

■ **Description**

Urine glucose.

■ **Symptoms**

May be asymptomatic.

■ **Diagnosis**

Urine analysis, dip-stick tests (Clinitest, Testape).

■ **Pathology**

Urinary glucose after renal threshold is exceeded (may indicate diabetes). Also noted with **renal glycosuria: normal serum glucose with disorder of glucose reabsorption** (congenital, drug/heavy metal induced or associated with Fanconi syndrome).

■ **Treatment**

Blood glucose control.

D. **Azotemia**

■ **Description**

Elevated blood nitrogen compounds.

■ **Symptoms**

Multisystem abnormalities with renal failure (skeletal, metabolic, cardiovascular, hematologic, etc). See Chapter 17, Renal System and Urology.

■ **Diagnosis**

History and physical examination, urine analysis, laboratory studies, cystoscopy, Foley catheter insertion (may treat and define obstruction), x-ray studies.

■ **Pathology**

Renal failure may be **prerenal** (dehydration), **renal, or postrenal** (obstruction).

■ **Treatment**

Prerenal—fluids.
Renal—treat primary renal injury (stop offending medication; for rhabdomyolysis, give mannitol).
Postrenal—remove obstruction.

Additional Information. **Prerenal azotemia: urinary osmolality (over 500) greater than plasma osmolality,** with urine sodium under 20).

E. **Proteinuria**

■ **Description**

Elevated urinary protein, indicating renal parenchymal disease.

■ **Symptoms**

Asymptomatic.

■ **Diagnosis**

Urine analysis, dipstick method, followed by 24-hour urine protein study (over 400 mg/24 h is abnormal).

■ **Pathology**

A result of **abnormal proteins (Bence Jones), inadequate reabsorption, glomerular permeability disorder, or renal flow dysfunction.**

■ **Treatment**

Treat primary condition.

Additional Information. **Consider specific gravity: minimal proteinuria on dipstick of dilute urine may reflect marked protein loss.**

F. **Nephrotic Syndrome**

■ **Description**

Syndrome involving glomerular dysfunction.

■ **Symptoms**

Edema, ascites, and possibly hypertension.

■ **Diagnosis**

History and physical examination, **24-hour urine protein collection (over 3.5 g/day proteinuria),** laboratory studies (**reduced albumin,** hyperlipidemia), urine analysis **(casts, oval fat bodies), renal biopsy.**

■ Pathology

Wide etiology in glomerular disease, often secondary to other systemic disorders (cancer, heavy metals, systemic lupus erythematosus [SLE], medications, etc).

■ Treatment

Treat specific cause when possible.

G. Renal Colic

■ Description

Ureteral spasm and pain.

■ Symptoms

Flank or testicle pain—upper ureter stone.

Flank/abdomen pain, nausea/vomiting—pelvic-brim-level stone.

Groin pain—distal ureter stone.

Dysuria/urgency—vesical stone.

Also chills, fever, muscle spasm, and signs of bladder irritation.

■ Diagnosis

History and physical examination, x-ray (KUB, IVP), urine analysis, ultrasound.

■ Pathology

Obstructive ureteral pain secondary to hyperperistalsis (etiology including infection, metabolic, and renal disorders).

■ Treatment

When stone will not pass, stone removal or lithotripsy. Metabolic work-up.

H. Urinary Incontinence

■ Description

Loss of urinary retention control.

■ Symptoms

Atonic bladder—urinary retention and overflow incontinence.

Spastic neuropathic bladder—incontinence.

Infection—incontinence, symptoms of infection.

Stress incontinence—incontinence with exertion and straining.

■ Diagnosis

History and physical examination, urine analysis and culture, urodynamic evaluation (cystometry, uroflowmetry), and x-ray studies (excretory urography, CT, ultrasound, etc).

■ Pathology

Causes of incontinence: neurologic, stress incontinence, outlet obstruction with overflow incontinence, inflammation, medications, trauma, dementia, and infectious etiology.

■ Treatment

As per individual condition (includes medication, surgery, catheterization, etc).

I. Urinary Retention

■ Description

Loss of ability to fully empty the bladder.

■ Symptoms

Abdominal **pain, urgency** (without results), nocturia, bladder spasm.

■ **Diagnosis**

History and physical examination, urine analysis and culture, urodynamic evaluation, x-ray studies (retrograde urethrography), ultrasound, and obtain laboratory studies (blood urea nitrogen [BUN], creatinine, electrolytes, and glucose).

■ **Pathology**

A result of medication (anticholinergics and sympathomimetics), obstruction (cancer, benign prostatic hypertrophy [BPH], stone, valves, etc), or neurologic disease.

■ **Treatment**

Remove obstruction, dilate stricture, stop offending medication.

Additional Information

Retention complications—hydronephrosis, renal failure.

Most frequent cause of retention in older men—benign prostatic hypertrophy.

In child—rule out posterior urethral valves (voiding cystourethrogram).

J. **Oliguria**

■ **Description**

Reduced urine production.

■ **Symptoms**

As described, **urine volume 100 to 400 mL/day,** renal failure (lethargy, hypertension, hematuria, and/or proteinuria).

■ **Diagnosis**

History and physical examination, urine analysis, laboratory studies (BUN, creatinine, calcium, electrolytes, ABGs, urinary osmolality/electrolytes, etc).

■ **Pathology**

Typically secondary to prerenal pathology (hypovolemia, congestive heart failure [CHF], burns, etc), renal pathology (renal failure/disease), or obstruction.

■ **Treatment**

Treat hypovolemic oliguric renal failure with volume expansion, mannitol/furosemide [Lasix], and dialysis.

Additional Information

Anuria—urinary output under 100 mL/day.

Prerenal oliguria—urinary osmolality over 500, and urine sodium under 20.

Renal oliguria—urinary osmolality under 350; urine sodium over 40.

VI. **GENERAL**

A. **Fever of Unknown Origin**

■ **Description**

Fever greater than 101° for more than 3 weeks, unexplained even after a 1-week hospital evaluation.

■ **Symptoms**

May be non-specific (lethargy, hot/cold flashes, sweating), or symptoms associated with the primary disorder.

■ **Diagnosis**

History and physical examination. Further testing as history and/or physical findings dictate (culture blood/urine/sputum/stool, chest/gallbladder x-rays, laboratory testing: CBC, heterophile, rapid plasma reagin [RPR], HIV, etc), bone scan, CT scan chest/abdomen, and others.

■ **Pathology**

Fever induced by very wide variety of disorders (infection, fungal, medication, tumor, connective tissue, viral, psychogenic, metabolic disorders, etc).

■ **Treatment**

Treat individual disorder.

B. **Lymphadenopathy**

■ **Description**

Enlarged lymph nodes.

■ **Symptoms**

Asymptomatic or local tenderness. May demonstrate signs/symptoms of associated disorder.

■ **Diagnosis**

History and physical examination, laboratory studies as indicated (heterophile, HIV, blood culture, serologic testing, etc), **biopsy.**

■ **Pathology**

Lymphadenopathy may be secondary to tumor, infection, and other conditions (sarcoid, phenytoin sodium [Dilantin], etc).

■ **Treatment**

Treat specific disorder.

BIBLIOGRAPHY

Geokas MC. *The Medical Clinics of North America, Vol. 72, No. 5. Difficult Diagnoses.* Philadelphia, Pa: WB Saunders Co; 1988.

Hurst JW. *Medicine for the Practicing Physician.* 3rd ed. Boston, Mass: Butterworth-Heinemann; 1992.

Pryse-Phillips WE. *Essential Neurology.* 4th ed. New York: Medical Examination Publishing Co; 1992.

Rakel RE. *Textbook of Family Practice.* 4th ed. Philadelphia, Pa: WB Saunders Co; 1990.

Schroeder SA. *Current Medical Diagnosis and Treatment.* 30th ed. Norwalk, Conn: Appleton & Lange; 1991.

Tanagho EA. *Smith's General Urology.* 13th ed. Norwalk, Conn: Appleton & Lange; 1992.

Weiner WJ. *Emergent and Urgent Neurology.* Philadelphia, Pa: JB Lippincott Co; 1992.

Woodley M. *Manual of Medical Therapeutics.* 27th ed. Boston, Mass: Little, Brown and Co; 1992.

Common Things to Think of . . .

HECTOR STELLA, MD

The following is not intended as a sole reference, nor as a bank of data, but should be used in conjunction with your knowledge acquired over the last 3 or 4 years in medical school, to help you remember these few things. These things should pop in your head during the test, which might key you into the proper answer. But remember, there is much more to consider and learn. Watch for those red herrings!

I have provided some blank space under the first column, for you to add or make your own notations, since none of us think identically.

Chest Pains

Anginal pain, musculoskeletal, esophagitis, other GI complaints, valvular problems, aortic dissection, myocardial infarction, arrhythmias, pericarditis.

Shortness of Breath (SOB!!!)

Pulmonary problems: asthma, COPD, bronchitis, pneumonia, upper airway infections, aspirations, foreign object aspirations/airway obstruction, pulmonary embolism, pleural effusions, cor pulmonale. Cardiac problems: angina, valvular, CHF, left ventricular dysfunction, cardiomyopathy, pericarditis, MI, arrhythmias. Other systems: severe anemia, peripherovascular problems such as claudication/vascular insufficiency, severe epiglottitis, severe liver disease, pregnancy, metabolic disorders such as DKA and others, certain acute intoxications.

Abdominal pains

Gastroenteritis, indigestion, gastritis, PUD, pancreatitis, gallbladder disease, esophagitis, viscous perforations, post-trauma, IBD, Crohn's disease, ulcerative colitis, spastic colon, psychogenic (might be an indication of a BIGGER problem such as sexual abuse, child abuse), mechanical bowel obstruction, ischemic bowel, foreign bodies, malignancies, volvulus, kidney problems such as kidney stones, acute renal infarcts, renal vein thrombosis, severe pyelonephritis, PID (in females), cystitis; myocardial infarction, some anginal pains, aortic dissections, adrenal infarcts could also present as abdominal pain, intoxications, metabolic disease, and other entities not as common.

Headaches

Vascular and non-vascular, stress/muscle, cluster, migraine, secondary to hypoxic episodes (OSA), aneurysms (actively bleeding or not), severe uncontrolled hypertension, subarachnoid bleeds/hematomas, subdural bleeds/hematomas, post-trauma (contusion), meningitis, encephalitis, primary CNS malignancies (space-occupying lesions), certain pre- or post-seizure episodes/auras, intraparenchymal bleeds, strokes, vasculitis, pseudotumor cerebri, SV thrombosis, skull fractures; visual disturbances such as decreased visual acuity, glaucoma, eye trauma, and others; severe otitis media, myringitis, mastoiditis, in some instances tympanic membrane perforation; sinusitis, nasal septum fractures, TMJ, psychogenic.

NOW, FROM THE BIG PICTURE TO THE NOT SO BIG "?"

Sign or Symptom	Think of
Loss of consciousness (LOC)/Change of mental status	Drugs (illicit as well as prescribed and OTC), not necessary OD; oversedation as one of the many iatrogenic causes; and do not forget intoxications such as ETOH; metabolic disorders such as DKA, myxedema, hyperosmolar state, uremia, liver encephalopathy, Wernicke's and/or Korsakoff and others; trauma to the head (SAH, SDH), contusion; massive primary CNS events such as certain types of strokes (with specific anatomic locations), encephalitis, meningitis, seizure disorders, space-occupying lesions (malignancies) and others less frequent; SLE, vasculitis in general with CNS involvement such as temporal arteritis; neuropsychiatric causes such as all types of dementias including Alzheimer's and HIV dementia, psychiatric disorders such as schizophrenia and major depression to mention only some of them, and don't forget hysteria.
Dizziness	There are many specific entities in the differential for this symptom as well as on the work-up for vertigo (which we can discuss forever but not for the test!). Now THINK OF SIMPLE THINGS such as inner ear infections (otitis media), side effects of medications, some metabolic disorders such as hyperglycemia and more likely hypoglycemia, Ménière's disease, and others less frequently.
Blurred vision	Hyper- or hypoglycemia; hypertensive episode; ophthalmologic problems such as glaucoma, cataracts; trauma to the eye causing blood accumulation, scratch of lens, orbit fracture (producing a trapped muscle preventing any of the necessary eye movements); myasthenia gravis; certain migraines and others; intoxications as well as primary CNS events; metabolic problems; nutritional deficiencies and/or psychiatric problems, usually give other type of visual disturbances such as transient blindness, field cuts, diplopia, hallucinations, and others.

Sign or Symptom	Think of
Epistaxis	**Common things first**—nose picking!; coagulopathies (or anticoagulation); other trauma besides nose manipulation; severe hypertension; dry mucosa; iatrogenic (eg, NG tube placement); AVMs, less frequently but need to think of it; Goodpasture's, Wegener's, and others less frequent such as ectopic pregnancy, etc.
Cough	Sinusitis; bronchitis; asthma; pneumonia; CHF; malignancy; pleural effusions; drugs such as ACE inhibitors and many others; other infectious sources such as TB and PCP are frequent in the HIV+ population; pulmonary embolism; hemorrhagic syndromes, and others less common.
Hemoptysis	First need to figure out if it is true hemoptysis or if it is epistaxis or hematemesis. Some of the common causes of hemoptysis you need to be aware of for the test include: bronchitis; infectious process such as with fungal infections, TB, and others; status post-endotracheal intubation; pulmonary embolus; pulmonary infarct; valvular diseases (MS); Goodpasture's, Wegener's, less frequently Churg–Strauss and others. Lung contusion, post-chest trauma, lung cancer, vasculitis/collagen-vascular disease (SLE), post-transplant (probably due to infectious process).
Wheezing	**All that wheezes is not asthma!** Asthma, CHF, airway hyperactivity (postinfectious), foreign object (especially in children), pseudoasthma (vocal cord asthma), and a few others that are not as common.
Palpitations	Important to define if they are atrial or ventricular in origin. Think of cardiac ischemia, thyroid disease, medication-induced, stress, drugs, post-MI, pulmonary embolism, MVP, panic attacks; other less frequent but you need to be aware of: Wolff–Parkinson–White (WPW), MAT, and prolonged QT just to mention a few.
Nausea and vomiting	Gastroenteritis, gastritis, PUD, certain types of cardiac ischemias (eg, IWMI), intoxication (various), DKA, pancreatitis, gallbladder disease, kidney stone, uremia, pregnancy (not always), bowel obstruction, medications (side effects), renal failure.

Sign or Symptom	Think of
Hematemesis and lower GI bleed	Defined as bleeding above or below the ligament of Trietz, respectively: UGIB (gastritis, PUD, Mallory–Weiss tear, cancer, esophageal varices, to mention only a few of the most common ones); LGIB (AVMs, malignancies, hemorrhoids, trauma, diverticulitis, colitis [Crohn's disease, ulcerative, pseudomembranous], and a few others).
Diarrhea or muddy waters	**Always think of the common ones first:** gastroenteritis, food intoxication/poisoning, infections (bacterial—*Salmonella, Shigella, Vibrio, Clostridium*), parasitic (*Giardia, Entamoeba*), as well as HIV-related; absorption syndromes (sprue, tropical sprue, lactulose intolerance), and many others that I will suggest for you to learn—if not for this test, for the near future.
Back pain	Musculoskeletal, DJD, arthritis, pancreatitis, PUD, pyelonephritis, renal infarct, kidney stones, sometimes renal vein thrombosis as well as cholecystitis, dissecting aortic aneurysms, ectopic pregnancy, spinal canal stenosis, radiculopathies (disc problems) and others.
Hematuria	Kidney stones, cystitis, menstrual cycle, anticoagulation/coagulopathy, bladder cancer, trauma, Foley catheter manipulation, infections (common as well as uncommon, such as *Schistosoma haematobium*), renal failure (in some ways).

A FEW HINTS

Look at your laboratory values.

Calculate your anion gap.

Check your sputum for WBC.

Check your urine analysis for bacteria and crystals, as well as for WBC, and correlate clinically.

Look carefully at x-rays, and remember: CXR—look for heart size, infiltrates, and their locations and for volume loss, masses, diaphragms (positions), hardware (ET tube, NGT). Look for pneumothorax and free air under the diaphragm. KUB—look for gas patterns, stones, and REMEMBER: the rule of 20/80% (20% of gallstones are seen on KUB and 80% of kidney stones are seen on KUB).

Don't forget common BUGS give you common THINGS. Think of *Streptococcus pneumonia, Escherichia coli, Haemophilus influenzae, Mycobacteria*; not so common such as *Klebsiella* (in those specific situations), *Listeria, Ichenela*, DF-2.

With HIV+, there is a lot to remember, but always remember—low WBC, low CD4 count, Kaposi's sarcoma, by definition autoimmunosuppression; affects all organs in one way or another, eg, dementia, parasitic invasions, CNS/GI/lung/eye, etc; infections, common PCP, TB, *Cryptococcus*, MAI, *Toxoplasma histolyticus.*

ONLY answer what they are asking you! Don't try to complicate the questions.

Always, but always, do CLINICAL CORRELATION.

Go with your first instinct and try not to change your answers.

Pay attention to physical exam findings.

Watch those hemodynamics—don't blow them off; they are trying to tell you something (eg, high CO/low SVR suggests sepsis; low CO/high SVR/high wedge pressure suggests cardiogenic shock; equalization of pressures suggests tamponade; high wedge, your patient could be wet; low wedge, your patient might be intravascularly depleted; high RA/high PAP with pad-wedge > 5 suggests pulmonary hypertension).

Always look at the whole picture. Don't blind yourself with one detail. Answer as many questions as you can, and GOOD LUCK!!

INDEX

Appleton & Lange USMLE Step 2 Reviews

Comprehensive

Go, *First Aid for the USMLE Step 2,* 150 pp., paperback, A2591-4

Goldberg, *The Instant Exam Review for the USMLE Step 2, 2/e,*
250 pp., paperback, A4328-0

Catlin, *A&L Review for the USMLE Step 2, 2/e,* 287 pp., paperback, A0266-5

Internal Medicine

Goldlist, *A&L Review of Internal Medicine,* 275 pp., paperback, A0251-7

Obstetrics & Gynecology

Julian, *A&L Review of Obstetrics and Gynecology, 5/e,* 416 pp.,
paperback, A0231-9

Pediatrics

Hansbarger, *MEPC: Pediatrics, 9/e,* 248 pp., paperback, A6223-0

Lorin, *A&L Review of Pediatrics, 5/e,* 222 pp., paperback, A0057-8

Public Health

Hart, *MEPC: Preventive Medicine and Public Health,*
350 pp., paperback, A6319-6

Penalver, *Public Health and Preventive Medicine Review, 2/e,*
120 pp., paperback, E5936-9

Surgery

Metzler, *MEPC: Surgery, 11/e,* 317 pp., paperback, A6195-0

Wapnick, *A&L Review of Surgery, 2/e,* 156 pp., paperback, A0220-2

See reverse side for more A&L review titles